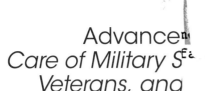

Advanced
Care of Military S...
Veterans, and

"Ambitious yet effective, scholarly yet jammed with practical tools, this comprehensive manual is a must-read for anyone providing medical, mental health, or pastoral care for military service members, veterans, or their families. Its chapter authors include top leaders in thought, research, and practice, and their subjects span the entire spectrum of war-related distress and dysfunction, from physical and brain injuries to social, cultural, and spiritual challenges of many kinds. This book will be a valuable reference for many years to come."

> *William P. Nash, M.D., CAPT, MC, USN (Retired); Boston VA Research Institute; former director, Marine Corps Combat and Operational Stress Control programs*

"From the values of military culture, to frequent moves and separations, to the stressors of the deployment cycle, service members and their families face a unique context of influence on their well-being and mental health. This edited text brings together experts in these contextual factors and military mental health to highlight the latest science in ways that provide practical suggestions for the practitioners who serve these individuals. Armed with the knowledge in this book, clinicians will be in a much better position to ask the right questions and provide the most effective resources and support for military families."

> *Sonja V. Batten, Ph.D., Department of Veterans Affairs Central Office and Uniformed Services University of the Health Sciences*

"One out of every five Americans is either a service member, a veteran, or a member of their family, yet few clinicians routinely ask patients 'Have you or someone close to you served in the military?' This reflects provider insecurity about what to do with the answer as well as profound reticence inherent in military culture. This book, written by experts spanning the military/ VA/community continuum of care, provides a field manual for making sense of and acting upon a military history in clinical settings. After more than a decade of war, this book should be required reading for every health care professional in America."

> *Harold Kudler, M.D., Duke University, Durham, North Carolina*

"This is a timely and compassionate book. In a succinct but comprehensive manner, it offers a guide for those providing care to our nation's service members and their families and a roadmap for understanding military culture and the military health care system. The book is a compendium of current knowledge on a range of practice-related issues including psychiatric and substance use disorders, combat injuries and bereavement, suicidal thoughts and behaviors, and deployment-related adjustment challenges."

Abigail Gewirtz, Ph.D., L.P., Associate Professor, Department of Family Social Science & Institute of Child Development, University of Minnesota

Care of Military Service Members, Veterans, and Their Families

Care of Military Service Members, Veterans, and Their Families

Edited by

Stephen J. Cozza, M.D.
Matthew N. Goldenberg, M.D.
Robert J. Ursano, M.D.

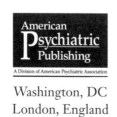

American **P**sychiatric Publishing

A Division of American Psychiatric Association

Washington, DC
London, England

If you would like to buy between 25 and 99 copies of this or any other American Psychiatric Publishing title, you are eligible for a 20% discount; please contact Customer Service at appi@psych.org or 800–368–5777. If you wish to buy 100 or more copies of the same title, please e-mail us at bulksales@psych.org for a price quote.

Copyright © 2014 American Psychiatric Association
ALL RIGHTS RESERVED
Manufactured in the United States of America on acid-free paper
17   16   15   14   13   5   4   3   2   1
First Edition

Typeset in Adobe's Janson Text Lt Std and ITC AvantGarde Std.

American Psychiatric Publishing
A Division of American Psychiatric Association
1000 Wilson Boulevard
Arlington, VA 22209-3901
www.appi.org

Library of Congress Cataloging-in-Publication Data
Care of military service members, veterans, and their families / edited by Stephen J. Cozza, Matthew N. Goldenberg, Robert J. Ursano. — First edition.
        p. ; cm.
    Includes bibliographical references and index.
    ISBN 978-1-58562-424-9 (pbk. : alk. paper)
    I. Cozza, Stephen J., 1958– editor of compilation. II. Goldenberg, Matthew, N., 1978– editor of compilation. III. Ursano, Robert J., 1947– editor of compilation. IV. American Psychiatric Association, issuing body.
    [DNLM: 1. Military Medicine—United States. 2. Family—United States. 3. Mental Disorders—therapy—United States. 4. Military Personnel—United States. 5. Veterans—United States. 6. Wounds and Injuries—therapy—United States. WB 116]
    UB369
    362.1086'970973—dc23   2013036887

British Library Cataloguing in Publication Data
A CIP record is available from the British Library.

To Kelly, Vincent, and Cecilia—my constant source of love,
encouragement, and inspiration — S.J.C.

Contents

PART I

Fundamentals for Treating Military Service Members, Veterans, and Families

 Derrick Hamaoka, M.D., LtCol, USAF, MC, FS
 Mark J. Bates, Ph.D.
 James E. McCarroll, Ph.D., M.P.H.
 William L. Brim, Psy.D.
 Travis K. Lunasco, Psy.D., Maj, USAF, BSC
 Jeffrey E. Rhodes, D.Min.

PART II

Military Service–Related
Conditions and Interventions

PART III
Meeting the Needs of Military and Veteran Children and Families

Contributors

Alvi Azad, D.O., M.B.A., Maj USAF MC
Medical Director and U.S. Air Force Staff Physician, Armed Forces Pacific

Paul Ban, Ph.D.
Chief, Program Management Section, U.S. Army Medical Command, Child, Adolescent, and Family Behavioral Health Office, Tacoma, Washington

Mia Bartoletti, Ph.D.
UCLA Nathanson Family Resilience Center, FOCUS Headquarters, Semel Institute for Neuroscience and Human Behavior, Los Angeles, California

Mark J. Bates, Ph.D.
Director, Resilience and Prevention, Defense Centers of Excellence for Psychological Health and Traumatic Brain Injury (DCoE), Silver Spring, Maryland

William R. Beardslee, M.D.
UCLA Nathanson Family Resilience Center, FOCUS Headquarters, Semel Institute for Neuroscience and Human Behavior, Los Angeles, California

David M. Benedek, M.D.
Professor and Deputy Chair, Department of Psychiatry, School of Medicine, Uniformed Services University of the Health Sciences, Bethesda, Maryland

William L. Brim, Psy.D.
Deputy Director, DOD Center for Deployment Psychology, Bethesda, Maryland; Associate Professor, Uniformed Services University of the Health Sciences, Bethesda, Maryland

David E. Cabrera, Ph.D., LTC, USA, MSC (deceased)
Assistant Professor, Department of Family Medicine, School of Medicine, Uniformed Services University of the Health Sciences, Bethesda, Maryland

Jesse Calohan, DNP, PMHNP-BC
Graduate School of Nursing, Uniformed Services University of the Health Sciences, Bethesda, Maryland

Judith Cohen, M.D.
West Penn Allegheny Health System, Pittsburgh, Pennsylvania

Christina Collins, M.S.
Military Family Research Institute at Purdue University, West Lafayette, Indiana

Daniel W. Cox, Ph.D.
Counselling Psychology Program, Department of Educational and Counselling Psychology and Special Education, University of British Columbia, Vancouver, British Columbia, Canada

Stephen J. Cozza, M.D.
Associate Director, Center for the Study of Traumatic Stress, Uniformed Services University of the Health Sciences, Bethesda, Maryland

Justin Curry, Ph.D.
Deployment Health Clinical Center, Bethesda, Maryland

Tricia D. Doud, Psy.D.
Neuropsychiatric Institute, University of California–Los Angeles, Los Angeles, California

Charles Engel, M.D., M.P.H.
Deployment Health Clinical Center, Bethesda, Maryland; Department of Psychiatry, Hébert School of Medicine, Uniformed Services University of the Health Sciences, Bethesda, Maryland

Michael Faran, M.D., Ph.D.
Chief, U.S. Army Medical Command, Child, Adolescent, and Family Behavioral Health Office, Tacoma, Washington

Matthew N. Goldenberg, M.D.
Department of Psychiatry, Uniformed Services University of the Health Sciences, Bethesda, Maryland

Jamie B. Grimes, M.D.
Chair, Department of Neurology, Uniformed Services University of the Health Sciences, Bethesda, Maryland

Derrick Hamaoka, M.D., LtCol, USAF, MC, FS
Staff Psychiatrist, Uniformed Services University of the Health Sciences, Bethesda, Maryland

Jill Harrington-LaMorie, D.S.W., LCSW
Senior Field Researcher/Clinician, Center for the Study of Traumatic Stress, Uniformed Services University of the Health Sciences, Bethesda, Maryland

Patti L. Johnson, Ph.D.
Deputy Chief, U.S. Army Medical Command, Child, Adolescent, and Family Behavioral Health Office, Tacoma, Washington

Larry G. Knauss, Ph.D.
Clinical Psychologist, U.S. Army Medical Command, Child, Adolescent, and Family Behavioral Health Office, Tacoma, Washington

Gregory A. Leskin, Ph.D.
UCLA National Center for Child Traumatic Stress, Los Angeles, California

Patricia Lester, M.D.
UCLA Nathanson Family Resilience Center, FOCUS Headquarters, Semel Institute for Neuroscience and Human Behavior, Los Angeles, California

Travis K. Lunasco, Psy.D., Maj, USAF, BSC
Chief, Mental Health Resiliency, Ramstein AFB, Germany

Shelley MacDermid Wadsworth, Ph.D.
Military Family Research Institute at Purdue University, West Lafayette, Indiana

James E. McCarroll, Ph.D., M.P.H.
Research Professor, Department of Psychiatry, Center for the Study of Traumatic Stress, Uniformed Services University of the Health Sciences, Bethesda, Maryland

Kimberly S. Meyer, APRN
Clinician, Defense and Veterans Brain Injury Center, Walter Reed National Military Medical Center, Bethesda, Maryland; Nurse Practitioner, Department of Neurosurgery, University of Louisville, Louisville, Kentucky

DeAnna L. Mori, Ph.D.
VA Boston Healthcare System (116-B), Boston, Massachusetts

James A. Naifeh, M.D.
Department of Psychiatry, Uniformed Services University of the Health Sciences, Bethesda, Maryland

Barbara L. Niles, Ph.D.
National Center for PTSD, VA Boston Healthcare System (116-B-2), Boston, Massachusetts

Matthew K. Nock, Ph.D.
Department of Psychology, Harvard University, Cambridge, Massachusetts

Robert M. Perito Jr., M.D.
Assistant Chief, Psychiatry Consult Liaison Service, Walter Reed National Military Medical Center, Bethesda, Maryland

Kris Peterson, M.D.
Child, Adolescent and Family Assistance Center, Madigan Army Medical Center, Tacoma, Washington

Jeffrey E. Rhodes, D.Min.
Contract Support for the Resilience and Prevention Directorate, Defense Centers of Excellence for Psychological Health and Traumatic Brain Injury (DCoE), Silver Spring, Maryland

Elspeth Cameron Ritchie, M.D., M.P.H.
Chief Medical Officer, District of Columbia Department of Mental Health, Washington, D.C.; Professor of Psychiatry, Uniformed Services University of the Health Sciences, Bethesda, Maryland

William R. Saltzman, Ph.D.
UCLA Semel Institute for Neuroscience and Human Behavior, Los Angeles, California; College of Education, California State University, Long Beach, California

Patcho Santiago, M.D., M.P.H., CDR, USN, MC
Assistant Professor, Department of Psychiatry, School of Medicine, Uniformed Services University of the Health Sciences, Bethesda, Maryland

Paula P. Schnurr, Ph.D.
National Center for PTSD (116D), VAMC, White River Junction, Vermont

Antonia V. Seligowski, B.A.
National Center for PTSD, VA Boston Healthcare System (116-B-2), Boston, Massachusetts

Robert J. Ursano, M.D.
Professor of Psychiatry and Neuroscience, Chairman, Department of Psychiatry, and Director, Center for the Study of Traumatic Stress, Uniformed Services University of the Health Sciences, Bethesda, Maryland

Susan L. Van Ost, Ph.D.
Center for the Study of Traumatic Stress, Uniformed Services University of the Health Sciences, Bethesda, Maryland

Harold Wain, Ph.D.
Chief, Psychiatry Consult Liaison Service, and Professor, Department of Psychiatry, Walter Reed National Military Medical Center, Bethesda, Maryland

Doug Zatzick, M.D.
University of Washington School of Medicine, Seattle, Washington

Disclosure of Interests

The following contributors to this book have indicated a financial interest in or other affiliation with a commercial supporter, a manufacturer of a commercial product, a provider of a commercial service, a nongovernmental organization, and/or a government agency, as listed below:

Judith Cohen, M.D.   *Royalties:* Guilford Press. *Grants:* SAMHSA, Annie E. Casey Foundation, NIMH. *Contracts:* Pennsylvania and New York State Offices of Mental Health

Kris Peterson, M.D.   *Speakers bureau:* Otsuka Pharmaceutical, AstraZeneca

The following contributors have indicated that they have no financial interests or other affiliations that represent or could appear to represent a competing interest with their contributions to this book:

Paul Ban, Ph.D.; William R. Beardslee, M.D.; David M. Benedek, M.D.; William L. Brim, Psy.D.; Christina Collins, M.S.; Daniel W. Cox, Ph.D.; Stephen J. Cozza, M.D.; Justin Curry, Ph.D.; Tricia D. Doud, Psy.D.; Charles Engel, M.D., M.P.H.; Michael Faran, M.D., Ph.D.; Matthew N. Goldenberg, M.D.; Jamie B. Grimes, M.D.; Derrick Hamaoka, M.D., Lt-Col, USAF, MC, FS; Jill Harrington-LaMorie, D.S.W., LCSW; Patti L. Johnson, Ph.D.; Larry G. Knauss, Ph.D.; Gregory A. Leskin, Ph.D.; Patricia Lester, M.D.; Shelley MacDermid Wadsworth, Ph.D.; James E. McCarroll, Ph.D., M.P.H.; James A. Naifeh, M.D.; Barbara L. Niles, Ph.D.; Matthew K. Nock, Ph.D.; Elspeth Cameron Ritchie, M.D., M.P.H.; Patcho Santiago, M.D., M.P.H.; Paula P. Schnurr, Ph.D.; Robert J. Ursano, M.D.; Susan L. Van Ost, Ph.D.; Harold Wain, Ph.D.; Doug Zatzick, M.D.

Dedication

During preparation of this book, **LTC David E. Cabrera, Medical Service Corps, United States Army,** one of our chapter authors, was killed in combat on October 29, 2011 in Kabul, Afghanistan from a suicide bombing of his convoy. Dave was a well-respected member of the Army behavioral health community who died in the line of duty doing what he was so skilled at, caring for those who serve in harm's way. He is survived by his wife, August Cabrera, and his four children, Corbin, Gillian, Maxwell, and Roanin, as well as a large and loving extended family. It is a reminder to the reader that those individuals who face the challenges described in these pages are not nameless and faceless; they require our nation's greatest care and attention. As Dave's son Maxwell described him, Dave Cabrera was "a soldier of kindness." It is to him, his wife, and his children that this book is dedicated.

Stephen J. Cozza
Matthew N. Goldenberg
Robert J. Ursano

Preface

SINCE 2001, more than two million military service men and women have deployed to combat operations in Iraq and Afghanistan. They come from every military service branch, hail from every state in the country, and represent the active duty, National Guard, and Reserve components of the military. These service members are from the Army, Navy, Air Force, and Marines. Just over half of all military service members are married, and nearly half are parents. Most of their children are young (approximately 40% of children of active duty service members are 5 years old or younger). Many families have faced repeated deployments, some as many as five or more. Since the start of combat operations, more than 6,000 service members have died in combat theater, tens of thousands have suffered combat injuries, and hundreds of thousands continue to suffer with traumatic brain injury (TBI) and posttraumatic stress disorder (PTSD) of varying severity. As this volume goes to publication, combat operations have slowed and many service members are returning from duty in war zones. Although combat experiences are decreasing, future exposure of military service men and women is likely given ongoing worldwide operations of the U.S. military. In addition, the sequelae from these combat-related experiences and conditions will continue to impact service members' health and functioning, as well as the health and functioning of their families, for years to come.

This volume offers essential information to health care (mental health and others) and community service providers who will work with service members, veterans, and their families in the coming years and includes critical information that should inform health care practice and decision making. Successful treatment of service members and veterans requires understanding three fundamental factors. First, *combat exposure impacts service member and veteran physical and mental health* and must be understood in order to better identify risk and to accurately diagnose and effectively treat patients. Second, the *deployment and combat-related experiences of service members are linked to the health and well-being of their family members.* As a result, effective treatments for service members and veterans require *family-focused care,* which addresses family impact and needs and includes family members in the care of service members. Third, despite the tendency to view the military force as monolithic and unchanging, *the composition of the*

U.S. military is constantly changing and transitioning between military and civilian communities. Approximately 10% of the force separates from service (voluntarily, involuntarily, or by retirement) every year and returns to civilian neighborhoods around the country. Veterans often move into communities where there are fewer resources to address their postcombat lives and where professionals likely have very little experience in the care of combat veterans or their families. The health of military service members, veterans, and their families must therefore be a focus for all health care providers, regardless of practice type or location, and should be considered a national health concern, not just of interest to the U.S. Department of Defense (DOD) and the U.S. Department of Veterans Affairs (VA).

The present volume provides information to clinicians and service providers whether they are skilled in caring for military service members and veterans or entirely new to their treatment. The volume is divided into three parts. Part I, "Fundamentals for Treating Military Service Members, Veterans, and Families," provides important information on military culture and the systems that resource them. Chapter 1, "An Introduction to Military Service," gives an overview of military culture, basic information about the military life cycle, and a review of military service branches and components. The authors offer practical information and guidelines for effectively connecting with, supporting, and addressing the needs of military service members, veterans, and their families. Chapter 2, "Understanding Military Families," summarizes information about military families, examining family constellation, marriage, divorce, parenthood, and challenges of military life. The authors also describe the unique inherent strength of military families, as well as opportunities available to them. Chapter 3, "Military Children and Programs That Meet Their Needs," describes military dependent children, underscoring that most are very young and that their common set of experiences leads to challenges, strengths, and opportunities in this population. Finally, Chapter 4, "Military Health Care System and the U.S. Department of Veterans Affairs," gives an overview of the health care systems in which service members and veterans are cared for.

Part II, "Military Service–Related Conditions and Interventions," describes service-related physical and mental health conditions and their treatment in military service members and veterans. Chapter 5, "Health Consequences of Military Service and Combat," reviews the research examining the impact of trauma and PTSD on physical health problems and highlights the mediating effect of PTSD on health outcomes. The authors also provide strategies for addressing the medical and psychiatric needs of combat veterans. Chapter 6, "Combat Stress Reactions and Psychiatric Disorders After Deployment," describes the range of postdeployment responses common in combat veterans, recognizing that these may range from transient and normative responses to chronic and unremitting conditions, including PTSD and depression. Treatments are also reviewed. Chapter 7, "Substance Use Disorders," describes the relatively common occurrence of substance use problems in service member and veteran populations, particularly in combat-exposed populations. The author reviews unique military considerations, military regulations, and military and veteran treatment options, as well as psychotherapeutic and pharmacological treatment options. Chapter 8, "Care of Combat-Injured Service Members," focuses on the unique therapeutic needs of the physically injured population. The authors focus on the resultant physical, psychological, and interpersonal impact of combat injuries, factors that impact recovery, the important role of psychological defenses in injury recovery, and the use of effective psychological and pharmacological treatment approaches. Chapter 9, "Traumatic Brain Injury," reviews one of the signature injuries of the recent conflicts in Iraq and Afghanistan. The authors cover the epidemiology, classification, assessment, and treatment of TBI in the military and VA health systems, as well as approaches to care when TBI coexists with other disorders, particularly PTSD. Chapter 10, "Suicidal Thoughts and Behaviors in Military Service Members and Veterans," emphasizes the importance of distinguishing types of self-injurious thoughts and behaviors. The authors describe the vulnerability-stress model and efforts within the DOD and VA to develop a range of prevention strategies to address elevated rates of suicidal behavior in service members and veterans. Chapter 11, "Collaborative Care," outlines the contribution of barriers to care (particularly stigma) in decreasing treatment seeking and access to effective treatments for mental illness. The authors describe evolving collaborative care health service models within the DOD and VA that serve to enhance engagement within primary care settings.

Part III, "Meeting the Needs of Military and Veteran Children and Families," focuses on military and veteran families, addressing the unique family challenges related to combat deployment, injury, illness, and death. Chapter 12, "Deployment-Related Care for Military Children and Families," describes the challenges faced by military children and families and the resultant programmatic responses within the DOD to better address their needs over time. The authors argue for continued research and expanded systems of care to better meet military family needs. Chapter 13, "Children and Families of Ill and Injured Service Members and Veterans," describes the unique short-term and longer-term challenges faced by families and children resulting from service member and veteran visible or invisible injuries over the course of injury recovery. The authors outline effective family-focused strategies for sustaining these families in the face of injury- and illness-related stress. Chapter 14, "Caring for Bereaved Military Family Members," distinguishes the unique features of military death that may pose distinctive risks or protective factors to military family survivors. The authors emphasize the lack of research in the area of military bereavement and the need to be aware of both normative and clinical (or complicated) grief outcomes that require distinctive interventions for adults and children. Chapter 15, "Building Resilience in Military Families," differentiates *mechanisms of risk* from *mechanisms of resilience* as they relate to military families facing the challenges that they encounter. The authors also describe one promising family preventive intervention model, Families Overcoming Under Stress (FOCUS), and the developing evidence base supporting its use in military and veteran families.

This volume is the effort of a group of exceptional authors from a variety of backgrounds, including those with military, veteran, and civilian experience, representing academic expertise in the areas of military medicine, adult and child clinical practice, family therapy, and preventive medicine. The authors span the fields of psychiatry, neurology, psychology, social work, chaplaincy, and nursing. In a focused way, this volume brings together a critical collaboration to help our nation build a community of effort to support our service members, veterans, their families, and their children.

Stephen J. Cozza
Matthew N. Goldenberg
Robert J. Ursano

Acknowledgments

The editors would like to acknowledge the help of the following professionals in the production of this clinical manual.

Sara Pula, Ph.D., for her exceptional assistance maintaining communication with chapter authors, coordinating editing and proofing of all chapters, providing editorial input to chapters, and facilitating communication with the APPI editorial team.

Jamie Sullivan, Abby Ridge-Anderson, and Erin Beech for their assistance in making electronic changes to chapters, checking references, researching information at editors' request, creating tables, and assisting in updates to DSM-5 criteria.

APPI staff, including Robert Hales, M.D., Editor-in-Chief; John McDuffie, Editorial Director; Greg Kuny, Managing Editor; Bessie Jones, Acquisitions Coordinator; Carrie Farnham, Senior Editor; and Tammy Cordova, Graphic Design Manager, for their assistance, support, and direction through the development and editing of this manuscript.

PART I

Fundamentals for Treating
Military Service Members,
Veterans, and Families

Chapter 1

An Introduction to Military Service

Derrick Hamaoka, M.D., LtCol, USAF, MC, FS
Mark J. Bates, Ph.D.
James E. McCarroll, Ph.D., M.P.H.
William L. Brim, Psy.D.
Travis K. Lunasco, Psy.D., Maj, USAF, BSC
Jeffrey E. Rhodes, D.Min.

MORE THAN 2.5 MILLION Americans currently serve in the U.S. military either on active duty, in the Reserves, or in the National Guard, and more than 20 million civilians are veterans of military service. These current and former service members and their families seek health care in military, veteran, and civilian settings. Some health care providers may be familiar with the military, but others may be less familiar because it is an organization with its own language, rules, customs, and culture.

In this chapter we highlight various aspects of life in the military and provide a context for understanding the perspectives and experiences of service members and their families. We provide civilian medical and non-medical care providers practical information and guidelines for effectively connecting with, supporting, and addressing the needs of military service members and their families.

Organization of the U.S. Military

The U.S. Department of Defense (DOD) consists of three Service departments: Army, Navy (including Marine Corps), and Air Force. (The Coast Guard operates under the auspices of the Department of Homeland Security.) The total number of military personnel on active duty is approximately 1.5 million (U.S. Department of Defense 2011), with 550,000 Army personnel (U.S. Army 2012), 325,000 Air Force personnel (U.S. Air Force 2012), 333,000 Navy and Marine personnel (U.S. Marine Corps 2012; U.S. Navy 2012), and 42,000 Coast Guard personnel (U.S. Coast Guard 2012). The U.S. military also consists of intermittently activated components, the Reserves and National Guard. About 1.4 million Americans serve in these components, which consist of just under half of the military's ready force (U.S. Department of Defense 2011). Unlike their active duty counterparts, members of these organizations often have other nonmilitary occupations and work for the military only at designated times (e.g., one weekend per month and a few other weeks during the year). During their nonduty time, Reservists and Guardsmen and Guardswomen typically work and live in communities that may be remote from military installations. They frequently seek medical care in their home communities from civilian clinicians. The military includes a variety of demographic factors and subcultures such as military services, National Guard and Reserve component designations, occupational specialties, unit affiliations, unique service history, ranks, grades, genders, and family structures that can influence beliefs, perceptions, and behavior. Health care providers need to be alert to these subcultures.

Demographics and Culture of Military Personnel

Service members represent a large portion of the population, including nearly every demographic category and geographic region of the United States and its territories. The active duty force is predominantly male (85.6%) and relatively young (50% of enlisted members are 25 years old or younger). Thirty percent of active duty members identify themselves as a racial or ethnic minority (U.S. Department of Defense 2011). Military families include not only service members but also their dependents and total approximately 1.9 million people. More than half (56%) of all active duty members are married, 39% are married with children, and 8% are single parents (U.S. Department of Defense 2011). Nearly 94% of the enlisted force has a high school diploma or equivalent and/or some college experience. Almost 83% of officers have a bachelor's degree or higher (U.S. Department of Defense 2011).

There are two distinct populations in the military—officers and enlisted personnel—each with its own rank structure and with officers outranking all enlisted service members. Officers are responsible for all aspects of a military unit, including issuing orders, enforcing policies, and addressing both work-related concerns and individual personal issues (e.g., financial challenges, marital problems, legal troubles). The enlisted ranks make up approximately 83% of the active duty force, provide the bulk of the military's workforce (U.S. Department of Defense 2011), and often join the military out of high school. Once in the military, enlisted service members are trained in such specialty areas as combat, administration, engineering, and health care.

Rank and Grades

The military is a hierarchical organization, with each service member having a rank and pay grade. Rank is determined partially by time in service but also reflects a service member's performance and potential to the military organization. Each military service member is assigned a rank that usually advances during the course of an individual's career. Officers (O) and enlisted personnel (E) belong to separate rank structures. Often, active duty service members and veterans prefer to be called by their military rank.

In addition to official organizational positions, a person's rank determines who is subordinate to whom. Officers are the only service members who can "hold command" (directing orders to a unit) and are superior in the rank structure to enlisted personnel. Rank can also be thought of as a way to address a service member, such as "Private," "Airman," "Sergeant," or "Captain." Rank is indicated on paperwork and through uniform insignias. Although the military services have different names for ranks, the services share the same basic grades, and the customs and courtesies due to senior ranks apply across services. Service members often retain a sense of pride regarding their rank. It must be earned, is an important representation of an individual's time in service and expertise, and should be respected.

Grade (or pay grade) is a designation made for pay purposes. Pay grades are E1 through E9 for enlisted personnel and O1 through O10 for commissioned officers. Although grade is standard across services, rank is often idiosyncratic and may mean different things in different military branches. For example, an Army captain (whose grade is O3) should not be confused with a Navy captain (who is at a much higher grade O6).

At the lower enlisted ranks, promotion is nearly automatic provided that the member is a reasonably good performer and has a relatively clean record (e.g., no record of trouble, problems, or disciplinary actions). E4 or E5 is the transition point at which enlisted service members become leaders or supervisors or noncommissioned officers (NCOs) and begin to compete for promotion. To obtain a promotion, service members must meet time-in-service and time-in-grade criteria as well as accumulate promotion points for each rank. Points can be obtained through performance on physical fitness tests, school scores, awards, and standardized tests. Higher-ranking NCOs are promoted on the basis of merit and points, with each higher rank being more selective and difficult to achieve.

Officer promotions are similar to that of the enlisted, with initial promotions (O1 through O3) being nearly automatic. To achieve officer "field grades," O4 and above, promotion becomes more competitive, is through recommendation, and involves a thorough record review by higher-ranking officers. In rare circumstances, service members may be demoted to a lower rank, usually as punishment for rules violations. Service members whose rank seems lower than it should be given his or her time in service should be asked about any adverse job actions.

Military Occupational Specialties

Distinct from rank, every member of the military is assigned to at least one occupation or specialty, known as military occupational specialties (MOS). These range from administrative fields to infantry, pilot, explosive ordnance disposal, security forces (military police), medical providers, and chaplains and can also be associated with a unique culture. It is common for service members to refer to their MOS, and health care providers may develop better relationships with service member or veteran patients by recognizing their occupational identities.

Gender Issues

Females in the military often have commonly held experiences as a result of their gender and being in the minority in a male-oriented culture. Although women's roles have been expanded and an increasing number of women have been promoted to the top officer ranks, a female in the military can face a range of challenges including 1) feeling as if she has to perform to a higher standard than male counterparts, 2) facing potential ostracism from her peers if she becomes pregnant (which may result in an extended period of absence during which coworkers must cover her duties), 3) facing traditional views of many people from within the military culture who still believe females are the weaker gender and should not be in military service, 4) feeling the need to change personal interaction styles in order to appear more masculine and fit in with her male peers, and 5) being less likely to ask for help for fear of being labeled weaker or less capable than her male counterparts (e.g., Ghahramanlou-Holloway et al. 2011).

Principles of Military Culture

When working with members of the military, it is important to understand both the general military culture and subculture memberships. Military members come from all ethnic, educational, and socioeconomic backgrounds but nevertheless belong to a distinct culture that is formed around shared beliefs and values. The military is generally a collectivistic culture that stresses the necessity of cooperation, communalism, interdependence, and conformity. For military members, a collectivist mentality is evident in issued uniforms, a requirement to conform to grooming standards, and the learning of a unique "language." In the military system, collectivistic beliefs and values are expressed as an identity that is based in the social system and being part of a group and involves emotional dependence on others in the group and self-sacrifice for the group.

The unequal distribution of power, in contrast to a more egalitarian organizational structure, is another characteristic of military culture. The military is a system of hierarchical relationships involving social authority, which determines a person's role and is required for control and prevention of disorganization (Hofstede 2001). While sometimes perceived as rigid, military social hierarchy and rank create a climate of harmony through norms and expectations (Kapoor et al. 1996). The military is organized with chains of command that describe the line of authority and responsibility along which orders are passed. Military culture also favors careful planning and structure, using rules and guidance to help manage and reduce uncertainty and risk (Hofstede 2001, p. 149). Each service is guided by regulations, instructions, and standard operating procedures.

Service Subcultures

Members of each military service branch have great pride in their service and typically believe that their service's mission is the best the military has to offer. Military branches have a strong influence on many other aspects of military service culture, including operational job specialties, training and operations, types of equipment and uniforms, and popular terms and slogans. (The appendix to this chapter provides resources for locating common terms, acronyms, rank structures, and military installations throughout the DOD.)

Army Service Culture

The U.S. Army is the nation's principal land force (U.S. Department of Defense 2010a) and the largest service and usually has the largest number of troops engaged in combat. Army service members, called soldiers, are not limited to land missions but perform a large amount of transport of troops on the sea and in the air. The Army has a high operational tempo, and it is not uncommon for soldiers to be deployed in a 2- or 3-year cycle that involves a year or more deployment and then 1 or 2 years "in garrison" (at their home base) before the cycle begins again. The Army has been on the ground in Iraq and Afghanistan since 2003, so many soldiers have deployed overseas numerous times. The Army espouses seven organizational values that guide expected behaviors among all soldiers: loyalty, duty, respect, selfless service, honor, integrity, and personal courage.

Marine Corps Service Culture

The U.S. Marine Corps' mission includes serving as an expeditionary force-in-readiness and conducting expeditionary and amphibious operations to include close air support for ground forces, crisis response, and power projection (U.S. Department of Defense 2010a). Marines are the smallest service but have the largest percentage of service members exposed to combat. The Marine Corps is structured around a Marine Air-Ground Task Force, organizations consisting of ground, aviation, and combat service support and command elements. Operating forces are organized for war fighting and then adapted for peacetime. The Marine Corps lives and breathes by its service motto "Semper Fidelis," which translates to "always faithful" and describes the love that Marines have for the Marine Corps, their unit, and their brothers and sisters in arms in combat and garrison alike.

Navy Service Culture

The U.S. Navy's primary mission is to "conduct offensive and defensive operations associated with the maritime domain" (U.S. Department of Defense 2010a, p. 31). Navy personnel are known as sailors, and although there is no official motto, "Non Sibi Sed Patriae," translated as "not self but country," has been used. Navy values include honor, courage, and commitment.

In the Navy, there are multiple and diverse communities, such as air, sea, submarine, and many "land-locked" bases and stations. Aircraft carriers have been described as floating cities whose residents include mail workers, cooks, repair staff for thousands of different machines and engines, painters, carpenters, gas station attendants, firefighters, doctors, clergy, and pilots. Given the diverse environments in which they may work, sailors may not know what personnel in other divisions on the ship do. Each of these divisions on a carrier has a culture of its own. The Navy also supports the Marine Corps by providing staff corps and support officers, including health care providers and chaplains, and acts as the major sea transport delivery systems for forward-deployed Marines who embark on Navy ships.

Air Force Service Culture

The U.S. Air Force is the newest of the military services. Created in 1947 as a separate branch, it was previously incorporated under the Army. Air Force doctrine stresses its role and unique capability to project national influence anywhere in the world on very short notice. Given its air assets, the Air Force emphasizes speed, range, flexibility, and precision to create effects where and when needed. Air Force deployment missions include security forces, explosive ordnance disposal (also known as bomb disposal), and medical and chaplain support as well as surveillance and intelligence missions, search and rescue, national air defense, delivery of satellites and materiel to outer space, and nuclear weapons operations. The Air Force's set of core values are integrity first, service before self, and excellence in all we do.

Reserve Components and National Guard

The Reserve component includes the U.S. Army Reserve, U.S. Navy Reserve, U.S. Marine Corps Reserve, U.S. Air Force Reserve, U.S. Coast Guard Reserve, Army National Guard, and Air National Guard. Members of the military Reserves and National Guard face unique challenges: 1) the challenge of dual identity as a result of living simultaneously in civilian and military communities (Griffith 2011a); 2) a dramatic increase in activation and deployments since the start of combat operations in Iraq and Afghanistan, constituting a significant shift in job expectations for Reserve or Guard members and their families (usually accustomed to serving in stateside units for one weekend a month and 15 annual training days); and 3) challenges associated with availability of personnel, preparation for deployments, and adjustments during and after deployments (Griffith 2011b) as a result of the increase in activation and deployments. Reserve forces often do not have access to the same support structure as their active duty counterparts and often rely on civilian providers for mental health needs (Institute of Medicine 2010).

Military Life Cycle: Recruitment to Separation or Retirement and Beyond

Joining the Military

For nearly the past four decades, the U.S. military has been an all-volunteer force; service members have chosen to join the military. An enlistee must choose a branch of service at the time of enlistment. Regardless of the branch of service they choose, individuals must meet a set of standards set by individual services. Age is the one of the first requirements; individuals must be at least 18 years of age (or in some cases, at least 17 years of age with parental consent). Enlistees must be either citizens of the United States or legal, permanent residents who are physically living in the country. A high school diploma or its equivalent is generally required. Applicants may also be excluded for a history of "questionable moral character," including a history of criminal behavior. Applicants must also meet certain height and weight standards that vary between services. Each applicant must undergo medical screening, including a physical examination to determine the presence or history of a medical or mental health condition that would prohibit entry. Prospective military enlistees take the Armed Services Vocational Aptitude Battery (ASVAB), a multiple-choice test that examines several domains, including verbal and mathematics knowledge. The test is offered regularly at many high schools and other locations throughout the country. A subset of the ASVAB known as the Armed Forces Qualifying Test (AFQT) determines whether an applicant qualifies for enlistment. Applicants scoring in the bottom 10th percentile are legally barred from military service, and most services accept only applicants who score above the 30th percentile.

Life in the Military

Military service is unlike any other job. A certain degree of freedom is lost by wearing the uniform. Service members become part of an organization in which they must follow specific rules and obey and execute the lawful orders of their superiors. Every activity is meant to serve the goal of personal and unit readiness, to serve and protect the country in peacetime and in war.

The military sets behavioral expectations that service members must meet. Service members must live in areas and work in fields as authorized by the military; meet standards of personal appearance, including restrictions on hair length and requirements for the proper wearing of their uniform; meet physical fitness standards to include both physical traits (e.g., weight, height) and functions (e.g., running, push-ups); and meet standards for appropriate conduct at all times, even when off duty. The use of illicit drugs is strictly forbidden. Certain physical injuries and medical or psychiatric illnesses are incompatible with continued military service.

Training and Education

After a recruit meets enlistment requirements and is sworn into the military, he or she goes to basic training for a period of 8–12 weeks. Basic training is a rite of passage for enlisted corps and is an intense period of instruction and indoctrination into military skills, rules, and customs, including saluting, proper wearing of the uniform, physical fitness, marksmanship, and some combat procedures. Emphasis is placed on obeying the operational hierarchy, following the direction of superiors, and executing orders efficiently and without question. The training period can be physically and emotionally demanding and is designed to imbue new service members with the physical stamina, discipline, and respect for authority necessary to succeed in the military.

Following the completion of basic training, the enlistee enters a second phase of training or schooling to provide necessary instruction and experience for a particular specialty. The length of these trainings can range from several weeks to months. Each service uses AFVAB results to determine an enlistee's specialty. Certain specialties also require particular physical, psychological, or character qualifications. With basic training and other schooling complete, the service members are moved to their first duty station, where they will begin work in their specialty. This move is referred to as a permanent change of station (PCS). A PCS refers to any permanent change of duty location and is distinguished from deployments and temporary duty (TDY) assignments.

On-the-job training and more formalized instruction through hands-on, simulation, classroom, and field modalities occur in all specialties. For most members of the military, their job training is short-term and specialty-specific and is conducted within the military. Certain career fields require long-term, highly specialized education, and the military supports such education both at military sites and through civilian routes. The military also provides scholarships to students to train at civilian institutions.

In addition to training specific to their day-to-day military work, service members are encouraged to further their education. The Post-9/11 GI Bill provides educational benefits military members can use during or after their time in the service. The amount of benefit varies depending on length of active duty service, but the full benefit covers 4-year tuition and fees (at in-state rates), a book and supply allowance of up to $1,000 per year, and a living stipend (equivalent to that of an E5). Enlisted service members may also have preexisting education debt paid through the Loan Repayment Program.

Benefits and Opportunities

Pay and Allowances

Military service members are employees of the federal government, and there are many forms of regular pay, special pay, and bonuses they can earn. On entry into the military, members begin to receive a salary, known as base pay. This varies by the member's military grade (e.g., E1 or O4), time in the military, and particular skills or duties. Members also receive allowances, which are considered reimbursements and are not taxed or garnished. Officers and enlisted personnel receive a basic allowance for housing, which is dependent on pay grade, location, and number of dependents. Enlisted soldiers also receive a basic allowance for subsistence (to offset the cost of meals) and a clothing allowance for military uniforms. Bonuses are offered for reenlisting and are given to personnel in high-demand special skills areas. Bonus size depends on number of years of reenlistment, specialty type, and need.

Life on Base

Members of the military live and work in a variety of locales around the globe, although many live and work on or near military installations. Installations are referred to by different names, including base, fort, camp, shipyard, post, or station. These installations vary in size, with the largest ones the size of small American cities. Installations frequently include work space and training facilities for service members and civilian employees, housing options (from barracks to single-family homes), schools for service members' children, health care facilities, recreational facilities, and shopping and dining options. Military members, retirees, and their families have access to the military commissaries (military grocery stores) and base exchanges (department stores) that offer a large selection of brand name foods, household goods, and clothing at or slightly below cost without associated sales tax.

Health Care

Active duty members, retired military, and their dependent family members receive largely free medical benefits with the exception of an annual deductible and small enrollment fee. Active duty military members and their dependents (as well as some reservists and retirees) are also eligible for civilian health benefits through a program known as TRICARE.

Challenges of Military Life: Service Members and Family

Military life, with its frequent moves, deployments, and separations from extended family and friends, can be difficult for service members and their families. Military families are often young and may be particularly vulnerable to the challenges of military life. Each branch of the military has established free support services for members and their families, such as the Army Community Services, Navy's Fleet and Family Support Centers, and Air Force Family Support Centers. These support services offer assistance for relocation or moving, coordination of special needs family care, home visits for expectant mothers, parenting classes, safety courses, stress management classes, relationship classes, and adjustment for spouses of newly enlisted service members.

Moves

Frequent moves are a way of life for service members and their families. Service members can receive notification to move at any time, giving them little time to prepare, reestablish, and adjust to a new location, and then receive new orders to move again. Although the military attempts to assign members to a single location for 2–3 years, this consistency is not guaranteed. Moves can introduce a host of challenges and opportunities, such as establishing new support systems, securing affordable housing, enrolling children in new schools, changing health care providers, and finding new jobs for spouses. Sometimes service members and their families relocate to places other than the continental United States with significantly different cultures, and acculturation to these places provides both opportunities and challenges.

Deployments

A deployment is an extended work assignment to an area away from home base and includes routine support to another installation or unit, military training, humanitarian crisis intervention or peacekeeping, or work in an operational or combat area. Deployments can vary in length, and recently, combat deployments have lasted between 6 and 15 months. A train-up and preparation period usually precedes the deployment and often means additional time away from family and home. Deployment experiences can vary considerably. Some service members are directly involved in combat, are exposed to harsh conditions, witness frequent injury or death, or may themselves incur injuries (physical, psychological, or both), whereas others spend their deployments in less threating assignments. Some service members feel their deployment is rich and rewarding, while others find the quality and pace of the work and/or the separation from family and friends more challenging.

Deployments can place a particular burden on the families of service members and strain family relationships. Technology allows for frequent communication between a deployed service member and his or her family; however, spouses and children of deployed service members must continue with their daily activities and responsibilities without the immediate help of the deployed member.

Although redeployment (returning from deployment) is generally a welcomed event, some service members have a difficult time readjusting to life at home. Such difficulties may result from physical or psychological injuries, and other difficulties include reintegration into relationships with family and friends. Because the experience is so variable, inquiring about a service member's particular deployment—what he or she did or witnessed, where he or she was stationed, how he or she felt about the experience—can be an important part of a clinical evaluation.

After the Military

Reenlistment Versus Separation

At some juncture through the first enlistment and later at midlevel (between 8 and 12 years of service), the service member must decide whether to stay in the military or be discharged. Officers may also choose to continue service after their obligation is complete, or they may resign their commission. If a service member leaves the military prior to retirement, he or she is considered to be separated. This can occur voluntarily or involuntarily. Involuntary separations can occur as an honorable discharge (laying off service members) or as a general discharge (given to members who have had significant behavioral problems or a personality disorder). Dishonorable or bad conduct discharges are punitive measures taken against members who have been convicted by court-martial of significantly bad acts. Such discharges cause members to lose eligibility for veterans' benefits or reenlistment opportunities.

Medical Separation or Medical Retirement

When health conditions are deemed incompatible with military service, members may be separated or retired through a Medical Evaluation Board process. Disability compensation may be paid to service members whose medical conditions developed while on active duty. In addition to military-connected medical retirement benefits, a disability determination is also rated by the U.S. Department of Veterans Affairs, resulting in monthly tax-free compensation based on the degree of disability.

Retirement

A service member is eligible for retirement after 20 years and must retire after 30 years. A pension amounting to 50% of the service member's base salary is paid for the remainder of the retiree's life upon 20 years of service and increases to 75% if the length of service reaches 30 years (basic allowance for housing and subsistence pay are not included in calculating retirement pay). Reservists can also receive retirement benefits, although the amount is based on other factors, such as years of active and inactive service and age. Retirees often enjoy continued access to shopping on military installations and, to some degree, access to health care.

Military Mental Health, Stigma, and Help-Seeking Resources

Military medical and mental health services provide critical support roles for service members by ensuring the fitness of all service members; however, military medical providers are also responsible for evaluating a person's fitness for duty. As a result, service members may be demotivated to report symptoms if they believe this will influence their ability to do their job or stay in the military.

In addition, the mental health culture can be at odds with the military culture in several ways. The value of collectivism in the military can be associated with service members not wanting to seek help because it might impact the unit, take time away from supporting the unit, or cause the service member to be pulled out of the unit. In this way, collectivistic values can contribute to stigma and hinder help seeking. Masculine values are often similarly associated with stigma because service members fear being seen as weak for seeking help. Stigma-related barriers are likely to be present even after a service member has left the military. Further, traditional mental health models promote individualism and an internal locus of control and subscribe to a pathology-based model, all of which can be experienced as conflicting with core military values. It is incumbent on a provider to be aware of and respect these issues. Practitioner models that use a team perspective and focus on strength and resilience are likely to be more successful with military members.

These stigma-related barriers are being addressed aggressively through such means as providing public service announcements from senior leaders, professional athletes, and popular actors; changing policies, such as altering the impact receiving psychotherapy has on security clearances; developing a public education campaign featuring testimonies from military personnel and their spouses about dealing with psychological issues; and creating services that can be accessed by phone or Internet. In addition, innovations in care include enhancing training for primary care providers on identification and treatment of psychological health issues (Engel et al. 2008), putting mental health providers in primary care (Hunter et al. 2010), embedding mental health providers in units (Hoyt 2006), and developing a specialty track for operational psychology (Staal and Stephenson 2006). Clinicians must work to provide strength-based care through established and accepted systems that will minimize stigma-related concerns.

Cultural Assessment Resources and Tools for Providers Working With Military Members or Veterans

An accurate assessment of a patient's military history can help the provider develop an understanding of how the military experience affected the member, either positively or negatively, thus enhancing the assessment, case conceptualization, and treatment planning process. In this section we describe practical considerations and suggest helpful questions that can be used during the assessment process and throughout therapy with service members, veterans, and their families. These valuable tools can help diminish stigma, build rapport, and develop a collaborative therapeutic relationship with the service member, veteran, or military or veteran family member.

Table 1–1 provides sample questions that health care providers working with a military service member or veteran should ask themselves in order to better assess their own attitudes and possible prejudices regarding military culture. Table 1–2 provides a list of general recommendations for building and maintaining a successful therapeutic relationship with service members, veterans, and their families. (Table 1–2 was based on the practical experience of the coauthors and on tips attributed to Col (Dr.) Landry by King 1999.)

Finally, a list of suggested questions is presented in Table 1–3 and is meant to be a practical tool to assist in the assessment of service members and veterans. The questions are intended to provide a systematic review of the individual's military background, the potential role of military culture in the expression of symptoms and dysfunction, and the effect that cultural differences may have on the therapeutic relationship. These questions are

TABLE 1–1.	Sample self-assessment questions

What are my preconceived notions about military culture?

What stereotypes do I have about the military?

What are my beliefs about the military and its role in our country?

How were my beliefs about the military and its role in our country formed?

What are my beliefs about the people who join the military?

How do I feel about the current conflicts?

Regardless of my feeling about the current conflicts, negative or positive, can I separate these feelings from how I feel about those who serve and who wear the military uniform?

TABLE 1–2.	General recommendations for interviewing military members

Acknowledge military service.
> Recognizing a member or veteran or military or veteran family member's sacrifice initially is important. Whether this is done in the waiting room with a sign that says, "Are you a military member or veteran?" or in the initial paperwork or interview, this is the first step in a conversation about the military culture and its impact on the patient.

Set clear goals and expectations.
> Military members are often used to clear goals and structure, so it may be helpful to approach interactions in a goal-driven and step-by-step fashion. For example, a semistructured interview can fit with their experiences with checklists and standard operating procedures.

Find ways to identify and leverage skills and strengths, especially those associated with military training experience, as opposed to illness and vulnerability.
> Consider the value of explaining the biological basis of symptoms, persistent distress, and functional impairment as literal injuries to the brain and body. This approach can potentially reduce stigma by explaining why these injuries are similar to other medical conditions involving the mind and the body (Nash et al. 2009).

Ask the extent to which the service member relates his or her symptoms and concerns to his or her military service.

If you are working in a nonmilitary or non-VA clinic or hospital, attempt to understand why the service member has not accessed care in the military or through the VA if eligible.

Create a safe environment to explore potential moral concerns and listen for themes like survivor guilt.

Source.   King 1999.

intended to be a guide for the clinician rather than a definitive review of all necessary information. They may be helpful for initiating discussion before getting into more diagnostically focused questions.

TABLE 1–3. **Sample questions**

What branch of service were you in?

Were you ever in the Guard or Reserve?

What years did you serve?

What was your rank?

What was your occupation(s) in the military?

How many duty assignments did you have and where were they?

What were some of the reasons you decided to join the military originally? Were they different from the reasons you stayed in the military (if the patient served more than 1–4 years)?

What were the major milestones in your career?

What was the impact of military service on your family?

What does it mean to you to be a service member or veteran?

Were you ever deployed?

What was most rewarding part of deployment?

What was most difficult part of deployment?

When did you deploy? Where?

How many times did you deploy and how long were the deployments?

What were your duties in theater?

Did you see combat? How often were you "outside the wire?"

Did you deploy with your unit or were you an individual augmentee?

If Guard or Reserve, what was impact on life of being deployed versus impact when you came home and returned to civilian life?

Did you feel supported by the unit?

Were you exposed to blasts while deployed?

What was your exposure to death of unit members, enemy combatants, or civilians?

Do you feel that there are any lasting physical or psychological effects of your exposure to these potentially traumatic events?

What is the possibility that you will get deployed again?

How was coming home from deployment; was it different from what you expected?

What was the impact of deployment on your family?

SUMMARY RECOMMENDATIONS FOR CIVILIAN CLINICIANS

- Use the same principles as working with a person from any different culture, realizing that a service member may or may not identify with the military culture in general or with specific subelements.

- Never make assumptions, but acknowledge one's own unfamiliarity and ask questions. Ensuring safety and openness is critical, especially in the first connection.

- Be attentive for any potential disruptions in the therapeutic relationship and address them in a proactive, collaborative, and respectful way.

- Consider ways to leverage what the military member is already familiar with and what is meaningful to the military member. Ask military members about their reasons for concern and satisfaction with different aspects of their experiences in the military.

- Consider approaching deployment-related issues initially as an adaptive response to occupational stress rather than a clinical disorder.

- When working with service members who are on active status, consider involving the chain of command as part of the support network if the service member is willing to sign a release and believes his or her superior officer will be helpful.

- When working with service members who are on active status, consider supporting the service member by leveraging resources that may be available throughout the military system such as chaplains and military medical, family support, and legal professionals.

- Consider if existing resources could be used to augment treatment such as recommending that a service member view specific vignettes on the Real Warriors Campaign Web site and giving the service member a handout describing the Defense Centers of Excellence for Psychological Health and Traumatic Brain Injury Outreach Center and AfterDeployment.org Web site for themselves and their family members.

References

Engel CC, Oxman T, Yamamoto C, et al: RESPECT-Mil: feasibility of a systems-level collaborative care approach to depression and post-traumatic stress disorder in military primary care. Mil Med 173(10):935–940, 2008

Ghahramanlou-Holloway M, Cox DW, Fritz EC, et al: An evidence-informed guide for working with military women and veterans. Prof Psychol Res Pr 42:1–7, 2011

Griffith J: Contradictory and complementary identities of U.S. Army Reservists: a historical perspective. Armed Forces Soc 37(2):261–283, 2011a

Griffith J: Decades of transition for the US Reserves: changing demands on Reserve identity and mental well-being. Int Rev Psychiatry 23(2):181–191, 2011b

Hofstede G: Culture's Consequences: Comparing Values, Behaviors, Institutions, and Organizations Across Nations, 2nd Edition. London, Sage, 2001

Hoyt GB: Integrated mental health within operational units: opportunities and challenges. Mil Psychol 18(4):309–320, 2006

Hunter CL, Goodie JL, Oordt, MS, et al: Integrated Behavioral Health in Primary Care: Step-by-Step Guidance for Assessment and Intervention. Washington, DC, American Psychological Association, 2010

Institute of Medicine: Returning Home from Iraq and Afghanistan: Preliminary Assessment of Readjustment Needs of Veterans, Service Members, and Their Families. Washington, DC, National Academies Press, 2010

Kapoor S, Comadena ME, Blue J: Adaptation to host cultures: an individualist-collectivist approach. Intercultural Communication Studies VI 1:35–54, 1996

King R: Aerospace Clinical Psychology. Aldershot, UK, Ashgate, 1999

Nash WP, Silva C, Litz B: The historic origins of military and veteran mental health stigma and the stress injury model as a means to reduce it. Psychiatr Ann 39(8):789–794, 2009

Staal MA, Stephenson JA: Operational psychology: an emerging subdiscipline. Mil Psychol 18(4):269–282, 2006

U.S. Air Force: United States Air Force, 2012. Available at: http://airforce.com. Accessed February 1, 2012.

U.S. Army: Go Army, 2012. Available at: http://www.goarmy.com/cl5.html. Accessed February 15, 2012.

U.S. Coast Guard: Coast Guard Reserve opportunities, 2012. Available at: http://www.gocoastguard.com/find-your-career/reserve-opportunities. Accessed February 29, 2012.

U.S. Department of Defense: Secretary Gates at the Pentagon, press transcript, April 11, 2007

U.S. Department of Defense: Functions of the Department of Defense and Its Major Components. Department of Defense Directive Number 5100.01. Washington, DC, U.S. Department of Defense, 2010a

U.S. Department of Defense: Department of Defense Dictionary of Military and Associated Terms. Joint Publication 1-02. Washington, DC, U.S. Department of Defense, 2010b

U.S. Department of Defense: Demographics 2010: profile of the military community, Washington, DC, U.S. Department of Defense, 2011

U.S. Marine Corps: U.S. Marine Corps: Marine recruiting, 2012. Available at: http://www.marines.com. Accessed February 15, 2012.

U.S. Navy: America's Navy: a global force for good, 2012. Available at: http://navy.com. Accessed February 15, 2012.

Appendix: Department of Defense Terms, Acronyms, Ranks, and Installations

DOD reference guide	
Military terms and definitions	For military terms and definitions, refer to the DOD Dictionary Web site, which is managed by the Joint Education and Doctrine Division, J-7, Joint Staff. All approved joint terms, definitions, acronyms, and abbreviations are contained in U.S. Department of Defense (2010b), as amended through May 15, 2011. • General Web site: http://www.dtic.mil/dtic/customer/acronyms.html • DOD Dictionary of Military and Associated Terms: http://www.dtic.mil/doctrine/new_pubs/jp1_02.pdf • Search capability for acronyms: http://www.dtic.mil/doctrinedod_dictionary?zoom_query=TDY&zoom_sort=0&zoom_per_page=10&zoom_and=1
Ranks and insignias	• Enlisted ranks: http://www.defense.gov/about/insignias/enlisted.aspx • Officer ranks: http://www.defense.gov/about/insignias/officers.aspx
Military installations	MilitaryInstallations is a companion Web site to DOD Military Homefront that lists names and locations of military installations. • Web site: http://www.militaryinstallations.dod.mil/

Chapter 2

Understanding Military Families

Their Characteristics, Strengths, and Challenges

Christina Collins, M.S.
Shelley MacDermid Wadsworth, Ph.D.

MILITARY FAMILIES are a numerical minority in U.S. society and are largely misrepresented, stereotyped, and misunderstood, particularly in the media (Lofty 2006; Spell 2011). During World War II, 1 in 10 members of the civilian population served in the active or Reserve components of the military (Bureau of Labor Statistics 2011; U.S. Census Bureau 2012). The percentage of adolescents willing to even consider military service has fallen below 20% for males and 10% for females (Bachman et al. 2000), and the number of members of Congress with military experience fell to only 20% during the 2010–2011 session, its lowest level since WWII, compared

Preparation of this manuscript was supported by *Strengthening Supports for Military and Veteran Families in Indiana and Beyond* (MacDermid Wadsworth, principal investigator). We wish to thank all of the staff and students at MFRI for their support and assistance. Some of the material in this chapter was developed for use in training interns preparing to work on military installations; our thanks to the Military-Extension partnership for including us in that effort. We also thank Mark Bates for generously sharing relevant information.

with more than 70% during the 1960s and 1970s (Military Officers Association of America 2011). Military members are sometimes portrayed as poorly educated, disproportionately from low-income backgrounds, or poorly paid relative to members of the civilian population (Rall 2007; Travers 2009). Each of these portrayals is either incorrect or incomplete. Military members are more likely than those in the civilian population to have earned a high school diploma or the equivalent but less likely to have earned a college degree (Table 2–1). Further, regular military compensation has exceeded comparable civilian pay, including allowances and in-kind benefits, since 2002 (Murray 2010). National Guard and Reserve members experience an average income increase of nearly $20,000 when facing long deployments (Hosek 2011).

Few people, even those *in* the military, know everything about military life. The goal of this chapter is to help civilian mental health practitioners increase their "cultural competence" for serving members of military families (Bean et al. 2001; Livingston et al. 2008). Cultural competence for professionals incorporates four key elements: 1) being knowledgeable about their own values and stereotypes, 2) using effective techniques in their work, 3) being knowledgeable and accepting of culturally diverse clients, and 4) appreciating the strengths and differences displayed by diverse others.

Demographic Characteristics of Military Families

Family members of service members (spouses, children, and legal dependents) outnumber service members in both the active duty and Reserve components. Within the active duty force there are 1.4 million service members and close to 2 million family members; the Reserve component comprises more than 800,000 service members and 1.2 million family members (Deputy Under Secretary for Defense for Military Community and Family Policy [DUSD] 2012).

On average, members of the active component are younger than members of the Reserve component (27.3 versus 30.8 years for enlisted members and 34.7 versus 40.1 years for officers for the active and Reserve components, respectively). Among spouses of service members on active duty ($N=725,377$), almost one-third (29.8%) are 25 years of age or younger, and only 13.3% are 41 or older. Reserve component spouses are older, with almost the reverse proportions: 14.1% ages 25 or younger and 32.5% ages 41 or older.

TABLE 2–1.   **Educational attainment of military members and civilians, 2010**

	Military	**Civilian**
High school diploma	97.6% enlisted accessions[a]	82.6% civilians ages 18–24[a]
High school or beyond	99.5% active duty force[b]	88.4% civilians ages 25–44[c] 91.1% civilian labor force[d]
BA or beyond	17.7% active duty force[b]	33.0% ages 25–44[c] 34.6% civilian labor force[d]

[a]Under Secretary of Defense, Personnel and Readiness 2010.
[b]Deputy Under Secretary of Defense for Military Community and Family Policy 2012, Figure 2.38.
[c]U.S. Census Bureau 2012, Table 231.
[d]U.S. Census Bureau 2012, Table 593.

Marriage

Overall, 56.4% of military members on active duty are married; the proportion of Reserve component personnel who are married is slightly lower, at 48.2% (DUSD 2012). In both the active and Reserve components, officers are more likely than enlisted members to be married (70% versus 53.7%, respectively) (DUSD 2012). A recent age-adjusted comparison of marriage among male civilians and military members showed that between 2002 and 2005, military members were significantly more likely than civilians to have married at some point in their lives (Karney et al. 2012).

Women serving in the military are substantially less likely to be married than their male counterparts, a pattern not observed among civilians of similar age. In the civilian population in 2010, 43.5% of males and 50.1% of females ages 18–44 were married (U.S. Census Bureau 2012). In the military, 72.5% of male officers and 51.0% of male enlisted personnel were married in 2005, compared with 51.0% of female officers and 42.8% of female enlisted personnel (Karney and Crown 2007). Female active duty service members are several times more likely than their male counterparts to be married to a fellow service member (22.3% and 4%, respectively), and the same is true of women serving in the Reserve component (8.7% and 1.3%, respectively) (DUSD 2012). Among married female service members, 48.2% of active duty members and 23.3% of Reserve component members are married to other service members. Thus, women in the military are far more likely than men to be in dual-military marriages.

Divorce

Several media outlets have reported a large jump in divorce rates as a result of deployment-related stressors (Alvarez 2007; Associated Press 2004; Parsons 2008). A recent analysis comparing military and civilian divorce rates showed that the percentages of male enlisted members and officers who were currently divorced were either the same or lower than the percentages of civilian men with comparable education, age, race or ethnicity, and employment status both prior to (1998–2001) and during (2002–2005) the wars in Iraq and Afghanistan (Karney et al. 2012).

Divorce rates within the military are lower among officers than enlisted personnel: among officers, the divorce rate was 1.9% in 2010, up from 1.4% in 2000. Enlisted members divorced at a rate of 2.9% in 2000, rising to 3.5% in 2005 and 4.1% in 2010 (DUSD 2012). In contrast, the civilian divorce rate fell noticeably, from 4.1 divorces per 1,000 members of the population in 2000 to 3.4 in 2007 (U.S. Census Bureau 2012). The marriages of female service members appear to be more vulnerable to divorce than those of males (Karney and Crown 2007). In 2006, 6.6% of married women in the active military experienced a marital dissolution, compared with 2.6% of married men. Enlisted women seem to be especially at risk for divorce. In 2005, 7.3% of married enlisted women experienced a divorce, compared with 2.8% of married enlisted men. The comparable rates among officers were 3.6% and 1.5% for women and men, respectively (Karney and Crown 2007). For both enlisted personnel and officers, women were more than twice as likely as men to experience divorce.

Parenthood

Overall, 44.1% of active duty and 43.2% of Reserve component members were parents in 2010, and officers were more likely than enlisted members to have children (DUSD 2012). Active duty members had a total of 1.2 million children in 2010, the single largest group of whom were children younger than 5 (see Table 2–2) (DUSD 2012). Among the 745,533 children of members of the Reserve component, the two largest groups were school-age and adolescent children.

Active duty military personnel tend to be younger than members of the Reserve component when they have their first child (24.9 versus 26.6 years); both groups of parents have 2.0 children on average. Military members are about twice as likely as civilians to have their first child between the ages of 20 and 24 (47% versus 25%), and they are less likely to have their children when they are younger than 20 (7% versus 10%) or 30 or older (18% versus 37%) (DUSD 2011; U.S. Census Bureau 2012).

TABLE 2-2.   **Age distribution of service members' children, 2010**

	Active duty	Reserve component
0–5 years	42.3%	27.9%
6–11 years	30.7%	30.1%
12–18 years	22.8%	30.3%
19–22 years	4.2%	11.7%

Source. Deputy Under Secretary of Defense for Military Community and Family Policy 2012.

TABLE 2-3.   **Distribution of service members by family type, 2010**

	Active duty	Reserve component
Single, no children	38.8%	42.5%
Single, with children	5.3%	9.0%
Married to civilian, no children	13.8%	13.1%
Married to civilian, with children	35.9%	32.5%
Dual military, no children	3.7%	1.2%
Dual military, with children	2.9%	1.4%

Source. Deputy Under Secretary of Defense for Military Community and Family Policy 2012

Compared with members serving on active duty, Reserve component members are slightly more likely to be single or to be single parents, as Table 2–3 shows. Among service members married to civilians, those on active duty are more likely than Reserve component members to be parents (DUSD 2011).

In the active duty military in 2010, there were 51,491 single fathers (4.2% of all male service members) and 24,463 single mothers (12.0% of all female service members). Although the number of single parents overall has decreased from its 2000 peak of 85,552, the number of single mothers set a new record in 2010 (DUSD 2012). Single parents are more common in the Reserve component (7.6% of male and 16.8% of female service members). The *likelihood* of being a single parent is much higher among women than men in both the civilian and military populations.

Military Spouses

Spouses of service members in both the active duty and Reserve components are primarily women (93.1% and 88.1%, respectively). The Air Force has the highest percentage of male spouses (10%), followed by the Navy (7.4%), Army (6.3%), and the Marine Corps (2.1%). Higher percentages of male spouses are found in the Reserve component, with 19.3% in the Air Force, 18.5% in the Army, and 15.1% in the Navy (DUSD 2012).

Compared with civilian populations, higher percentages of active duty military spouses report that they are either unemployed or not in the labor force. Among spouses of active duty officers, 37% report that they are employed in the civilian labor force; 11% are military members; 8% are unemployed but seeking work; and 45% are not in the labor force, meaning they are neither employed nor seeking employment. Similarly, among spouses of enlisted members, 36% report that they are in the civilian labor force, and 37% are not in the labor force (DUSD 2012). In the civilian population in 2010, 59.7% of all married couples had both partners in the labor force, and 61.0% of all married women participated in the labor force (U.S. Census Bureau 2012).

In summary, although the prevalence of marriage has fallen in both military and civilian populations in recent decades, members of the military are more likely than civilians with similar characteristics to marry. Although divorce rates have recently risen in the military, service members are no more likely than civilians to divorce, and this has not changed during the course of the current conflicts. Female service members are more likely to divorce than their male peers. Military members tend to bear their children during their 20s, and although there are more single fathers than mothers in the military, the likelihood of being a single parent is substantially higher for women, as is true in the civilian population. Labor force participation rates among military spouses are similar to those reported by civilian spouses, but unemployment rates are higher in the military.

Challenges of Military Life

Military culture imbues a strong sense of mission, readiness to be asked to serve anywhere at a moment's notice, and a commitment to get the job done no matter what is required. The work is often physically demanding, with long and unpredictable hours, heavy training responsibilities, and a heavy workload. Service members are reassigned frequently, as are their co-workers and superiors, leading to chronic "churn" in the work environment. Service members must pass regular fitness, weight, drug, and health tests and are open to scrutiny regarding financial and other matters in order to maintain their security clearances. Each of these elements of military service has the potential to affect the lives of family members.

Family Separation

Deployment is a defining feature of military life regardless of whether a war is being fought and is just one type of family separation in the military. Routine training, schooling, and temporary duty (often referred to as TDY) are other types of assignments that require the service member to temporarily relocate from his or her home station. These family separations may range from days to more than a year with varying levels of advance notice (Aldridge et al. 1997). More than 2 million service members have deployed to the wars in Iraq and Afghanistan since 2001, and the effects of frequent and lengthy combat deployments on military family members has emerged as an issue for practitioners and researchers.

Characteristics of the deployment and of family members affect a family's adjustment to separation. The length and frequency of separations in addition to whether or not the mission is a wartime or peacekeeping operation are influential, as are the age and sex of children. Parental attitudes, access to social support, coping skills and adaptability, and past experiences with separation all predict a family's response to deployment (McCarroll et al. 2005).

In a study of recently returning service members (Sayers et al. 2009), family concerns cited included feeling like guests in their households, having trouble with their relationship with their children, feeling uncertain about their role in the family, and experiencing conflict with and/or aggression toward their spouses. Service members who experienced mental health concerns following deployment were more likely to report family reintegration issues.

Spouses also experience individual effects of deployment. A study of more than 250,000 U.S. Army wives' medical records revealed that when compared with spouses of nondeployed soldiers, wives of soldiers deployed to Operation Enduring Freedom/Operation Iraqi Freedom experienced higher rates of depressive disorders, sleep disorders, anxiety, acute stress reactions, and adjustment disorders. Deployments lasting longer than 11 months were associated with even higher rates of spousal distress (Mansfield et al. 2010). In terms of marital stability, Karney and Crown (2007) found that as the number of days deployed increased, the likelihood of a couple divorcing decreased.

Although deployments and family separations can be sources of stress, mental health concerns, and family difficulties, service members and their spouses also report positive effects of deployment, including financial gain, a sense of pride and patriotism, and, for family members, a sense of confidence and independence (Castaneda et al. 2008). Not having enough personal time, having too many responsibilities at home, changing marital roles, growing apart from their partner, and experiencing parenting hassles due to children's problematic behavior at school and at home are some of the most commonly reported challenges facing spouses during deployment (Chandra et al. 2011). Another common challenge is boundary ambiguity, in which service members and family members are uncertain about the degree to which the service member is fully "present" psychologically in the family (Faber et al. 2008).

Deployment may differentially affect active duty and Guard or Reserve families (Castaneda et al. 2008; Chandra et al. 2011). Reserve and Guard samples report poorer emotional well-being, more relationship problems during deployment, and more deployment and reintegration challenges with their children than active component families (Chandra et al. 2011). These difficulties are due to more complex transitions into and out of civilian life, changes in health care and services as families transition into and out of active duty military status, and belonging to a civilian community that is less prepared to meet the challenges of military members (Faber et al. 2008; MacDermid Wadsworth 2010).

Relocation

Geographic mobility, or frequent relocation, represents one of the most often mentioned features of military life, especially as it relates to children's adjustment. In 2010, military members were more than twice as likely as civilians to move (31% versus 13%, respectively) (U.S. Census Bureau 2011). Moving can affect family well-being, financial well-being, spousal employment, and social support (Burrell 2006). On average, relocation occurs every 2–3 years for military families, although there are wide variations (Burrell 2006). In the 2006 Survey of Active Duty Spouses, among spouses whose partners had served between 3 and 5 years, 25% had moved once, 18% had moved twice, and 10% had moved three or more times. Among those whose spouses had served 6–9 years, 27% had moved three or more times (Defense Manpower Data Center 2006). Within military populations, frequent relocation is often reported as one of the most stressful aspects of military life (Ender 2006; Kelley et al. 2003). Kelley et al. (2003) found that such factors as low family cohesiveness or family problems present before the move are exacerbated during a stressful move, but frequent relocations alone did not appear to cause psychopathology. Lyle (2006) found that children's scores on academic achievement tests dropped slightly as a function of both household relocations and parental deployment.

Spouse Employment

Military spouses choose similar occupations to their civilian peers, often working in such fields as administration, teaching, and health care. They often choose to work for financial reasons but also note such motives as achieving personal fulfillment, keeping busy, using their education, and maintaining their career status (Harrell et al. 2004). Among military spouses who do not work, the primary reason cited for being out of the labor force is parenting demands; less common responses include attending school and volunteering. Even spouses who are out of the labor force by choice indicate reluctance to enter the labor force because of frequent moves, feeling like a single parent because of the service member's military career demands, and child care concerns (Harrell et al. 2004). A 2010 study of underemployment found that when military wives are compared with civilian wives who are similar on many demographic factors, military wives are more likely to be out of the labor force, involuntarily working part time, underemployed, or underearning (Lim and Schulker 2010).

Spouses cite several reasons for the military's negative effects on their employment, including frequent and disruptive moves, the military member's absence because of deployments, inconsistent and intensive military work schedules, and the demands of parenthood. Some spouses perceive stigma or bias in their communities against hiring military spouses (Castaneda and Harrell 2008). Researchers have described military husbands and wives as "tied migrants" who often sacrifice their own occupational potential to follow the migration of their spouse's military career. Findings indicate that both men and women in a tied migrant status suffer in terms of employment status, earnings, and hours worked (Cooke and Speirs 2005; Little and Hisnanick 2007).

The relationship between the employment status of military spouses and their sense of well-being is complex. Research has found that underemployment does not seem to correlate with satisfaction as a military spouse. Lim and Schulker (2010) suggested that military spouses may be more willing to accept underemployment and note that factors other than employment may be more important predictors of their well-being. However, other research suggests that adverse employment opportunities for military spouses can have significant negative effects on both the spouse and the military's ability to retain service members. Career development satisfaction has been linked to military wives' general well-being (Rosen et al. 1990), and the majority of military spouses perceive that the military has a negative effect on their employment (Harrell et al. 2004). Castaneda and Harrell (2008) argued that recruiting and retention efforts of active duty personnel are contingent on the military's ability to support both service members and spouses in achieving both occupational and life satisfaction. Spousal employment concerns predict service members' intentions to reenlist in the military (Schwartz et al. 1991), and military wives also believe they have a strong influence on their active duty husbands' reenlistment decisions (Lim and Schulker 2010). Spouses interviewed about their employment experiences cited several suggestions for increasing their employment opportunities: improving child care, promoting awareness and utilization of military-sponsored employment assistance programs, culti-vating government employment opportunities for military spouses, requiring less frequent moves, and addressing interstate licensing and certification constraints (Castaneda and Harrell 2008).

Intimate Partner Violence

Child maltreatment is addressed in Chapter 3, "Military Children and Pro-grams That Meet Their Needs," so the focus here is only on intimate part-ner violence (IPV). Intimate partner violence in military families has been studied somewhat less than child maltreatment. In a review, Rentz et al. (2006) found 11 studies of child maltreatment but only 3 addressing spouse abuse and 1 focusing on both. The literature on family violence in military populations lacks rigorous studies on the prevalence of intimate partner vi-olence and spouse abuse (Clark and Messer 2006).

Researchers have found elevated rates of domestic violence among mil-itary couples relative to civilian populations (Clark and Messer 2006; Rentz et al. 2006), especially among veterans who struggle with combat stress, de-ployments, and posttraumatic stress disorder (PTSD; Sherman et al. 2006). Younger couples and lower enlisted couples are at the greatest risk for IPV (Newby et al. 2005). In a side-by-side comparison of rates in the Army and civilian populations, Heyman and Neidig (1999) found no differences in rates of moderate husband-to-wife violence (reported by 10% of respon-dents) but a higher rate of severe violence in the Army versus a comparable civilian sample (2.5% versus 0.7%).

Evidence is mixed, however, regarding the relationship between deploy-ment and IPV. For example, one study of U.S. Army soldiers indicated that a 6-month deployment to Bosnia did not increase the likelihood of domes-tic violence (Newby et al. 2005). Similarly, Bradley (2007), studying veter-ans and nonveterans in the National Survey of Families and Households, found that veteran status was not significantly related to the likelihood of spousal aggression. In contrast, McCarroll and colleagues (2010) examined rates of spousal aggression in data gathered from more than 25,000 service members between 1990 and 1994 and found that the probability of moder-ate aggression rose from 17.6% with no deployment to 18.5% in the pres-ence of deployments lasting 6–12 months. The chance of severe aggression rose from 3.7% to 5.0%. A clearer pattern may emerge when psychological symptoms are taken into account. In a multigroup study of 179 veterans, Sherman and colleagues (2006) contrasted groups of veterans dealing with PTSD or depression relative to a control group. On the basis of veterans' self-reports (spouse reports were higher), members of the PTSD group were 5.4 times more likely to commit violence and 26.4 times more likely to commit severe violence than members of the control group. The comparable figures for members of the depression group were 4.0 and 8.6. Physical health problems also increased the likelihood of violence.

Protective factors against IPV are built into the military system. A military member maintains mandatory stable employment with a steady income, and the federal government provides health care, housing, and family support programs (Rentz et al. 2006). Military members also risk discharge and serious consequences from the military for the discovery of family violence or its risk factors, including mental health problems, substance abuse, and criminal actions (Raiha and Soma 1997).

Financial Difficulties

The high level of military activity during the past 11 years has prompted increased attention to the financial circumstances of military families. Specific concerns have arisen in Congress and the U.S. Department of Defense regarding "predatory lending," in which lenders aggressively seek out military members with questionable loan products. This is of particular concern in the military because financial problems can make it impossible for service members to hold a security clearance, which is a prerequisite for continuing their military careers.

A 2006 Department of Defense report concluded that some lenders target young and/or financially inexperienced service members by locating near military installations or marketing through the Internet. In response, the Department of Defense has aggressively educated service members about financial management and less problematic options, such as loans available through military aid societies.

Self-report data from the Survey of Active Duty Service Members indicate a downward trend between 2003 and 2006 in the percentage of service members reporting financial problems, particularly bouncing checks (which fell from 13% to 7%); failing to make minimum credit card payments or receiving pressure from creditors (both of which fell from 17% to 11%); and having telephone, cable, or Internet shut off (which fell from 10% to 7%). Levels of other financial problems (falling behind in rent or mortgage payments, having utilities shut off, or having large items repossessed) were much lower and changed little.

Access to Services

Although military members and their families are eligible for a wide array of services provided by the Department of Defense, including health care; housing; subsidized child care; programs for children and youth, including extensive resources for families with special needs children; spousal employment programs (Karney and Crown 2007); and other services, there are gaps in access to these services. For example, the Department of Defense Task Force on Mental Health (Arthur et al. 2007) described gaps in the continuum of care for psychological health that disadvantage military spouses and children who do not have access to military hospitals. Family members and service members who rely on the military TRICARE system of civilian providers also may experience gaps in care. For example, a study assessing the participation of mental health care providers from the TRICARE list indicated that only 25% of the providers were accepting new patients, and the likelihood of accepting new patients was *negatively* related to the number of deployed service members in the market area (Avery and Wadsworth 2011).

Opportunities for Families in Military Life

The structure and requirements of military service mean that service members and their spouses and children avoid many of the serious risk factors that threaten civilian families, such as lack of education, poverty, and homelessness. While serving, every military member meets a minimum educational standard and has a job with benefits, including health care coverage for family members; housing; strong incentives to remain drug-free, physically fit, and financially responsible; access to a variety of formal family supports, including subsidized high-quality child care, parent education, and youth programs; and support for continued education and spouse employment. Nonetheless, as documented in this chapter, some military families do experience problems with finances, spousal employment, violence, or other serious challenges.

Strengths of Military Families

Using an ecological perspective, Harrison et al. (1990, p. 350) argued that ethnic minority families in the United States have developed "adaptive strategies" or "cultural patterns that promote the survival and well-being of the community, families, and individual members of the group" in response to the challenges of living as minority groups. Common adaptive strategies across ethnic minority groups include role flexibility, family extendedness, ancestral worldviews, and biculturalism. Even though military families as a group differ from ethnic minority groups in several ways, the authors of this chapter suggest that there are important shared elements of their experiences that have led military families to become adept at some of the same adaptive strategies.

Role Flexibility

The structure of military life requires that families develop role flexibility even when their preference is to follow a particular kind of role arrangement. Because service members are frequently assigned to training or temporary duty at distant locations, as well as longer deployments for peacekeeping, combat, or natural disasters, all family members must repeatedly reallocate domestic responsibilities. Service members may need to adjust to having less control over daily family events, and other family members must take over many of the tasks service members are unable to perform. Management of resources and thus family power also may shift in response to family separations, giving spouses periods of intermittent "leadership" of the family.

Family Extendedness

In ethnic minorities, family extendedness takes many forms, including clan-based family structures, matriarchal structures, and creation of "fictive kin." Harrison et al. (1990, p. 351) suggested that "the extended family is a problem-solving and stress-coping system that addresses, adapts, and commits available family resources to normal and non-normal transitional and crisis situations." Although military culture emphasizes nuclear families, it also attempts to promote exchanges of mutual support among families. Family readiness groups in the Army are intended to be a "front line" of mutual support for spouses, bringing them together to provide emotional and instrumental assistance and essentially encouraging them to act as fictive kin for one another. There are also many examples of extended family members providing substantial assistance in response to the demands of military service, including caring for grandchildren during deployments or relocating to provide full-time care to a wounded service member.

Ancestral Worldviews

Harrison argued that a third adaptive strategy of minority groups is to understand that the well-being of the individual is tightly connected to the well-being of the group and thus to value loyalty to the group. This value manifests in military culture in several ways. First, loyalty to the military and their unit is expressly required of service members, who pledge it in their service oaths. In addition, the extensive and elaborate rituals of military culture, including ceremonies, language, artifacts, and dress, serve to reinforce a sense of belonging to the group and a strong connection to "ancestors" in the form of heroes or heroic actions in the past. Finally, military service often runs in families, providing a literal ancestral connection to the group.

Biculturalism

Members of most minority groups must learn to function successfully in the dominant culture as well as in their traditional culture through such accommodations as shifting their behavior to fit whichever culture they happen to be functioning in at that moment. Members of military families also must develop this skill. A profound skill that service members and their families develop is that of being self-aware and filtering information they share with a constant eye on what is safe to share given security concerns, as well as what is personally safe to reveal (e.g., controversial or shocking information). A common example is service members who are questioned as to whether or not they killed someone while deployed. In their bicultural role, service members can deny or refuse to answer the question, which may seem like a rejection of peers, or they can affirm the question, which opens the possibility of being judged negatively and becoming an object of derision. The challenges of biculturalism intensify when service members leave active military service because they may not know how to communicate their occupational experiences to civilian employers or how to navigate their way around communities that are organized very differently from military communities.

Conclusions

In this chapter, we have provided a description of available demographic data about military families, described some of the seminal challenges and opportunities of military life, and proposed some specific family strengths that apply to military families. Significant gaps remain in our understanding of military families, however. For example, because the focus of most programs, practices, and policies is the traditional nuclear family, knowledge about other family forms—such as unmarried partners, stepfamilies, gay and lesbian headed families, or families with nonresidential children—is limited. Although there has been considerable attention to the quality and stability of military marriages, less attention has been devoted to the formation of families in the military, which is a potentially important topic given the youth of the force. Because the substantial majority of military members are male, relatively little attention is devoted to male spouses, which is troubling given the relative fragility of female service members' marriages. In addition, awareness of predatory lenders and other "bad actors" can make military families wary of seeking assistance even when they are eligible. All of these gaps constitute potential hurdles that professionals may need to be prepared to surmount in order to provide effective service to individuals who have served the United States with such commitment and loyalty.

SUMMARY POINTS

- In 2010, active duty members had a total of 1.2 million children, the single largest group of whom were children younger than 5.

- Women serving in the military are substantially less likely to be married than their male counterparts but when married are far more likely than their male counterparts to be married to a fellow service member. The marriages of female service members appear to be more vulnerable to divorce than those of males.

- Divorce rates within the military are lower among officers than enlisted personnel. The percentages of male divorced enlisted members and officers were either the same or lower than the percentages of civilian men with comparable education, age, race or ethnicity, and employment status as recently as 2005.

- Challenges to military families include separation, characteristics of deployment, change in marital and family roles, relocation, spousal employment, financial difficulties, and access to services.

- Strengths of military families include a sense of confidence and independence, a sense of pride and patriotism, financial gain, role flexibility, family extendedness, ancestral worldviews, and biculturalism.

References

Aldridge DM, Sturdivant TT, Smith CL, et al: Background Characteristics of Military Families: Results From the 1992 Surveys of Officer and Enlisted Personnel and Military Spouses. Arlington, VA, Defense Manpower Data Center, 1997

Alvarez L: Long Iraq tours can make home a trying front. New York Times, February 23, 2007. Available at: http://www.nytimes.com/2007/02/23/us/23military.html?pagewanted=all. Accessed September 9, 2013.

Arthur DC, MacDermid SM, Kiley K, et al: An achievable vision: report of the Department of Defense Task Force on Mental Health. Falls Church, VA, Defense Health Board, 2007

Associated Press: Army seeks to save war-torn marriages. USA Today, December 19, 2004. Available at: http://www.usatoday.com/news/nation/2004-12-29-army-marriage_x.htm. Accessed September 9, 2013.

Avery GH, Wadsworth SM: Access to mental health services for active duty and National Guard TRICARE enrollees in Indiana. Mil Med 176(3):261–264, 2011

Bachman JG, Freedman-Doan P, O'Malley PM: Youth attitudes and military service: findings from two decades of monitoring the future national samples of American youth. Arlington, VA, Defense Manpower Data Center, 2000. Available at: http://www.dtic.mil/cgi-bin/GetTRDoc?AD=ADA386284. Accessed September 9, 2013.

Bean RA, Perry BJ, Bedell TM: Developing culturally competent marriage and family therapists: guidelines for working with Hispanic families. J Marital Fam Ther 27(1):43–54, 2001

Bradley C: Veteran status and marital aggression: does military service make a difference? J Fam Violence 22:197–209, 2007

Bureau of Labor Statistics: Economic news release: employment situation. Washington, DC, U.S. Department of Labor, 2011. Available at: http://www.bls.gov/news.release/empsit.t01.htm. Accessed April 25, 2012.

Burrell LM: Moving military families: the impact of relocation on family well-being, employment, and commitment to the military, in Military Life: The Psychology of Serving in Peace and Combat, Vol 3: The Military Family. Edited by Castro C, Adler A, Britt T. Westport, CT, Praeger, 2006, pp 39–63

Castaneda LW, Harrell MC: Military spouse employment: a grounded theory approach to experiences and perceptions. Armed Forces Soc 34:389–412, 2008 doi:10.1177/0095327X07307194

Castaneda LW, Harrell MC, Varda DM, et al: Deployment Experiences of Guard and Reserve Families: Implications for Support and Retention. Santa Monica, CA, RAND, 2008

Chandra A, Lara-Cinisomo S, Jaycox LH, et al: Views From the Homefront: The Experiences of Youth and Spouses From Military Families. Santa Monica, CA, RAND, 2011

Clark JC, Messer SC: Intimate partner violence in the U.S. military: rates, risks, and responses, in Military Life: The Psychology of Serving in Peace and Combat, Vol 3: The Military Family. Edited by Castro C, Adler A, Britt T. Westport, CT, Praeger, 2006, pp 193–219

Cooke TJ, Speirs K: Migration and employment among civilian spouses of military personnel. Soc Sci Q 86:343–355, 2005 doi:10.1111/j.0038-4941.2005.00306.x

Defense Manpower Data Center: Survey of active duty spouses. Arlington, VA, Defense Manpower Data Center, 2006

Deputy Under Secretary of Defense for Military Community and Family Policy (DUSD): Profile of the military community: DoD 2009 demographics. Alexandria, VA, ICF International, 2011. Available at: http://www.militaryonesource.mil/12038/MOS/Reports/2009_Demographics_Report.pdf. Accessed September 9, 2013.

Deputy Under Secretary of Defense for Military Community and Family Policy (DUSD): Profile of the military community: DoD 2010 demographics. Alexandria, VA: ICF International, 2012. Available at: http://www.militaryonesource.mil/12038/MOS/Reports/2010_Demographics_Report.pdf. Accessed September 9, 2013.

Ender MG: Voices from the backseat: demands of growing up in military families, in Military Life: The Psychology of Serving in Peace and Combat, Vol 3: The Military Family. Edited by Castro C, Adler A, Britt T. Westport, CT, Praeger, 2006, pp 138–166

Faber A, Willerton E, Clymer S, et al: Ambiguous absence, ambiguous presence: a qualitative study of military reserve families in wartime. J Fam Psychol 22: 222–230, 2008 doi:10.1037/0893-3200.22.2.222

Harrell MC, Lim N, Castaneda LW, et al: Working Around the Military: Challenges to Military Spouse Employment and Education. Santa Monica, CA, RAND, 2004

Harrison AO, Wilson MN, Pine CJ, et al: Family ecologies of ethnic minority children. Child Dev 61:347–362, 1990 doi:10.2307/1131097

Heyman RE, Neidig PH: A comparison of spousal aggression prevalence rates in U.S. Army and civilian representative samples. J Consult Clin Psychol 67:239–242, 1999

Hosek JR: How is Deployment to Iraq and Afghanistan Affecting U.S. Service Members and Their Families?: An Overview of Early RAND Research on the Topic. Santa Monica, CA, RAND, 2011

Karney BR, Crown JS: Families Under Stress: An Assessment of Data, Theory, and Research on Marriage and Divorce in the Military. Santa Monica, CA, RAND, 2007

Karney BR, Loughran DS, Pollard MS: Comparing marital status and divorce status in civilian and military populations. J Fam Issues 33(12):1572–1594, 2012

Kelley ML, Finkel LB, Ashby J: Geographic mobility, family, and maternal variables as related to the psychosocial adjustment of military children. Mil Med 168(12):1019–1024, 2003

Lim N, Schulker D: Measuring Underemployment Among Military Spouses. Santa Monica, CA, RAND, 2010

Little RD, Hisnanick JJ: The earnings of tied-migrant military husbands. Armed Forces and Society 33:547–570, 2007

Livingston J, Holley J, Eaton S, et al. Cultural competence in mental health practice. Best Practices in Mental Health 4:1–14, 2008

Lofty: Military (family life) myths, part I [Web log]. Blogspot, March 16, 2006. Available at: http://porttampa.blogspot.com/2006_03_01_archive.html. Accessed September 9, 2013.

Lyle DS: Using military deployments and job assignments to estimate the effect of parental absences and household relocations on children's academic achievement. J Labor Econ 24:319–350, 2006

MacDermid Wadsworth SM: Family risk and resilience in the context of war and terrorism. J Marriage Fam 72:537–556, 2010 doi:10.1111/j.1741-3737.2010.00717.x

Mansfield AJ, Kaufman JS, Marshall SW, et al: Deployment and the use of mental health services among U.S. Army wives. N Engl J Med 362(2):101–109, 2010

McCarroll JE, Hoffman KJ, Grieger TA, et al: Psychological aspects of deployment and reunion, in Military Preventive Medicine: Mobilization and Deployment, Vol 2. Edited by Kelley PW. Falls Church, VA, Surgeon General of the Army, 2005, pp 1395–1424

McCarroll JE, Ursano RJ, Liu X, et al: Deployment and the probability of spousal aggression by U.S. Army soldiers. Mil Med 175(5):352–356, 2010

Military Officers Association of America: Declining military experience in Congress. Military Officers Association of America, 2011. Available at: http://www.moaa.org/lac/lac_resources/lac_resources_tips/lac_resources_tips_decline.htm. Accessed April 26, 2012.

Murray CT: Evaluating military compensation: testimony before the Subcommittee on Personnel Committee on Armed Services United States Senate. Washington, DC, Congressional Budget Office, 2010

Newby JH, Ursano RJ, McCarroll JE, et al: Postdeployment domestic violence by U.S. Army soldiers. Mil Med 170(8):643–647, 2005

Parsons C: U.S. military marriages strained by long deployments. Reuters, May 6, 2008. Available at: http://www.reuters.com/article/2008/05/06/idUSN22289468. Accessed September 26, 2013.

Raiha NK, Soma DJ: Victims of child abuse and neglect in the U.S. Army. Child Abuse Negl 21(8):759–768, 1997 doi:10.1016/S0145-2134(97)00037-9

Rall T: Poor and uneducated, like we thought: debunking the military debunkers. Boise Weekly, August 1, 2007. Available at: http://www.boiseweekly.com/boise/poor-and-uneducated-like-we-thought/Content?oid=933196. Accessed April 21, 2012.

Rentz ED, Martin SL, Gibbs DA, et al: Family violence in the military: a review of the literature. Trauma Violence Abuse 7(2):93–108, 2006 doi:10.1177/1524838005285916

Rosen LN, Ickovics JR, Moghadam LZ: Employment and role satisfaction: implications for the general well-being of military wives. Psychol Women Q 14:371–385, 1990

Sayers SL, Farrow VA, Ross J, et al: Family problems among recently returned military veterans referred for a mental health evaluation. J Clin Psychiatry 70(2):163–170, 2009

Schwartz JB, Wood LL, Griffith JD: The impact of military life on spouse labor force outcomes. Armed Forces and Society 17:385–407, 1991

Sherman MD, Sautter F, Jackson MH, et al: Domestic violence in veterans with posttraumatic stress disorder who seek couples therapy. J Marital Fam Ther 32(4):479–490, 2006

Spell K: Military family stereotypes debunked. BabyCenter.blog, June 11, 2011. Available at: http://blogs.babycenter.com/mom_stories/military-family-stereotypes-debunked/. Accessed September 9, 2013.

Travers K: Exclusive: Michelle Obama's emotional meeting with military families. ABC News, March 12, 2009. Available at: http://abcnews.go.com/GMA/Politics/story?id=7067528&page=1. Accessed April 21, 2012.

Under Secretary of Defense, Personnel and Readiness: Population representation in the military services, Table B-6. Non-prior service active component enlisted accessions, FY10: by education tier, service, and gender with civilian comparison group. U.S. Department of Defense, 2010. Available at: http://prhome.defense.gov/rfm/MPP/ACCESSION%20POLICY/PopRep2010/appendixb/appendixb.pdf. Accessed September 13, 2013.

Under Secretary of Defense, Personnel and Readiness: Population representation in the military services. U.S. Department of Defense, 2010. Available at: http://prhome.defense.gov/RFM/MPP/ACCESSION%20POLICY/PopRep2010/. Accessed April 21, 2012.

U.S. Census Bureau: Statistical abstract of the United States (129th edition), U.S. Census Bureau, 2011. Available at: http://www.census.gov/compendia/statab/. Accessed September 13, 2013.

U.S. Census Bureau: Statistical abstract of the United States (130th edition), U.S. Census Bureau, 2012. Available at: http://www.census.gov/compendia/statab/. Accessed April 20, 2012.

Chapter 3

Military Children and Programs That Meet Their Needs

Patti L. Johnson, Ph.D.
Larry G. Knauss, Ph.D.
Michael Faran, M.D., Ph.D.
Paul Ban, Ph.D.

MILITARY CHILDREN and families have made critical contributions to the success and functioning of the U.S. Armed Forces. The life experiences of these children and families, the subculture in which they live, and the challenges and benefits of this lifestyle have transformed over time. Understanding the multifaceted culture of the military family is critical to working with military children and families. Aspects of military living and experiences shared by all military children and adolescents affect their identity as "military brats." Although characteristics of this culture may also be shared by their nonmilitary counterparts, military children share a common set of experiences that distinguish them from nonmilitary children.

History

From the time of the Revolutionary War, a constituency of military wives and children—"campfollowers"—have accompanied their spouses on military assignments and missions (Alt and Stone 1991). They were not generally regarded as a responsibility of the military and were discouraged from joining soldiers. When they did, living conditions were quite poor, with limited housing options, poor food rations, and no amenities available. Through World War II and into the Vietnam era, a majority of service members were single, partly because of mandates against marriage for enlisted personnel. For those who were married, family members were increasingly allowed to accompany military members to both stateside and overseas assignments, and the military began to provide such basic services as housing and other modest benefits to families. It was not until after the Vietnam War that the military as an organization began to seriously acknowledge and provide targeted support for military families and their children. This was particularly true when the military transformed to an all-volunteer force in the 1970s and included older members who were married and had children. The cultural changes of the 1960s and 1970s impacted the military in similar ways (Martin and McClure 2000; Paden and Pezor 1993): there were more women in the uniformed services, more dual-career military couples, more single parents, more ethnic minorities, and fewer "traditional" family units. The military became a "professional" fighting force requiring greater technical skills and more highly educated personnel; therefore, the quality of life in the military was viewed as an important consideration in recruiting and retaining highly qualified service members. The life satisfaction of family members was shown to be critical to a service member's military performance, readiness, and retention (Griffith et al. 1993), highlighting the fact that the military family was an integral part of the success of the mission. Thus, the military began to initiate policies and programs to address the needs and quality of life of military children and families.

Beginning in the early 1980s, Congress and the military enacted policies and legislative acts to improve the lifestyle of the military child and family. The U.S. Department of Defense Family Advocacy Program (FAP), which mandates the identification and prevention of child and spouse abuse, was initiated in 1981. In 1985, the Military Family Act was passed to support such family programs as child care and other support services. The Exceptional Family Member Program, which ensures that the special needs of family members are considered in assignment decisions, began in the late 1980s. Service members have since been preferentially assigned to installations in locations where services are available for their special needs family members. Within the Army, the culminating commitment to provide for the needs of family members occurred in 2007 with adoption of the Army Family Covenant, a pledge to provide support to ensure the optimal health and well-being of military family members. These various programs have helped children and family members gain a sense of acceptance, belonging, and assistance in the military system.

The al-Qaeda terrorist attacks on September 11, 2001 were a defining moment for the military as a whole, including family members. Since then the United States has engaged in the longest war in its history. Service members have been impacted by multiple deployments and the stresses of wartime missions. The challenges of being a military child have been exacerbated by this decade-long conflict, with frequent, lengthy, and repeated family separations as well as the threat of harm to a parent. These stresses have impacted the life experiences and social and emotional well-being of military children and families (e.g., Chartrand et al. 2008; Flake et al. 2009) and are discussed at length in Chapter 12, "Deployment-Related Care for Military Children and Families."

Challenges Facing the Military Child

Numerous aspects of the military lifestyle may present stressors and/or challenges for the military child. These include frequent moves, discontinuity in friendships and other social relationships, educational challenges of changing schools, isolation from the civilian community, family separations both within the nuclear family and from extended family members, and threat of harm to the service member (Booth et al. 2007; Ender 2002; Hall 2008).

Members of the military move on average every 3 years (Booth et al. 2007). This stressor is often experienced as a sense of loss for military children: a loss of their school, friends, and familiar environments. This is particularly challenging for peer relationships, with the need for children to emotionally distance themselves from their current relationships in preparation for a move and then to forge new friendships at the next assignment location. Moves also disrupt children's adult social relationships, such as with teachers, coaches, clergy, and counselors, all of whom contribute to the health and well-being of youth. High school students appear to have more adjustment issues in terms of social and emotional problems, peer difficulties, and academic struggles than younger children (Orthner 2002).

Frequent moves also present significant and unique educational challenges to military children (Military Child Education Coalition 2001), such as educational discontinuities with differences in curriculum, academic rigor, and graduation requirements. Students find that they must adjust their expectations and academic programs to fit each new educational system. These differences are likely to be particularly difficult for children with special needs because there are often disruptions in the educational services they receive. Initiatives have begun (e.g., Military Child Education Coalition, Operation Military Kids) to remedy these obstacles by educating families and promoting school policies that ease transition problems.

Because of the fact that military children move frequently, often live in on-post military housing and/or may overidentify with the military system, they may feel disconnected from the broader community in which they live

(Hall 2008). Some military children report that their civilian counterparts cannot relate to the experiences of being a military dependent. Some children may even feel unwelcome in certain communities because of perceptions that they are different and do not fit in. This may lead to a feeling of isolation from the larger community, decreasing opportunities for social support or experiences outside the military culture.

Family separations for military children pose yet another challenge (Booth et al. 2007). Studies suggest that the absence of a parent is experienced as a stressful event for military children (Jensen et al. 1989, 1996). Because of the war on terror, these separations are frequent, long, and recurring. The impact on the military child is only now being evaluated (e.g., Chartrand et al. 2008; Flake et al. 2009). The studies seem clear that recurrent wartime deployments create a difficult and stressful life situation and may lead to negative outcomes for children and adolescents that include increased anxiety, depressive symptoms, behavioral problems, and academic difficulties (see Chapter 12 for more detailed information). Further, most active duty military families do not live near extended family members; therefore, family support systems to assist with child care, domestic support, and social support are not readily available. This may be particularly stressful for dual-military couples, single-parent military members, or young spouses. In addition, children from divorced families are often geographically separated from their noncustodial parent. Geographic separations from extended family make these traditionally supportive family relationships difficult to access, nurture, and maintain.

Children of National Guard and Reservist parents face additional and somewhat different challenges. When National Guard and Reserve members are called to extended active duty, their children are suddenly "military brats" who experience increased anxiety, depression, and academic difficulties. However, formal and informal services and structures that are available for active duty military families who live near or on military installations are often not as readily available to these family members. Although National Guard and Reserve dependents may not move or change schools when their parent is activated and are more likely to live near extended family, they are not likely to be immersed in the military culture and may not feel as supported or understood by their peers or other social support systems. Programs such as Operation Military Kids were developed specifically to help these children understand the military culture and expectations, to connect them with local resources, to help them achieve a sense of community support, and to enhance their well-being.

The current literature indicates that, at least during peacetime, military children have fewer social and emotional problems than their civilian peers (Jeffries and Leitzel 2000; Jensen et al. 1995; Watanabe 1985; Watanabe and Jensen 2000). Wartime stressors may complicate the typically healthy responses of military children (see Chapter 12). Thus, it is important to understand aspects of military life that provide protective experiences and resilience for children as well as other experiences that may incur greater risk.

Cultural Strengths and Current Opportunities for Military Children

Military children and families experience a host of positive experiences and opportunities that may strengthen their resilience and protect against military-specific stressors or risk factors (Booth et al. 2007; Ender 2002). These include stable family income, housing, and medical care; exposure to diverse experiences, populations, and cultures; opportunities to adapt to new situations and friendships; military-sponsored recreational activities and support services; exposure to positive values such as patriotism; and a sense of belonging to a close-knit community.

With some exceptions, most military members' pay and benefits are fairly competitive with their civilian counterparts and provide sufficient financial income to support a family (Booth et al. 2007; Hall 2008). Although some lower enlisted service members may require additional public assistance depending on the size and needs of their families, they do have the benefit of job security and predictable earnings. In addition, all service members are able to either live in on-post military housing or receive a housing allowance. Another critical benefit to military families is free or low-cost medical care that includes primary care, behavioral health care, and other specialty care. The military offers significantly lower dental and life insurance premiums in comparison with civilian prices. Military members are also able to take advantage of commissary and post exchange discount pricing for food and other products. And in the past decade the military has allowed service members to contribute to retirement funds (Thrift Savings Plan), which is particularly beneficial to service members who may not choose the military as a career. All of these financial benefits and allowances guarantee that military children and adolescents are likely to have a reasonable standard of living that, at a minimum, supports their basic needs.

The military sponsors a variety of recreational activities and programs that give military children opportunities to be active and involved in prosocial endeavors (Booth et al. 2007; Rosen and Durand 2000). Such services include after school programs, sports programs, youth centers, on-post recreational facilities (movie theaters, bowling alleys, parks, swimming pools, boat rentals, etc.), and discounted community recreational events (e.g., professional sports tickets, amusement parks, water parks, skiing, snowboarding). Although geographic mobility may present a challenge for some military children, the opportunity to travel and be exposed to various subcultures within the United States, as well as international cultures and populations, can also be viewed as a positive experience for many military children. In a qualitative study of a group of military adolescents living in Germany (Tyler 2002), the participants reported that their interactions with the local population helped them broaden their views of the world and that these experiences were very positive. Many military children become bilingual on the basis of their experiences living in foreign countries or because of the fact that one of their parents is a non-U.S. citizen or nonnative English speaker. The military itself is a very diverse organization (Deputy Under Secretary of Defense for Military Community and Family Policy 2010), providing a range of experiences to military children. Children who live on military installations are often exposed to diverse populations, which include a range of socioeconomic statuses, races, religions, and ethnic backgrounds. Military children learn to interact and deal with people who are different from themselves. Living within a diverse subculture is likely to help military children and teenagers build tolerance and acceptance, broaden their ability to adapt to new situations, and become more resilient.

Although frequent moves and parental absences were initially considered detrimental to military children (LaGrone 1978), a number of positive benefits have been reported. Other reported benefits, such as the opportunity to develop strong personal resources and social skills, include developing higher self-esteem (Ender 2006); learning to interact with a variety of social groups and forge friendships quickly (Jeffries and Leitzel 2000); and instilling responsibility, independence, tolerance, and maturity (Hall 2008; Jeffries and Leitzel 2000; Park 2011).

Further, positive values propagated by the military organization, such as patriotism, honesty, selflessness, and honor, are often transmitted to and embraced by the children of military service members. The adoption of positive core values, when not blindly adhered to, is thought to contribute to enhanced self-worth and to promote healthy social and emotional development in children (Hall 2008).

Finally, many military children and families report a strong sense of belonging to the military community. This may be particularly true for those children living on a military installation or attending a school with a high enrollment of other military children. The families often have a strong sense of identification with and pride in this community. One study examining the effects of deployment on children found that those families who felt supported by the military community were less likely to express concern regarding their children's adjustment (Flake et al. 2009). A strong sense of purpose and connection is likely to contribute to the resilience of many military children and adolescents.

Military Child and Family Programs

Numerous programs have become part of the military culture and are believed to contribute to the overall wellness of military children and adolescents. During the mid-twentieth century the military intensified the organizational emphasis on the quality of life for family members when research documented the critical contributions military children and families make to mission success and retention of service members (Albano 1994). This organizational shift in focus resulted in the development and implementation of a great number of programs aimed at improving the quality of life for military families (Brown 1993). Extending to families basic privileges that were historically reserved only for service members contributed to some of the first benefits families enjoyed. These early benefits included on-post housing for married service members and some "space available" medical care within the military medical system. In 1956, Congress passed the Dependents' Medical Care Act, which allowed family members to obtain medical care not only through military treatment facilities where service members received care but also through civilian health care providers. This initial health care program transformed into the Civilian Health and Medical Program of the Uniformed Services (CHAMPUS) in 1966 and eventually evolved into TRICARE, the current managed care medical model for military dependents (see Chapter 4, "Military Health Care System and the U.S. Department of Veterans Affairs," for details). Current military medical insurance benefits are highly valued by family members (Booth et al. 2007).

Consistent with an overall emphasis on health and well-being, the military has sought to decrease incidents of domestic violence and instituted the Family Advocacy Program in 1981. FAP was designed to develop programs to prevent family violence, investigate reports of family violence, and provide monitoring and intervention services. FAP offers educational and counseling programs regarding strategies to decrease the risk of domestic violence (e.g., parent training and communication skills training), as well as monitoring and therapeutic services for those families who have a confirmed case of domestic violence. The military also maintains a central registry of domestic violence cases in order to monitor and track confirmed cases. Although some military members are charged with criminal conduct or discharged for documented cases of domestic violence, this generally occurs in extreme or repeat cases. More typically, families are offered services through the Family Advocacy Clinical program or through TRICARE providers to help treat and prevent future incidents.

Data suggest that the rate of child maltreatment within the military is lower than within the civilian community (U.S. Department of Defense 2004a, 2004b). As reported by Booth et al. (2007), the estimated rate of child abuse in the civilian population in 2004 was 12.4 per 1,000, in comparison with the military rate of 7.0 per 1,000 in the same year. This lower rate of documented child abuse appears to be due in part to lower rates of child neglect within the military in comparison with the civilian sector. Several aspects of military service, such as steady employment, housing benefits, and available medical care, may mitigate some of the known risk factors related to child maltreatment. However, no level of child abuse is acceptable, and support for the mission of the FAP to prevent, identify, monitor, and treat those families affected by family violence continues to be a high priority within the military system.

Another vulnerable population identified by the military as worthy of dedicated attention and resourcing is family members with special needs. The Exceptional Family Member Program (EFMP) enrolls adult and child family members with chronic physical, emotional, developmental, or intellectual disabilities whose medical needs cannot be met in primary care or who require special education services. It is mandatory that service members enroll their special needs family members in this program and update enrollment every 3 years or whenever there is a change in the health status of the exceptional family member. Approximately 120,000 military family members are enrolled in this program, and approximately two-thirds of these are children or adolescents (R. Posante, personal communication, April 2012). The military utilizes EFMP enrollment information to ensure that duty assignments are made with the special medical or educational needs of these family members in mind. This prevents family members enrolled in EFMP from being sent to locations that do not have the required services to meet their needs.

Another critical basic service undertaken by the uniformed services was the education of military children and families, particularly those living overseas. The Department of Defense Dependent School (DODDS) for minor dependents was instituted in 1946 in overseas areas where many military children continue to receive their schooling when in non-U.S. assignments. Currently, the Department of Defense Education Activity, which has subsumed DODDS school systems, continues to operate schools on several military posts outside the continental United States (previously DODDS schools) as well as on several stateside military installations.

As a result of the Military Family Act passed in 1985, all branches of the military have implemented family support services, offering a variety of programs to assist children and family members such as child care services, recreational activities, and financial and employment counseling. One of the largest programs is Child and Youth Services, which includes on-installation child care centers as well as certification of on-installation, in-home family child care. Youth services are also provided to preadolescent and adolescent family members, including after school programs, teen centers, extracurricular activities, and recreational services. These child care and youth programs are regularly utilized and are reported to help service members fulfill their mission by decreasing job time lost because of family demands and by increasing family satisfaction (Booth et al. 2007). Family Support Services also offer financial planning, transition (relocation or transition to civilian life) planning, and spousal employment services (Brown 1993). All of these programs help families cope with challenges presented by the military lifestyle and help maintain a healthy, functional family.

In addition to organized child and youth programs, the military offers on-post recreational activities and facilities such as movie theaters, bowling alleys, parks, and golf courses that add to the quality of life for military children. Most posts have outdoor recreation centers where families can rent equipment for a variety of activities such as boating, skiing, hiking, and camping. The Morale, Welfare, and Recreation office offers discounted tickets or trips to numerous commercial activities such as sporting events and amusement parks. Most branches in the military have also adopted strategies to provide unit support to family members through family readiness groups (FRGs). FRGs ensure that there is a support network that reaches out to all families within the unit and, especially during deployment, serve a critical communication role between the unit and family members. FRGs sponsor social events as well as educational activities, with the goal to provide a sense of "family cohesion" within the unit.

Other services and programs that have been developed for military children and families include Military OneSource—a comprehensive program offering referral services, online resources, educational resources, and short-term counseling—and the Army's Comprehensive Soldier Fitness Program—an online assessment and educational program that helps service members and spouses become aware of and enhance their personal coping resources. Another Army program contracts social workers and other counselors to provide prevention and early intervention support services to family members. These military family life consultants function within the broad military community and provide targeted, short-term services to help families cope with deployment and other military stressors. Further, the Families Overcoming Under Stress (FOCUS) intervention program, developed by clinical researchers at the University of California, Los Angeles, has been implemented at several military installations. A myriad of chaplaincy programs also have been implemented throughout the military system. Finally, the Army Medical Department has developed and is implementing the Behavioral Health System of Care, which is devoted to providing quality behavioral health care to soldiers as well as children and families. This is only a brief sampling of the programs that have been developed for family members subsequent to the War on Terror. Many others exist and substantially benefit service members' children.

Conclusions

The sacrifices that children and adolescents make as a result of having a parent in the military are significant. Geographic moves, social transitions, lack of stability of social supports, educational discontinuities, and family separations are challenges that most military children must learn to cope with as part of their everyday life. These same stressors can lead to growth opportunities and positive experiences as these challenges are mastered and competence is gained in dealing with them. Exposure to diverse peoples and cultures, immersion in the military culture that embraces positive core values, provision of financial support and medical care, a variety of support programs and recreational activities, and opportunities to develop numerous prosocial skills such as responsibility, independence, and flexibility all generally lead to healthy emotional and social development in these youth. The military has developed and implemented many programs to support children and families aimed at offsetting the potentially negative effects of living within a military environment. These programs help improve the quality of life and healthy functioning of the military child and family. Ongoing recognition of the sacrifices made by family members and the maintenance of programs to support military children will continue to be critical to the optimal well-being and adjustment of these important and heroic members of our society.

SUMMARY POINTS

- The military as an organization has increasingly acknowledged the reciprocal nature of the relationship between family well-being and the well-being, performance, and retention of service members.
- Military children enjoy numerous benefits, such as stable housing; medical care; exposure to diverse populations; belonging to a close-knit community; the opportunity to become bilingual; the opportunity to live abroad; and access to after school programs, teen centers, recreational services, and extracurricular activities.
- Challenges to military children include frequent moves, discontinuity in peer relationships, separation from nuclear and extended family, changing schools, and disrup-

tions in relationships with supportive adults (coaches, clergy, teachers, counselors).

- Children who live on military installations are exposed to people of different races, religions, and ethnic backgrounds and learn to interact and deal with people who are different from themselves. Living within a diverse subculture is likely to help military children and teenagers build tolerance and acceptance, broaden their ability to adapt to new situations, and become more resilient.

References

Albano S: Military recognition of family concerns: Revolutionary War to 1993. Armed Forces and Society 20(2):283–302, 1994

Alt BS, Stone DM: Campfollowing: A History of the Military Wife. New York, Praeger, 1991

Booth B, Segal MW, Bell DB, et al: What We Know About Army Families: 2007 Update. Fairfax, VA, Caliber Associates, 2007

Brown RJ: Military family service centers: their preventive and interventive functions, in The Military Family in Peace and War. Edited by Kaslow FW. New York, Springer, 1993, pp 163–172

Chartrand MM, Frank DA, White LF, et al: Effect of parents' wartime deployment on the behavior of young children in military families. Arch Pediatr Adolesc Med 162(11):1009–1014, 2008

Deputy Under Secretary of Defense for Military Community and Family Policy: Demographics 2009: profile of the military community. Washington, DC, U.S. Department of Defense, 2010

Ender MG (ed): Military Brats and Other Global Nomads: Growing Up in Organization Families. Westport, CT, Praeger, 2002

Ender MG: Voices from the backseat: demands of growing up in military families, in Military Life: The Psychology of Serving in Peace and Combat, Volume 3, The Military Family. Edited by Castro CA, Adler AB, Britt TW. Westport, CT, Praeger, 2006, pp 138–166

Flake EM, Davis BE, Johnson PL, et al: The psychosocial effects of deployment on military children. J Dev Behav Pediatr 30(4):271–278, 2009

Griffith JD, Rakoff S, Helms RF: Report on family and other impacts on retention. Technical Report 986. Alexandria, VA, U.S. Army Research Institute for the Behavioral and Social Sciences, 1993

Hall LK: Counseling Military Families. New York, Routledge, 2008

Jeffries DJ, Leitzel JD: The strengths and vulnerabilities of adolescents in military families, in The Military Family: A Practice Guide for Human Service Providers. Edited by Martin JA, Rosen LN, Sparacino GL. Westport, CT, Praeger, 2000, pp 225–240

Jensen PS, Grogan D, Xenakis SN, et al: Father absence: effects on child and maternal psychopathology. J Am Acad Child Adolesc Psychiatry 28(2):171–175, 1989

Jensen PS, Watanabe HK, Richters JE, et al: Prevalence of mental disorder in military children and adolescents: findings from a two-stage community survey. J Am Acad Child Adolesc Psychiatry 34(11):1514–1524, 1995

Jensen PS, Martin D, Watanabe HK: Children's response to parental separation during Operation Desert Storm. J Am Acad Child Adolesc Psychiatry 35(4):433–441, 1996

LaGrone DM: The military family syndrome. Am J Psychiatry 135(9):1040–1043, 1978

Martin JA, McClure P: Today's active duty military family: the evolving challenges of military life, in The Military Family: A Practice Guide for Human Service Providers. Edited by Martin JA, Rosen LN, Sparacino GL. Westport, CT, Praeger, 2000, pp 3–23

Military Child Education Coalition: Secondary Education Transition Study (SETS) 2001. Arlington, VA, Military Family Resource Center, 2001

Orthner DK: SAF IV Survey Report: impact of PCS moves on high school students in Army families. Chapel Hill, U.S. Army Community and Family Support Center, University of North Carolina, 2002

Paden LB, Pezor LJ: Uniforms and youth: the military child and his or her family, in The Military Family in Peace and War. Edited by Kaslow FW. New York, Springer, 1993, pp 3–24

Park N: Military children and families: strengths and challenges during peace and war. Am Psychol 66(1):65–72, 2011

Rosen LN, Durand DB: Coping with the unique demands of military family life, in The Military Family: A Practice Guide for Human Service Providers. Edited by Martin JA, Rosen LN, Sparacino GL. Westport, CT, Praeger, 2000, pp 55–72

Tyler MP: The military teenager in Europe: Perspectives for health care providers, in Military Brats and Other Global Nomads: Growing Up in Organization Families. Edited by Ender MG. Westport, CT, Praeger, 2002, pp 25–34

U.S. Department of Defense: Family Advocacy Program child abuse data: 2004 report. Washington, DC, Office of the Secretary of Defense, 2004a

U.S. Department of Defense: Family Advocacy Program spouse abuse data: 2004 report. Washington, DC, Office of the Secretary of Defense, 2004b

Watanabe HK: A survey of adolescent military family members' self-image. J Youth Adolesc 14(2):99–107, 1985

Watanabe HK, Jensen PS: Young children adaptation to a military lifestyle, in The Military Family: A Practice Guide for Human Service Providers. Edited by Martin JA, Rosen LN, Sparacino GL. Westport, CT, Praeger, 2000, pp 209–22

Chapter 4

Military Health Care System and the U.S. Department of Veterans Affairs

An Overview

Elspeth Cameron Ritchie, M.D., M.P.H.

THE INTENT of this chapter is to quickly give the reader an overview of the Military Health System (MHS) and the U.S. Department of Veterans Affairs, often referred to as the VA. The chapter will cover the missions and structures of each organization. Although often seen from the outside as one organization, they are actually very different. In this chapter we highlight both the similarities and the differences. Some of the topics touched on here, such as transitions from the U.S. Department of Defense (DOD) to the VA for wounded service members and the two different disability systems, are extremely complex. Further details are provided in the references or at the relevant Web sites.

Disclaimer: The views expressed in this chapter are those of the author and do not necessarily represent the views of the U.S. Department of Veterans Affairs or the District of Columbia Department of Mental Health.

Military Health System

Overview

The medical departments in the U.S. military strive primarily to serve military members and their dependents and serve retirees when space is available. Retirees are service members who either have served long enough to receive retirement benefits (usually 20 years) or have been retired for medical reasons. The staff of the medical departments is a mix of uniformed personnel, DOD civilians, and contractors. All of the uniformed personnel are members of one of the military branches, Army, Navy, Air Force, or U.S. Public Health Service, and may be deployed to any conflict location. They often support humanitarian missions, such as the 2004 and 2011 tsunamis, and participate in smaller medical missions, such as supporting clinics in Honduras and Africa. Because they are service members, they must meet the standards of their branch and are subject to the Uniform Code of Military Justice. There is a robust teaching mission, as many of the larger hospitals train medical students, residents, and fellows, who are all active duty. Psychologists and social workers are also often trained by the teaching hospitals.

Brief History and Organization

The Army Medical Department and the Army Medical Corps were founded in 1775. The Army Nurse Corps dates from 1901, the Dental Corps from 1911, the Veterinary Corps from 1916, the Medical Service Corps from 1917, and the Army Medical Specialist Corps from 1947. The Army Surgeon General is both the commander of the Army's Medical Command and a medical staff officer, answering to the Army Chief of Staff. The Army Medical Command (MEDCOM) is headquartered in San Antonio, Texas, but the Office of the Army Surgeon General is in northern Virginia, near the Pentagon. MEDCOM has command and control over most medical military assets in the United States but not necessarily overseas.

The Navy's Bureau of Medicine and Surgery, established in 1775, is in downtown Washington, D.C., where the Navy Surgeon General also resides. Navy medical personnel also provide services to Marines. The Air Force is the newest service, and the Air Force Surgeon General is located at Bolling Air Force Base in Washington, D.C.

In addition to providing medical services, the Army and Navy also have large medical research missions. The Army has a separate research command, the Medical Research and Materiel Command in Fort Detrick, Maryland, and the Walter Reed Army Institute of Research in Forest Glen, Maryland, which sponsors research on behavioral health issues.

History of TRICARE

In 1956 the Department of Defense estimated that 40% of active duty dependents either did not have access to federal facilities because of distance or had incomplete medical coverage at the federal facility because of saturation. Congress responded by passing the Dependents' Medical Care Act of 1956 and the Military Medical Benefits Amendments of 1966. These acts created the program known as the Civilian Health and Medical Program of the Uniformed Services (CHAMPUS).

In the late 1980s, the CHAMPUS Reform Initiative (CRI) was initiated because of escalating costs, claims paperwork demands, and general beneficiary dissatisfaction. Under CRI, a contractor provided both health care and administrative-related services, including claims processing.

In 1993 the DOD announced plans for implementing a nationwide managed care program for the MHS to be implemented by 1997, TRICARE. TRICARE has undergone several restructuring initiatives, including realignment of contract regions, base realignment and closure, and the addition of "TRICARE for Life" and "TRICARE Reserve Select" in 2005. There are currently three TRICARE regions. There are three TRICARE plans: Standard, Extra, and Prime (Institute of Medicine 2012) (see Table 4–1).

Military Health Care System

The MHS is divided into the direct care system, military treatment facilities, and the purchased care system TRICARE. In the direct care system, the priority of services received is for active duty service members first, then dependents, then retirees. If there is no space available, dependents and retirees use TRICARE.

Direct Care

The military operates an immense array of hospitals, clinics, battalion aid stations, and other treatment centers. In the Army, the large hospitals are known as MEDCENs (Medical Centers) and the smaller ones as MEDDACs (Medical Department Activities). Army and Navy medical centers have recently consolidated to form the San Antonio Military Medical Center (SAMMC) in San Antonio, Texas, and the Walter Reed National Military Medical Center in Bethesda, Maryland. Other major Navy medical centers include the Naval Medical Center San Diego in San Diego, California, and the Naval Medical Center near Norfolk, Virginia. The Air Force's largest hospital is Wilford Hall Ambulatory Surgical Center in San Antonio, and it is currently consolidating with SAMMC.

TABLE 4–1.   TRICARE program descriptions

Program	Description	Enrollment	Access to care
TRICARE Prime (includes TRICARE Prime Remote for active duty family members)	Similar to managed care or health maintenance organization options Available in specific geographic locations	Enrollment required Annual enrollment fees paid by retirees, their families, survivors, and qualifying former spouses Lowest out-of-pocket costs	Care maximized by using a primary care manager at a military treatment facility or accessing services within the TRICARE network
TRICARE Prime Remote	Benefits akin to TRICARE Prime for active duty service members (ADSMs) who reside and work in remote locations, with the eligible family members living with the benefactor	Enrollment required	Care accessed through the TRICARE network (or a TRICARE-authorized nonnetwork provider if network providers are unavailable)
TRICARE Standard	Fee-for-service option for eligible non-ADSMs Available internationally	No enrollment required Annual deductibles and cost shares[a]	Care accessed through TRICARE-authorized nonnetwork providers No referrals necessary Prior authorization necessary for some services
TRICARE Extra	Preferred provider option available in established TRICARE network locations	No enrollment required Annual deductibles and discounted cost shares Unavailable internationally	Care accessed from TRICARE network providers No referrals necessary Prior authorization necessary for some services

TABLE 4-1. TRICARE program descriptions *(continued)*

Program	Description	Enrollment	Access to care
TRICARE Reserve Select (TRS)	Premium-based health care plan for qualifying Selected Reserve of the Ready Reserve members for themselves and/or family members. Similar coverage and costs to TRICARE Standard for active duty family members[a]	Enrollment required. Available internationally. Member-only and member-and-family coverage. TRS qualification and purchase required to participate. Monthly premiums, annual deductibles, and cost shares	Care accessed from any TRICARE-authorized provider (network or non-network). No referrals necessary. Prior authorization necessary for some services
TRICARE Retired Reserve (TRR)	Premium-based health care plan for qualified retired Reserve members for themselves and/or family members. Similar coverage and costs to TRICARE Standard for retirees[a]	Enrollment required. Available internationally. Member-only and member-and-family coverage offered. TRR qualification and purchase required. Monthly premiums, annual deductibles, and cost shares	Care received from any TRICARE-authorized provider (network or non-network). No referrals necessary. Prior authorization necessary for some services
TRICARE For Life	Available to all Medicare-eligible TRICARE beneficiaries regardless of age (provided that they have Medicare Part A and Part B). Serves as a Medicare wraparound coverage	No enrollment required. Must be eligible for premium-free Medicare Part A and have Medicare Part B	Care accessed from Medicare participating, nonparticipating, or opt-out providers, but opt-out provider services costly[b]. TRICARE pharmacy benefits included

[a]Authorized providers that are not part of TRICARE network may charge beneficiaries up to 15% above the TRICARE-allowable charge for services.
[b]Providers who opt out of Medicare enter into private contracts with patients and are not allowed to bill Medicare. Therefore, Medicare does not have to pay for health care services received from opt-out providers. Beneficiaries are responsible for paying remaining billed charges.
Source. Adapted from information found at www.tricare.osd.mil.

In Theater

The Army has a wide range of medical assets "in theater," the term used to describe the theater of war. These assets include combat support hospitals, area support medical battalions, and battalion aid stations. Specific to mental health are combat stress control detachments and companies, which have a blend of disciplines, including psychologists, psychiatrists, social workers, psychiatric nurses, occupational therapists, and enlisted mental health technicians. Each combat brigade also has a behavioral health officer, usually either a psychologist or a social worker, and an enlisted tech.

Outside of the United States

Finally, outside of the United States but not in the theater of war are many medical facilities. These are especially common in Germany, Japan, and Korea. The hospital at Landstuhl, Germany, currently receives all the casualties from the Middle East. Korea has an Army evacuation hospital with a small psychiatric ward and several Air Force bases. Japan has many Naval and some Army facilities. If evacuation is needed from Asia, most patients go to Tripler Army Medical Center in Hawaii.

Purchased Care

The purchased care system is managed by the TRICARE Management Activity, which is overseen by the Office of the Assistant Secretary of Defense for Health Affairs. There are a variety of different plans that serve dependents, retirees, and service members who live either too far away from a military treatment facility or where there is not "space available" (Table 4–2). Full details of the different plans may be obtained at http://tricare.mil.

Access to Care and Types of Care Available

The military has a wide variety of preclinical and clinical care available. In mental health, clinical care is generally delivered in either outpatient clinics or inpatient psychiatric wards. Many installations have started intensive outpatient programs. The therapies used are diverse, including psychotherapy and pharmacotherapy, and reflect best practices used in the civilian world. One continual challenge is the short course of treatment, dictated by the unit and service member's busy schedule. Service members may not deploy while taking certain psychiatric medications, such as mood stabilizers and antipsychotics, because of potentially harmful side effects in a combat setting. Certain jobs, such as aviation, have more restrictions than others. More details may be found in DOD policy guidance (U.S. Department of Defense 2006).

TABLE 4–2. Examples of VHA programs and services listed by mental health concern

Mental health concern	Programs and services available through VHA
Depression and anxiety	Medication (prescribed by either a primary care physician or a mental health professional) Talk therapies: Cognitive-behavioral therapy Acceptance and commitment therapy Interpersonal therapy
Homelessness	Homeless National Call Center Outreach to veterans living on the streets Drop-in centers Medical treatment for physical and mental disorders, including substance abuse Emergency shelter referral Transitional housing in community-based programs Referral to permanent housing (via rental assistance vouchers) Long-term assistance, case management, and rehabilitation Employment assistance Residential treatment
Military sexual trauma	Free treatment to male and female veterans for mental and physical health conditions related to military sexual trauma The veteran does not need to be service connected and may be eligible even if not eligible for VA care The veteran does not need to have reported the incident
Posttraumatic stress disorder	Medications Talk therapies: Cognitive-behavioral therapy Cognitive processing therapy Prolonged exposure therapy Residential care
Returning veterans	Readjustment counseling at Vet Centers

TABLE 4–2.   Examples of VHA programs and services listed by mental health concern *(continued)*

Mental health concern	Programs and services available through VHA

Substance abuse	Medications
	Talk therapies:
	    Motivational enhancement therapy
	    Cognitive-behavioral therapy
	Opioid treatment programs
	Residential treatment programs
	Work therapies

Severe mental illnesses	Medications Psychosocial rehabilitation and recovery services Work therapies Residential care Mental health intensive case management
Specialized services for female veterans	Women's inpatient units Women's residential treatment programs Special treatment tracks for women
Suicide prevention services	Suicide prevention coordinators Veterans crisis line Personalized safety planning
Justice-involved veterans	Mental health assessments for veterans charged with offenses that allow for community-based alternatives to jail or prison Assistance for veterans to connect with VA services
Services for older veterans	VA community living centers Home-based primary care Screening for dementia Assessments to help decide if a veteran can live safely at home and make informed medical decisions

Source.   Adapted from information found at U.S. Department of Veterans Affairs 2011f.

Preclinical care is often delivered by chaplains, counselors, or family support agencies, such as those found through Military OneSource. Although these interventions are quite popular, their effectiveness is largely unknown because no records are kept.

The MHS has been criticized for insufficient access to behavioral health care. Since 2007 they have been increasing the number of providers, with a 70% increase from 2007 to 2011.

Training

There are two principal pipelines for medical students to enter the service: the Uniformed Services University of the Health Sciences in Bethesda, Maryland, and the Health Professions Scholarship Program, which offers scholarships to medical schools for top-quality applicants. In the Army, psychiatry residency training is offered at Walter Reed and Tripler. The Navy trains psychiatric residents at Portsmouth, San Diego, and Walter Reed National Military Medical Center. The Air Force trains them at Wilford Hall and at Wright-Patterson Air Force Base in conjunction with Case Western Reserve University. Similarly, there are numerous psychology training programs and emerging social work programs. The Army offers a new social work training program through Fayetteville State University in Texas.

Transition of Care From DOD to VA

In the past, when patients left the DOD to seek care at the VA, there was a potential gap in services. Currently, there are numerous ongoing efforts to bridge this gap. The wounded, ill, and injured are extensively case managed and may be transferred directly from a military hospital to a VA one. Those who are discharged from the military at the end of their enlistment are more likely to fall through the cracks. Efforts to provide continuity of care include having VA staff at Transition Assistance Program classes and at the Post-Deployment Health Reassessment Program. (Full details are available at http://www1.va.gov/opa/publications/benefits_book/benefits_chap10.asp.)

There are numerous levels of priority for VA patients, with the highest priority given to service members who have deployed to Iraq or Afghanistan in the 5 years preceding discharge.

Eligibility for care at the VA is not the same as eligibility in a military treatment facility (MTF); some service members may be eligible for one and not the other. Service members on active duty can be seen at an MTF. In general, they have to have served in the military at least 6 months and have received an honorable discharge to be seen at the VA. Guard and Reserve soldiers may go back and forth. Soldiers who are retired from the military, either through length of service or a medical retirement, are eligible for both. Eligibility must be confirmed by the VA before service members can be seen there, and electronic medical records shared between the DOD and the VA are currently still limited.

The Disability System in the Military

If a service member is wounded, ill, or injured, he or she may receive a medical evaluation board. This is a review panel of physicians who recommend whether a service member should be medically separated from the service. If the board recommends separation, then the case is referred to a physical evaluation board, which makes the final decision about medical discharge and determines the disability rating. If the service member receives a 30% disability rating, he or she is medically retired and is eligible for care in the military health system. The process is complex; more information may be found at http://www.pdhealth.mil/downloads/Army_Physical_Disability_Evaluation_System_(APDES).pdf.

This disability system and rating is currently distinct from the VA disability rating. There are ongoing efforts to combine the DOD and VA physical exam processes. VA disability compensation is a benefit paid to veterans secondary to injuries or disease that occurred on or were made worse by active duty (U.S. Department of Veterans Affairs 2011a). In some cases these benefits are paid to individuals who become disabled secondary to VA health care (U.S. Department of Veterans Affairs 2011a). Individuals with a service-related disability (i.e., a disability that is the result of an injury, a disease, or an event in military service) may be eligible for such compensation. Veterans can apply for benefits by completing and submitting VA Form 21-526 (http://www.vba.va.gov/pubs/forms/vba-21-526-are.pdf). Veterans can also apply for benefits online at https://www.ebenefits.va.gov/ebenefits-portal/ebenefits.portal?_nfpb=trueand_portlet.async=falseand_pageLabel=ebenefits_myeb_vonapp1.

Research

There are multiple research efforts ongoing in the DOD. In the arena of posttraumatic stress disorder (PTSD), many of them were funded by Congressional support, starting in 2007. Mental health advisory teams have deployed to theater approximately every year since 2003 to obtain information on symptoms of anxiety and depression, barriers to care, and other mental health care issues (Hoge et al. 2011). There is a very large research project with the National Institute of Mental Health on suicide known as STARRS (Army Study to Assess Risk and Resilience in Service Members).

VA Health Care System

Veterans Health Administration Mission and Vision Statement

As will be discussed in the section "History of the VA," the Veterans Health Administration (VHA) is one branch of the Department of Veterans Affairs. The VHA's mission "is to honor America's Veterans by providing exceptional health care that improves their health and well-being" (U.S. Department of Veterans Affairs 2011b). As noted, the primary focus of the VHA is to improve the health and function of U.S. veterans (Kizer 1999). This is accomplished in part by reducing the "impact and burden of illness, injury, and disability of those conditions related to their service in the armed forces, especially those conditions resulting from combat" (Kizer 1999, p. 4). Additional missions of the VHA include education and training, research, and contingency support and emergency management.

As one of its statutory missions, the VHA educates and trains health professional students and residents with the goal of enhancing the quality of care provided to veterans (U.S. Department of Veterans Affairs 2011c). According to the VA Office of Academic Affiliations, each year more than 115,000 individuals receive some or all of their clinical training in a VA facility (U.S. Department of Veterans Affairs 2011c). The VHA is also mandated to conduct research aimed at bettering the lives of veterans. Finally, the VHA provides medical care system backup to the U.S. Departments of Defense and Public Health Service during times of war and/or disaster. The operations of the VA are currently guided by Secretary Eric Shinseki's Transformation 21 (T-21) Initiative, which is focused in part on such issues as homelessness, electronic medical records, and telehealth.

History of the VA

Following a long history of caring for the nation's veterans, in 1930 Congress authorized the creation of the Veterans Administration, which combined the formerly established Veterans Bureau, Bureau of Pensions of the Interior Department, and National Home for Disabled Volunteer Soldiers. The Veterans Administration grew extensively over time, with benefits associated with service increasing following World War II, and grew to include the National Cemetery System. In 1989 the VA was elevated to the cabinet-level Department of Veterans Affairs (U.S. Department of Veterans Affairs 2010a). The VA is the currently the second largest federal department and has more than 278,000 employees and an annual budget of $96 billion (Office of Human Resources and Administration [OHRA] 2010).

VA Contributions to General Medical Knowledge

As the largest integrated health care system in the United States, the VA can also serve as a "national laboratory" for health care quality management and improvement (Kizer 1999). In 1995 the VHA initiated a redesign of the health care system, which included efforts to ensure consistent and predictable health care from facility to facility (Kizer 1999). The VA created the Quality Enhancement Research Initiative (QUERI) to link research activities to clinical care with the goal of enhancing the adoption of best clinical practices and improving veteran outcomes (Stetler et al. 2008). QUERI is one of many resources within the VHA that have facilitated and continue to facilitate the implementation of quality care indicators with the goal of improving veterans' health care.

The VA also has an extensive history of developing and adopting information technology (IT) systems in order to support administrative and patient care services (Byrne et al. 2010). Currently, VA hospitals, nursing homes, outpatient clinics, and Vet Centers use the Veterans Health Information Systems and Technology Architecture (VistA) as an integrated electronic health records system (OHRA 2010). Among the many VistA systems are electronic health records, radiological imaging, and laboratory and medication ordering and administration (Byrne et al. 2010).

The Computerized Patient Record System, which was initially launched in 1996 and was nationally mandated in 1999, is a component of VistA that allows for patient-centered electronic medical charting (Brown et al. 2003). Because of VistA, the VA is "one of the few national, health IT-enabled, integrated delivery systems in the United States" (Byrne et al. 2010, p. 629). VistA has increased patient safety through such systems as automated allergy alerts and the use of bar code technology on patient armbands and medications (OHRA 2010).

Structure of the VA

Leadership within the VA includes the Secretary of Veterans Affairs, who is a member of the President's cabinet and advises him on veterans' affairs, and the Deputy Secretary of Veterans Affairs, who serves as the VA's chief operating officer. The VA includes 3 administrations, 7 assistant secretaries, and 14 staff offices. The three administrations (the Veterans Health Administration, Veterans Benefits Administration, and National Cemetery Administration) are responsible for the provision of services and benefits to veterans (OHRA 2010).

The Veterans Health Administration is the nation's largest integrated health care system (U.S. Department of Veterans Affairs 2011b). Just as the larger VA system has grown and developed over the years, the VHA has as well. In 1995, the VHA underwent significant organizational change with the decentralization of bureaucracy through the creation of regional networks throughout the country referred to as Veterans Integrated Service Networks (VISNs). The VHA began to focus on quality management (Kizer 1999), increasing accessibility through systems of care and health promotion and disease prevention (OHRA 2010). The VHA employs more than 239,000 staff at more than 1,400 locations, including, but not limited to, medical centers, nursing homes, and clinics (U.S. Department of Veterans Affairs 2011b).

The Veterans Benefits Administration (VBA) oversees financial compensation and other forms of benefits veterans can receive. The VBA also administers benefits to dependents and surviving family members of a service member or veteran who has died. Two of the five programs within this system are disability compensation and pension. Disability compensation is given because of injury or disease that was obtained or exacerbated in the person's military service. Pension is provided to support low-income wartime veterans with a nonservice-connected condition or their families. The Associate Deputy Under Secretary for Field Operations manages all field operations, the Records Management Center, and the Appeals Management Center. There are 57 regional offices within the VBA. The third central leadership position within the VBA is the Associate Deputy Under Secretary for Management, who oversees five staff offices responsible for the integration of programs to sustain VBA business and regional offices (OHRA 2010).

Another important component of the VA, which requires collaboration between the VHA and VBA, is assistance with the transition from active military service to civilian life. More than 150,000 active and Reservist service members separate from the military and become veterans each year (Office of the Secretary 2010). Many of these veterans transition their health care from the DOD to the VA or the private sector and may or may not have access to their health care records, which can impact the care they receive following discharge. In the Department of Veteran Affairs Strategic Plan for FY 2010–2014 (Office of the Secretary 2010), Secretary Eric Shinseki highlighted the need for seamless transfer of a veteran's medical records to VA or private health care providers. One of the major initiatives outlined in the strategic plan is for the creation of virtual lifetime electronic records (VLERs). VLERs would contain a veteran's lifetime history of medical care and would allow for a much easier and effective transition of care for veterans.

Another initiative set forth in the strategic plan is the modernizing of the Vocational Rehabilitation and Employment Program. One of the intended outcomes of this initiative is to provide veterans with training and education in order to ease the transition to civilian life following their military service. The strategic plan also highlights the overall importance of strong collaboration, including legal support, between the DOD and the VA to support the transition process (Office of the Secretary 2010).

Structure of VISNs

As mentioned in the section "Structure of the VA," the VHA was reorganized into VISNs during its redesign in 1995. This allowed funding and services to reach a greater number of veterans out in their communities rather than only those who had access to large facilities (Kizer 1999). VISNs serve as managers and budgeters of the smaller health care facilities they contain. They also integrate services to ensure that local needs are met, duplication of services and administration is reduced, and services are coordinated to increase the quality of health care veterans receive.

There are currently 23 VISNs spanning the United States, Philippines, American Samoa, and Guam (U.S. Department of Veterans Affairs 2011d). Figure 4–1 illustrates how VISNs fit into both the VHA and VA organizations and what VISNs may comprise: health care systems, medical centers, community living centers (CLCs), domiciliaries, Vet Centers, community-based outpatient clinics (CBOCs), and outpatient clinics. Variability exists between VISNs and what they contain. For example, VISN 19 (Rocky Mountain Network) contains 3 health care systems, 3 medical centers, 8 outpatient clinics, 38 CBOCs, and 15 Vet Centers. VISN 21 (Sierra Pacific Network), however, does not contain any health care systems but does have 8 medical centers, 21 outpatient clinics, 17 CBOCs, and 25 Vet Centers.

As noted in Figure 4–1, health care systems are regional bodies that may contain medical centers, domiciliaries, outpatient clinics, Vet Centers, CBOCs, or CLCs. They are responsible for integrating the care provided by these other facilities to offer efficient care to the veterans served in that area. Domiciliaries are homelike environments that provide care to veterans coping with a variety of medical, psychiatric, vocational, educational, or social concerns or illnesses.

Vet Centers offer readjustment counseling and outreach to any veteran who served in a combat zone, along with some services available to family members coping with military life. CBOCs offer outpatient services throughout communities so that veterans do not have to travel to the larger medical centers to receive care. Importantly, CBOCs are increasing in rural areas to provide more services to veterans in remote locations. CLCs offer nursing care to veterans with chronic, stable conditions that require rehabilitation or those needing care during the end of life (U.S. Department of Veterans Affairs 2011b).

Within the structure of the VHA, various Mental Health Centers of Excellence (MH COEs) are designed to meet the mental health needs of veterans. Multiple MH COEs exist around the country, and the National Center for PTSD, opened in 1989, was the first MH COE. Ten Mental Illness, Research, Education and Clinical Centers (MIRECCs; U.S. Department of Veterans Affairs 2011e) were then established, with two more opened to meet needs related to homelessness and integrated health care.

A number of factors are considered in determining an individual's eligi-

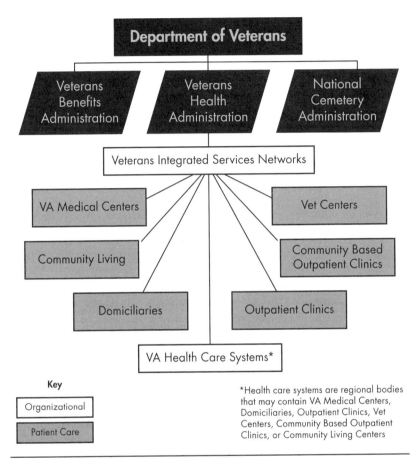

FIGURE 4–1. **Department of Veterans Affairs chart.**

bility for services within the VHA. These include military discharge status, length of service, and income level. Information regarding VHA care, eligibility, and enrollment is available at http://www.va.gov/healtheligibility/eligibility/.

Access to and Types of Mental Health Care Available Through the VHA

There are a variety of mental health services that can be accessed through the VHA in medical centers and CBOCs. Vet Centers also provide readjustment counseling for combat veterans, as described in the section "Structure of the VA." Mental health services where veterans receive medical health care, such as specialty clinics, primary care clinics, nursing homes, and residential care facilities can also be accessed. VHA mental health services and programs include inpatient care, intensive outpatient care, outpatient care in a psychosocial rehabilitation and recovery center, regular outpatient care (including telemedicine), residential care, and supported work settings (U.S. Department of Veterans Affairs 2011f). Table 4–1 provides examples of some programs and services specifically tailored to treat or address various mental health concerns faced by veterans.

As individuals return from Iraq and Afghanistan, many are seeking care within the VHA. According to the Office of Public Health and Environmental Hazards (2011), 53.6% (772,000) of the total separated Operation Enduring Freedom/Operation Iraqi Freedom/Operation New Dawn (OEF/OIF/OND) veterans have obtained health care from the VA since fiscal year 2002. To facilitate the transition from DOD to VA health care systems, every VA medical center has an OEF/OIF/OND care management team. These teams work to address the concerns of this unique population.

This cohort of veterans tends to be young; 46.8% of the 772,000 OEF/OIF/OND veterans seeking VA health care were born between 1980 and 1994. The OEF/OIF/OND cohort also presents with a wide range of medical and mental health concerns. Diagnoses for these veterans have spanned 8,000 different ICD-9 diagnostic codes. Most commonly, these veterans are diagnosed with musculoskeletal ailments (predominantly joint and back disorders), mental disorders, and symptoms, signs, and ill-defined conditions (Office of Public Health and Environmental Hazards 2011).

Part of the changing demographics of individuals now seeking care within the VHA is related to the increasing number of women who have served in the military. In fact, women are one of the fastest-growing cohorts among the veteran population. As such, the VA has developed a wide range of services and programs to respond to the unique needs of female veterans.

Research and the Way Forward

Much of the research funding within the VA is overseen by the Office of Research and Development (ORD). The organizational structure of ORD is presented in Figure 4–2. According to the ORD Web site, the office "aspires to discover knowledge, develop VA researchers and health care leaders, and create innovations that advance health care for our Veterans and the nation" (U.S. Department of Veterans Affairs 2010b). ORD comprises four research services (Biomedical Laboratory Research and Development Service, Clinical Science Research and Development Service, Health Services Research and Development Service Rehabilitation, and Research and Development Service) that together facilitate exploration regarding the wide range of health care issues faced by veterans.

In collaboration with ORD, researchers at COEs and MIRECCs are exploring issues of import for OEF/OIF/OND veterans as well as veterans from previous cohorts. Areas of focus include PTSD, neurorehabilitation, postdeployment mental health, and suicide prevention. For example, the National Center for PTSD (U.S. Department of Veterans Affairs 2011g) "aims to help U.S. Veterans and others through research, education, and training on trauma." The work of the VISN 2 COE and VISN 19 MIRECC (U.S. Department of Veterans Affairs 2011h) is focused on suicide prevention in terms of both public health (VISN 2) and clinical (VISN 19) approaches. Finally, the overarching goals of the VISN 6 MIRECC, which include "improving clinical assessment and treatment and development of novel interventions [for postdeployment mental health issues] through basic and clinical research," are complemented by the work being done at the VISN 19 COE regarding traumatic brain injury (U.S. Department of Veterans Affairs 2011i).

SUMMARY POINTS

- The Military Health System (MHS) serves military members, their dependents, and retirees and includes the Army Medical Command and the Navy's Bureau of Medicine and Surgery.
- In response to inadequate access to health care, Congress created CHAMPUS, the first attempt to provide complete medical coverage at federal facilities for active duty dependents.
- When CHAMPUS proved inefficient and resulted in overall dissatisfaction of beneficiaries, the MHS was then divided into two systems: a direct care system and a nationwide managed care program known as TRICARE.
- The transition from receiving DOD services to receiving VA services can lead to a gap in services. Problems include different eligibility criteria between the two systems and incompatible electronic medical records. Efforts to bridge this gap have included extensive case management.
- The Veterans' Health Administration (VHA) is the nation's largest integrated health system and is organized into regional networks, referred to as Veterans Integrated Service Networks (VISNs), which allows the VHA to reach out to a greater number of communities.
- The Veterans Benefits Administration (VBA) oversees fi-

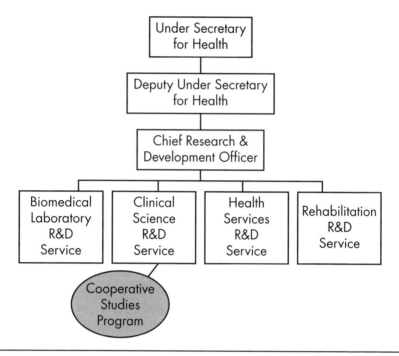

FIGURE 4–2.   Organizational chart, Office of Research and Development.

Source.   U.S. Department of Veterans Affairs 2010b.

nancial compensation and other veterans benefits. The VHA and VBA collaborate to help service members transition from active military service to civilian life.

References

Brown SH, Lincoln MJ, Groen PJ, et al: VistA: U.S. Department of Veterans Affairs national-scale HIS. Int J Med Inform 69(2–3):135–156, 2003

Byrne CM, Mercincavage, LM, Pan EC, et al: The value from investments in health information technology at the U.S. Department of Veterans Affairs. Health Aff (Millwood) 29(4):629–638, 2010 doi:10.1377/hlthaff.2010.0119

Hoge CW, Adler AB, Wright KM, et al: Walter Reed Army Institute of Research contributions during Operations Iraqi Freedom and Enduring Freedom: from research to public health policy, combat and operational behavioral health, Fort Sam Houston, TX, Borden Institute, 2011

Institute of Medicine: Treatment for Posttraumatic Stress Disorder in Military and Veteran Populations, Washington, DC, National Academies Press, 2012

Kizer KW: The "new VA": a national laboratory for health care quality management. Am J Med Qual 14(1):3–20, 1999 doi:10.1177/106286069901400103

Office of Human Resources and Administration (OHRA): Department of Veterans Affairs 2010 organizational briefing book. Office of Administration, 2010. Available at: http://www.va.gov/ofcadmin/docs/vaorgbb.pdf.

Office of Public Health and Environmental Hazards: Analysis of VA health care utilization among Operation Enduring Freedom (OEF), Operation Iraqi Freedom (OIF), and Operation New Dawn (OND) veterans, Washington, DC, Veterans Health Administration, Department of Veterans Affairs, 2011

Office of the Secretary: Department of Veterans Affairs strategic plan: FY 2010–2014. U.S. Department of Veterans Affairs, 2010. Available at: http://www.va.gov/op3/Docs/StrategicPlanning/VA_2010_2014_Strategic_Plan.pdf. Accessed February 19, 2012.

Stetler CB, Mittman BS, Francis J: Overview of the VA Quality Enhancement Research Initiative (QUERI) and QUERI theme articles: QUERI series. Implement Sci 3:8–16, 2008 doi:10.1186/1748-5908-3-8

U.S. Department of Defense: Policy guidance for deployment-limiting psychiatric conditions and medications. U.S. Department of Defense, 2006. Available at: http://www.health.mil/Libraries/HA_Policies_and_Guidelines/Guidance_20061107_deplo_limiting_psyc_cond.pdf. Accessed February 19, 2012.

U.S. Department of Veterans Affairs: History—VA history. U.S. Department of Veterans Affairs, 2010a. Available at: http://www.va.gov/about_va/vahistory.asp. February 19, 2012.

U.S. Department of Veterans Affairs: About the Office of Research and Development. Veterans Health Administration Research and Development, 2010b. Available at: http://www.research.va.gov/about/default.cfm. Accessed February 19, 2012.

U.S. Department of Veterans Affairs: VA disability compensation. U.S. Department of Veterans Affairs, 2011a. Available at: http://www.vba.va.gov/bln/21/compensation. Accessed February 19, 2012.

U.S. Department of Veterans Affairs: About VHA. U.S. Department of Veterans Affairs, 2011b. Available at: http://www.va.gov/health/aboutVHA.asp. Accessed February 19, 2012.

U.S. Department of Veterans Affairs: Mission of the Office of Academic Affiliations. U.S. Department of Veterans Affairs, 2011c. Available at: http://www.va.gov/oaa/OAA_Mission.asp. Accessed February 19, 2012.

U.S. Department of Veterans Affairs: Locations: Veterans Health Administration. U.S. Department of Veterans Affairs, 2011d. Available at: http://www2.va.gov/directory/guide/division_flsh.asp?dnum=1. Accessed February 19, 2012.

U.S. Department of Veterans Affairs: MIRECC centers: What is MIRECC? U.S. Department of Veterans Affairs, 2011e. Available at: http://www.mirecc.va.gov/index.asp. Accessed February 19, 2012.

U.S. Department of Veterans Affairs: Guide to VA mental health services. U.S. Department of Veterans Affairs, 2011f. Available at: http://www.mental-health.va.gov/docs/Guide_to_VA_Mental_Health_Srvcs_FINAL12-20-10.pdf. Accessed February 19, 2012.

U.S. Department of Veterans Affairs: National Center for PTSD: trauma and PTSD. U.S. Department of Veterans Affairs, 2011g. Available at: http://www.ptsd.va.gov/. Accessed February 19, 2012.

U.S. Department of Veterans Affairs: MIRECC centers: MIRECC of the VA Rocky Mountain Network (VISN 19 MIRECC). U.S. Department of Veterans Affairs, 2011h. Available at: http://www.mirecc.va.gov/visn19/. Accessed February 19, 2012.

U.S. Department of Veterans Affairs: MIRECC centers: MIRECC program overview. U.S. Department of Veterans Affairs, 2011i. Available at: http://www.mirecc.va.gov/national-mirecc-overview.asp. Accessed February 19, 2012.

PART II

Military Service–Related Conditions and Interventions

Chapter 5

Health Consequences of Military Service and Combat

Barbara L. Niles, Ph.D.
DeAnna L. Mori, Ph.D.
Antonia V. Seligowski, B.A.
Paula P. Schnurr, Ph.D.

MILITARY PERSONNEL deployed in a theater of war are typically exposed to a host of physical and psychological stressors. Physical trauma, such as losing a limb in a blast, has an obvious impact on health and postwar functioning. In recent decades it has become apparent that psychological trauma, such as witnessing a buddy being hit by a bullet, can also have a profound and lasting impact on both mental and physical health (Green and Kimerling 2004; Schnurr and Green 2004). More than 90% of service members and veterans are exposed to traumatic events either in the military or at some other point in their lives (Dedert et al. 2009), and approximately 14% develop posttraumatic stress disorder (PTSD; Ramchand et al. 2010). (See Chapter 6, "Combat Stress Reactions and Psychiatric Disorders After Deployment," for more information about PTSD in military service members and veterans.)

In this chapter we review the research on the associations between 1) trauma exposure and physical health problems and 2) PTSD and physical health problems. Evidence supporting the hypothesis that PTSD mediates the relationship between trauma exposure and physical health functioning is summarized, and the theory of allostatic load is introduced. Strategies for providers and clinics to use in addressing the specific needs of service personnel and veterans with ongoing medical problems and PTSD are offered.

Trauma Exposure and Physical Health

Evidence accrued over the past few decades has shown that exposure to combat and/or other traumatic events is associated with greater levels of self-reported health problems. A large-scale longitudinal study of male veterans showed that those who reported they had experienced both combat trauma *and* at least one noncombat trauma endorsed a greater number of symptoms than those who had experienced either combat trauma or noncombat trauma (but not both) or had experienced neither (Schnurr et al. 1998). In a sample of active duty male and female soldiers, a positive association was found between the number of violent traumas and sexual assaults experienced and self-reported physical health symptoms (Martin et al. 2000). Community studies have similarly demonstrated a positive association between trauma exposure and self-reported health problems (e.g., Flett et al. 2002; Ullman and Siegel 1996). In a study of women in a large HMO, those who had experienced childhood maltreatment had more medical diagnoses in their charts than those who did not have these experiences (Walker et al. 1999). Even mortality is linked to trauma exposure. A 7% higher mortality risk was observed over a 30-year period in Vietnam War veterans compared with veterans of the same era who did not serve in Vietnam (Boehmer et al. 2004). In this study, higher mortality was attributable to external causes (e.g., accidents, suicide) rather than disease. Other studies of veterans (Visintainer et al. 1995) and civilians (Sibai et al. 2001) exposed to war indicate increased mortality rates due to disease and illness compared with individuals not exposed to war.

PTSD and Physical Health

The studies summarized in the section "Trauma Exposure and Physical Health" illustrate a positive association between trauma exposure and health ailments. Other research has focused on the relationship between PTSD following a trauma exposure and subsequent health problems in military personnel from World War II through the conflicts in Iraq and Afghanistan. In a study of the effects of mustard gas exposure on World War II veterans, those who developed PTSD as a result of exposure reported more physical symptoms and illnesses than veterans exposed to mustard gas who did not develop PTSD (Schnurr et al. 2000a). Illnesses included coronary, urological, gastrointestinal, dermatological, and musculoskeletal disorders as well as chronic obstructive pulmonary disease. In addition, the veterans with PTSD were more likely to be disabled and to utilize U.S. Department of Veterans Affairs (VA) health services than those who were similarly exposed to mustard gas but did not have PTSD.

Research on Vietnam veterans over the past 30 years has shown that PTSD is associated with reports of increased health problems and health care utilization. In the National Vietnam Veterans Readjustment Study, Kulka and colleagues (1990) found that Vietnam theater veterans with PTSD reported more physical health problems than those without PTSD. Similar findings have been reported for female nurses (Wolfe et al. 1994) and Australian soldiers (O'Toole and Catts 2008) who served in Vietnam.

In Iraq and Afghanistan war veterans, PTSD is also linked to self-reported poor physical health (Engelhard et al. 2009; Jakupcak et al. 2008), and the unique contribution of PTSD in predicting physical health has been linked to specific diseases, such as the increased risk of diabetes onset (Boyko et al. 2010).

Taken together, the above research findings make a compelling case for the link between PTSD and subjective self-reports of poor health functioning in veterans and service members. There is increasing evidence that PTSD also is associated with *objective* indicators of physical health problems, such as mortality rates. Two large-scale studies indicate that Vietnam veterans with PTSD have "all cause" mortality rates that are 70%–100% greater than those of veterans without PTSD (Boscarino 2006; Bullman and Kang 1994). Deaths due to external causes, such as suicide, accidents, and homicide, are higher for veterans with PTSD than those without PTSD (Boscarino 2006; Bullman and Kang 1994). However, there is also evidence that there are higher rates of cardiovascular and autoimmune disorders, which contribute to higher rates of mortality in Vietnam veterans with PTSD (Boscarino 2008).

Morbidity rates related to specific diseases are also elevated for veterans with PTSD compared with those without PTSD. A longitudinal study of World War II and Korean War veterans found that PTSD was associated with increased incidence of arterial, lower gastrointestinal, dermatological, and musculoskeletal disorders (Schnurr et al. 2000b). A series of longitudinal studies on Vietnam theater and Vietnam era veterans has provided strong evidence of the association between PTSD and increased rates of cardiovascular diseases (Boscarino 2004, 2008) and autoimmune diseases such as rheumatoid arthritis, psoriasis, insulin-dependent diabetes, and thyroid disease (Boscarino 2004). In addition, veterans with more severe or complex PTSD were more likely to have clinically higher T cell counts, hyperreactive immune responses on standardized delayed cutaneous hypersensitivity tests, clinically higher immunoglobulin M levels, and clinically lower dehydroepiandrosterone levels (Boscarino 2004). These biological markers are consistent with a broad range of inflammatory disorders, including both cardiovascular and autoimmune diseases.

PTSD also is associated with greater cardiovascular risk factors even in younger veterans who are less likely to have yet developed cardiovascular disease. Using VA medical records of more than 300,000 Operation Enduring Freedom/Operation Iraqi Freedom (OEF/OIF) veterans with a mean age of 31 years, Cohen and colleagues (2009) found that a diagnosis of PTSD was associated with significantly increased risk for tobacco use, hypertension, dyslipidemia, and obesity compared with veterans with no mental health diagnoses, and veterans with PTSD had significantly more medical visits than those without a mental health diagnosis.

Mediating Role of PTSD

Injury and illness at the time of the traumatic event are *direct* and observable ways that trauma affects health. An acute physical trauma, such as a shrapnel wound, is clearly evident in the immediate aftermath of a combat event. Effects due to chemical exposure may be obvious immediately, such as respiratory problems in response to airborne contaminants following the collapse of the World Trade Center on 9/11 (Mauer et al. 2007), while other effects from chemical exposure may be more subtle and become evident only years after exposure, such as diabetes associated with Agent Orange exposure in Vietnam veterans (Kang et al. 2006; Michalek and Pavuk 2008).

A range of studies examining the *indirect* effects of trauma exposure have provided evidence that PTSD mediates the association between combat exposure and later physical health. In a study of Gulf War veterans, combat exposure assessed upon return from the war zone was a significant predictor of self-reported health status 18–24 months later (Wagner et al. 2000). This association was significantly reduced when PTSD was included in the regression model (see Table 5–1). Findings are similar in smaller studies of female veterans (e.g., Smith et al. 2011) and large path analytic studies of veterans (Schnurr and Spiro 1999; Taft et al. 1999), which indicate that PTSD may account for as much as 90%–100% of the association between exposure to military stressors and subsequent self-reported health problems.

A study of OEF/OIF service members diagnosed with traumatic brain injury (TBI) found that mild TBI is strongly associated with PTSD and later self-reported physical health problems in service members and that PTSD is an important mediator of the relationship between mild TBI and subsequent reports of physical health problems (Hoge et al. 2008). (See Chapter 9, "Traumatic Brain Injury," for more information on TBI.) Thus, outside of circumstances in which an illness or injury is a direct conse-

TABLE 5–1. Four mechanisms by which PTSD affects physical
health morbidity and mortality

Mechanism	Effects
Biological	Altered stress response, including changes in the locus coeruleus/norepinephrine sympathetic and hypothalamic-pituitary-adrenal systems
Psychological	Depression, hostility, and poor coping
Behavioral	Unhealthy lifestyle behaviors, such as substance abuse, tobacco use, risky sexual behavior, and refraining from exercise
Attentional	Methods to cope with PTSD symptoms, such as attending to physical or medical symptoms in order to avoid thinking about a traumatic event

quence of a traumatic event, PTSD plays a critical mediating role in the association between trauma exposure and subsequent physical health issues. It is the symptoms of PTSD and not the trauma exposure itself that most contributes to increased risk for later physical health problems.

Distinct Role of PTSD Compared With Other Mental Disorders

Several studies have examined whether the effects of PTSD on physical health are unique or attributable to the effects of other psychological disorders that commonly occur with PTSD, such as depression and substance abuse. In OEF/OIF service members, Hoge and colleagues (2008) found that TBIs associated with altered mental status were significantly associated with PTSD but not with depression. Studies of veterans who served during OEF/OIF (Boyko et al. 2010), Vietnam veterans (Boscarino 2008), and VA primary care patients (Possemato et al. 2010) support the finding that PTSD is associated with greater medical disease burden over time after accounting for other psychological disorders. These studies illustrate that PTSD has a strong and distinct association with the development of subsequent ill health even when other psychiatric disorders are considered.

Mechanisms and Allostatic Load

Schnurr and colleagues (Schnurr and Green 2004; Schnurr and Jankowski 1999; Schnurr et al. 2007) have proposed an allostatic load model to explain how traumatic events can affect physical health, both directly and indirectly via other mechanisms. These authors identified four hypothesized mechanisms by which PTSD can affect physical health morbidity and mortality: biological, psychological, behavioral, and attentional (see Table 5–1). These mechanisms combine and interact to contribute to poor health for individuals with PTSD.

The concept of *allostatic load* has been proposed to explain how numerous and sometimes subtle changes related to PTSD substantially impact health over time (Friedman and McEwan 2004; Schnurr and Green 2004; Schnurr and Jankowski 1999). Allostatic load is defined as "the strain on the body produced by repeated ups and downs of physiologic response, as well as the elevated activity of physiologic systems under challenge, and the changes in metabolism and wear and tear on a number of organs and tissues" (McEwen and Stellar 1993, p. 2094). This unifying concept explains how seemingly small alterations in biology, psychology, behavior, and attention can accumulate and interact over time to produce disease. For example, as shown in Figure 5–1, increased heart rate alone for an individual with PTSD may not be sufficient to produce cardiovascular disease. But when subtle changes in biology related to PTSD combine with behavioral changes associated with PTSD, such as smoking, alcohol use, and sedentary lifestyle, the allostatic load may become sufficient to produce disease. Only one study has examined the association between PTSD and allostatic load, however. Glover et al. (2006) studied mothers of pediatric cancer patients and found that allostatic load was higher in the mothers who developed PTSD relative to those who did not. Schnurr and Jankowski (1999) first proposed that PTSD may contribute to allostatic load more than other mental health disorders, but this remains an untested hypothesis that warrants further investigation. Future research should continue to evaluate the utility of the allostatic load model in understanding how PTSD may impact physical health.

Treatment of PTSD and Physical Health

Some recent studies suggest that treating PTSD may be helpful in decreasing health problems; however, the extent to which treatment of PTSD can impact physical health remains unclear. Two randomized trials examining empirically supported PTSD treatments for female physical and sexual assault survivors found that treatment had a positive effect on self-reported physical health status. Rauch and colleagues (2009) found that self-reported physical health problems were reduced in the two prolonged exposure treatment groups compared with a wait-list control. In a study that compared cognitive processing therapy and prolonged exposure treatment, Galovski and colleagues (2009) found reductions in health-related concerns for both groups, with relatively more improvement for the cognitive processing group. In both of these studies, the results were maintained through the follow-up period. Similarly, in a random-

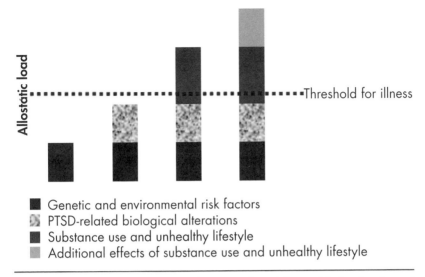

Genetic and environmental risk factors
PTSD-related biological alterations
Substance use and unhealthy lifestyle
Additional effects of substance use and unhealthy lifestyle

FIGURE 5–1. A hypothetical example of how biological and behavioral factors could combine to increase allostatic load in an individual with PTSD.

Source. From Schnurr PP, Green BL, Kaltman S: *Handbook of PTSD: Science and Practice.* New York, Guilford, 2007, p. 408. Copyright [2007] by Guilford. Adapted with permission.

ized controlled trial of cognitive-behavioral treatment for individuals with PTSD and serious mental illness, Mueser and colleagues (2008) found that physical health concerns were reduced in the intervention group as opposed to the control group, and these differences were maintained throughout the 6-month follow-up. However, other evidence suggests that treatment of PTSD may have little or no effect on health complaints (Malik et al. 1999; Schnurr et al. 2003, 2007). For example, in a study of female veterans and service members, Schnurr and colleagues (2007) found no improvement in self-reported health among women who received PTSD treatment relative to women who received a nonspecific comparison treatment, although there was a reduction in PTSD symptoms in the treatment group. More investigation is needed in this area to determine if the negative health effects associated with PTSD can be reduced if symptoms of PTSD are treated.

Implications for the Provision of Treatment to Service Members and Veterans

When veterans and service members with PTSD present to health and mental health clinics, clinicians must be sensitive to the relationship between trauma and poor health to enhance quality of care. Most individuals with PTSD do not seek mental health care and are likely to seek care in a medical setting instead (Samson et al. 1999), where their PTSD may go unrecognized (Magruder and Yeager 2008; Taubman-Ben-Ari et al. 2001). Thus, attention should be paid to the mental health needs of veterans and service members in medical settings. Building on prior work (Schnurr and Green 2004; Schnurr et al. 2007), we offer the following recommendations for providing high-quality care to veterans and service members who present in different settings.

Mental Health Care Settings

In a mental health setting, a clinician should conduct a comprehensive assessment to address the patient's mental health needs while taking physical health issues into account (Kilpatrick et al. 1997). Understanding the complex interrelationship between mental and physical health allows the clinician to develop a more complete conceptualization of a patient's experience and issues and will facilitate the clinician's ability to develop an effective treatment approach. Educating patients with PTSD or other trauma-related disorders about the relationship between their distress and their physical health can facilitate the management of both physical and mental health problems (Kilpatrick et al. 1997).

Given the high rates of unhealthy behaviors (e.g., physical inactivity, tobacco and alcohol use, obesity) and low rates of preventive behaviors (e.g., following through with regular medical screens) (Buckley et al. 2004), a careful assessment of health behaviors with trauma survivors can be useful to determine if the patient is properly addressing his or her health issues. Use of tobacco, alcohol, or recreational drugs; overeating; or eating unhealthy foods may be employed to cope with trauma-related stress. In these instances, the clinician should help patients identify alternative, more adaptive, and healthier methods of coping (Rheingold et al. 2004).

Some evidence suggests that individuals with PTSD are less adherent to their medical regimens (Delahanty et al. 2004; Shemesh et al. 2004; Zen et al. 2012) and that they are less likely to trust their medical providers (Bassuk et al. 2001). These factors make it more difficult for providers and patients with PTSD to form collaborative relationships. It is important for mental health clinicians to encourage and help patients with PTSD adhere to their medical regimens, communicate with their providers, and perhaps make medical adherence an independent treatment goal (see Chapter 11, "Collaborative Care").

Medical Care Settings

PTSD patients frequently present in primary care clinics, are high utilizers of health care, and show higher rates of functional impairment than those

TABLE 5–2. **Primary care PTSD screen**

In your life, have you ever had any experience that was so frightening, horrible, or upsetting that, in the past month, you...

Have had nightmares about it or thought about it when you did not want to?	No	Yes
Tried hard not to think about it or went out of your way to avoid situations that reminded you of it?	No	Yes
Were constantly on guard, watchful, or easily startled?	No	Yes
Felt numb or detached from others, activities, or your surroundings?	No	Yes

Source. Prins et al. 2004.

individuals who present to primary care without a psychiatric disorder (Deykin et al. 2001; Stein et al. 2000). In a study of women seeking VA health care, those with PTSD had more outpatient visits, diagnostic tests, hospitalizations, and surgical procedures than those without PTSD (Dobie et al. 2006). Unfortunately, medical providers may not always have an understanding of PTSD or the relationship between trauma and physical health, and PTSD can go undetected in these settings.

The first issue to be addressed is the proper identification of patients with PTSD. This can be done with one of several PTSD screens. The four-item Primary Care PTSD Screen (PC-PTSD) assesses each of the four DSM-IV-TR (American Psychiatric Association 2000) PTSD symptom clusters with a "yes" or "no" response. Endorsing three or more of the four items has shown optimal sensitivity and specificity for detecting PTSD (see Table 5–2) (Freedy et al. 2010; Prins et al. 2004). The PC-PTSD has been recommended in the U.S. Department of Veterans Affairs/Department of Defense Clinical Practice Guidelines for the management of PTSD (Management of Post-Traumatic Stress Working Group, 2010) and is used in both the Post Deployment Health Assessment (PDHA) and Post Deployment Health Reassessment (PDHRA) that are administered when service members return from deployment (PDHA) or after redeployment (PDHRA).

The PTSD Checklist (PCL; Weathers et al. 1993) is a widely used questionnaire that includes each of the 17 DSM-IV-TR symptoms of PTSD rated on a five-point Likert scale. Appropriate cutoff scores vary according to the settings and populations, with greater sensitivity being more desirable for screening purposes. Yeager and colleagues (2007) evaluated the performance characteristics of the PCL in VA primary care patients and recommended a cutoff score of 31 for primary care settings. Higher cutoffs are recommended for civilian settings (Freedy et al. 2010).

Mental health clinicians can help set up a system of screening and educate other medical care providers about PTSD and trauma reactions (see Chapter 11). It is important to provide medical care providers with information on what they can do when their patients screen positive. Access to mental health services is critical; therefore, pathways to care should be clearly delineated and obstacles to care eliminated as best as possible. The best screen available will not enhance clinical care if appropriate follow-up mechanisms are not adequately in place.

Integrated Care

Large medical systems can be difficult to negotiate and can be very confusing to patients, particularly those with complex needs (Uomoto and Williams 2009). Patients feel less overwhelmed by large medical centers when their medical and mental health needs can be addressed in the same clinic or geographic location and when providers collaborate to coordinate care. Care delivered in this integrated and coordinated manner has been shown to enhance access to services and treatment adherence, improve health outcomes, and lead to higher satisfaction among providers and patients (Blount 1998; Pomerantz et al. 2009). Integrated care can be delivered in different ways (e.g., mental health clinicians embedded in primary care clinics or primary care providers embedded in mental health clinics), but the most important elements are good communication and effective collaboration between the interdisciplinary providers. Patients respond well when care is provided by a cohesive team of providers who are working toward consistent, nonconflicting goals and when the patient is encouraged to be an active part of the treatment planning.

The VA and U.S. Department of Defense have been at the forefront of promoting integrated primary care. Since 2007, the VA has optimized medical care by including behavioral health prevention and treatment services in primary care settings. Specifically, behavioral health providers are embedded in primary care clinics to work collaboratively on interdisciplinary treatment teams with the goal of providing optimal physical and mental health care in a timely manner (often the same day). The behavioral health clinician is in an ideal position to offer mental health assessment and treatment services in this collaborative setting while also being able to promote healthy behaviors (e.g., healthy eating, physical activity, good sleep habits) that can prevent the onset or progression of physical and psychological problems.

Given the relationship between PTSD and physical health, clinics that provide integrated medical and mental health care can be the ideal place for individuals with PTSD to receive care.

Zatzick and colleagues (2011) have been able to show that it is feasible to implement this type of collaborative care, even in acute care settings (see

Chapter 11). Other studies that have investigated the effectiveness of trauma-focused treatment for PTSD in primary care settings have produced encouraging, but mixed, results. Engel and colleagues (2008) implemented 3CM, a collaborative care model developed by Dietrich et al. (2004), for managing PTSD and depression in Army soldiers. The Army project involved screening for PTSD and depression in primary care and providing a nurse care facilitator who ensured continuity of care for soldiers in need of mental health treatment. The authors found this model to be feasible to implement and acceptable to both military primary care providers and patients and also found that patients typically showed clinical improvements. Cigrang and colleagues (2011) reported pilot data on a brief PTSD intervention that was designed to be delivered to active duty service members in primary care. This intervention incorporated elements of prolonged exposure therapy and cognitive processing therapy, and preliminary results showed that PTSD severity, depression, and global mental health functioning all improved for the OEF/OIF service members who received it. However, the effectiveness of brief treatments for PTSD provided in primary care remains somewhat inconclusive, as is evidenced by the findings reported by the Coordinated Anxiety Learning and Management (CALM) study (Craske et al. 2011). Craske and colleagues investigated the effectiveness of a brief, multimodal treatment for anxiety disorders administered in a primary care setting but did not obtain significant results to support their treatment.

The VA and U.S. Department of Defense have taken steps forward in supporting integrated health care, and although this has been a very positive advance, issues remain before the effectiveness of treating PTSD in this context can be fully understood. Possemato and colleagues (2011) reported that most of the treatment for PTSD that is provided in VA primary care clinics is with medication or supportive therapy and that more intensive treatment of PTSD continues to occur in clinics with highly specialized PTSD services.

SUMMARY POINTS

- Exposure to a traumatic event is associated with increased physical health problems such as cardiovascular diseases, diabetes, gastrointestinal disorders, dermatological disorders, autoimmune diseases, increased risk for tobacco use, and obesity. In addition to physical trauma, illness, or injury directly resulting from an event, current evidence suggests that PTSD related to psychological trauma is the pathway by which trauma leads to subsequent physical health problems.

- Practitioners should consider the effect of allostatic load on the patient, such as PTSD-related biological changes combined with PTSD-related behavioral changes that may become sufficient to produce disease. The allostatic load model suggests that PTSD affects multiple body systems via various pathways.

- Practitioners in a medical setting should be especially vigilant in looking for signs of PTSD because individuals with PTSD often do not seek mental health care. Carefully assess the patient's health behaviors (overeating, alcohol use, tobacco use) and help him or her identify alternative, more adaptive, and healthier methods of coping with trauma-related stress.

- Practitioners should educate patients with PTSD on the relationship between distress and physical health.

- Wellness interventions that promote healthy behaviors and target both mind (psychological issues) and body (medical issues) are a logical approach to treatment for individuals with PTSD. Promotion of behaviors that slow the accumulation of allostatic burden may be particularly relevant for PTSD: exercise, healthy diet, stress management, and compliance with medical regimens. Targeting the cessation of behaviors that contribute to allostatic burden, such as smoking and alcohol use, is another useful strategy.

References

American Psychiatric Association: Diagnostic and Statistical Manual of Mental Disorders, 4th Edition, Text Revision. Washington, DC, American Psychiatric Association, 2000

Bassuk EL, Dawson R, Perloff J, et al: Post-traumatic stress disorder in extremely poor women: implications for health care clinicians. J Am Med Womens Assoc 56(2):79–85, 2001

Blount A: Introduction to integrated primary care, in Integrated Primary Care: The Future of Medical and Mental Health Collaboration. Edited by Blount A. New York, WW Norton, 1998, pp 1–43

Boehmer TK, Flanders WD, McGeehin MA, et al: Postservice mortality in Vietnam veterans: 30-year follow-up. Arch Intern Med 164(17):1908–1916, 2004

Boscarino JA: Posttraumatic stress disorder and physical illness: results from clinical and epidemiologic studies. Ann NY Acad Sci 1032:141–153, 2004

Boscarino JA: Posttraumatic stress disorder and mortality among U.S. Army veterans 30 years after military service. Ann Epidemiol 16(4):248–256, 2006

Boscarino JA: A prospective study of PTSD and early-age heart disease mortality among Vietnam veterans: implications for surveillance and prevention. Psychosom Med 70(6):668–676, 2008

Boyko EJ, Jacobson IG, Smith B, et al: Risk of diabetes in U.S. military service members in relation to combat deployment and mental health. Diabetes Care 33(8):1771–1777, 2010

Buckley TC, Mozley SL, Bedard MA, et al: Preventive health behaviors, health-risk behaviors, physical morbidity, and health-related role functioning impairment in veterans with post-traumatic stress disorder. Mil Med 169:536–540, 2004

Bullman TA, Kang HK: Posttraumatic stress disorder and the risk of traumatic deaths among Vietnam veterans. J Nerv Ment Dis 182(11):604–610, 1994

Cigrang JA, Rauch SAM, Avila LL, et al: Treatment of active-duty military with PTSD in primary care: early findings. Psychol Serv 8:104–113, 2011

Cohen BE, Marmar C, Ren L, et al: Association of cardiovascular risk factors with mental health diagnoses in Iraq and Afghanistan War veterans using VA health care. JAMA 302(5):489–492, 2009

Craske MG, Stein MB, Sullivan G, et al: Disorder-specific impact of coordinated anxiety learning and management treatment for anxiety disorders in primary care. Arch Gen Psychiatry 68(4):378–388, 2011

Delahanty DL, Bogart LM, Figler JL: Posttraumatic stress disorder symptoms, salivary cortisol, medication adherence, and CD4 levels in HIV-positive individuals. AIDS Care 16(2):247–260, 2004

Dedert EA, Green KT, Calhoun PS, et al: Association of trauma exposure with psychiatric morbidity in military veterans who have served since September 11, 2001. J Psychiatr Res 43(9):830–836, 2009

Deykin EY, Keane TM, Kaloupek D, et al: Posttraumatic stress disorder and the use of health services. Psychosom Med 63(5):835–841, 2001

Dietrich AJ, Oxman TE, Williams JW Jr, et al: Re-engineering systems for the treatment of depression in primary care: cluster randomised controlled trial. BMJ 329(7466):602–605, 2004

Dobie DJ, Maynard C, Kivlahan DR, et al: Posttraumatic stress disorder screening status is associated with increased VA medical and surgical utilization in women. J Gen Intern Med 21 (suppl 3):S58–S64, 2006

Engel CC, Oxman T, Yamamoto C, et al: RESPECT-Mil: feasibility of a systems-level collaborative care approach to depression and post-traumatic stress disorder in military primary care. Mil Med 173(10):935–940, 2008

Engelhard IM, van den Hout MA, Weerts J, et al: A prospective study of the relation between posttraumatic stress and physical health symptoms. Int J Clin Health Psychol 9:365–372, 2009

Flett RA, Kazantzis N, Long NR, et al: Traumatic events and physical health in a New Zealand community sample. J Trauma Stress 15(4):303–312, 2002

Freedy JR, Steenkamp MM, Magruder KM, et al: Post-traumatic stress disorder screening test performance in civilian primary care. Fam Pract 27(6):615–624, 2010

Friedman MJ, McEwan BS: Posttraumatic stress disorder, allostatic load, and medical illness, in Trauma and Health: Physical Health Consequences of Exposure to Extreme Stress. Edited by Schnurr PP, Green BL. Arlington, VA, American Psychological Association, 2004, pp 157–188

Galovski TE, Monson C, Bruce SE, et al: Does cognitive-behavioral therapy for PTSD improve perceived health and sleep impairment? J Trauma Stress 22(3):197–204, 2009

Glover DA, Stuber M, Poland RE: Allostatic load in women with and without PTSD symptoms. Psychiatry 69(3):191–203, 2006

Green BL, Kimerling R: Trauma, posttraumatic stress disorder, and health status, in Trauma and Health: Physical Health Consequences of Exposure to Extreme Stress. Edited by Schnurr PP, Green BL. Arlington, VA, American Psychological Association, 2004, pp 13–42

Hoge CW, McGurk D, Thomas JL, et al: Mild traumatic brain injury in U.S. soldiers returning from Iraq. N Engl J Med 358(5):453–463, 2008

Jakupcak M, Luterek J, Hunt S, et al: Posttraumatic stress and its relationship to physical health functioning in a sample of Iraq and Afghanistan War veterans seeking postdeployment VA health care. J Nerv Ment Dis 196(5):425–428, 2008

Kang HK, Dalager NA, Needham LL, et al: Health status of Army Chemical Corps Vietnam veterans who sprayed defoliant in Vietnam. Am J Ind Med 49(11):875–884, 2006

Kilpatrick DG, Resnick HS, Acierno R: Health impact of interpersonal violence. 3: Implications for clinical practice and public policy. Behav Med 23(2):79–85, 1997

Kulka RA, Schlenger WE, Fairbank JA, et al: The prevalence of physical health problems, in Trauma and the Vietnam War Generation: Report of Findings From the National Vietnam Veterans Readjustment Study. New York, Brunner, 1990, pp 189–199

Magruder KM, Yeager DE: Patient factors relating to detection of posttraumatic stress disorder in Department of Veterans Affairs primary care settings. J Rehabil Res Dev 45(3):371–381, 2008

Malik ML, Connor KM, Sutherland SM, et al: Quality of life and posttraumatic stress disorder: a pilot study assessing changes in SF-36 scores before and after treatment in a placebo-controlled trial of fluoxetine. J Trauma Stress 12(2):387–393, 1999

Management of Post-Traumatic Stress Working Group: VA/DoD clinical practice guideline for management of post-traumatic stress. Washington, DC, U.S. Department of Veterans Affairs, 2010

Martin L, Rosen LN, Durand DB, et al: Psychological and physical health effects of sexual assaults and nonsexual traumas among male and female United States Army soldiers. Behav Med 26(1):23–33, 2000

Mauer MP, Cummings KR, Carlson GA: Health effects in New York State personnel who responded to the World Trade Center disaster. J Occup Environ Med 49(11):1197–1205, 2007

McEwen BS, Stellar E: Stress and the individual: mechanisms leading to disease. Arch Intern Med 153(18):2093–2101, 1993

Michalek JE, Pavuk M: Diabetes and cancer in veterans of Operation Ranch Hand after adjustment for calendar period, days of spraying, and time spent in Southeast Asia. J Occup Environ Med 50(3):330–340, 2008

Mueser KT, Rosenberg SD, Xie H, et al: A randomized controlled trial of cognitive-behavioral treatment for posttraumatic stress disorder in severe mental illness. J Consult Clin Psychol 76(2):259–271, 2008

O'Toole BI, Catts SV: Trauma, PTSD, and physical health: an epidemiological study of Australian Vietnam veterans. J Psychosom Res 64(1):33–40, 2008

Pomerantz AS, Corson JA, Detzer MJ: The challenge of integrated care for mental health: leaving the 50 minute hour and other sacred things. J Clin Psychol Med Settings 16(1):40–46, 2009

Possemato K, Wade M, Andersen J, et al: The impact of PTSD, depression, and substance use disorders on disease burden and health care utilization among OEF/OIF veterans. Psychol Trauma 2:218–223, 2010

Possemato K, Ouimette P, Lantinga LJ, et al: Treatment of Department of Veterans Affairs primary care patients with posttraumatic stress disorder. Psychol Serv 8:82–93, 2011

Prins A, Ouimette P, Kimerling R, et al: The Primary Care PTSD Screen (PC-PTSD): Development and operating characteristics. Primary Care Psychiatry 9:9–14, 2004

Ramchand R, Schell TL, Karney BR, et al: Disparate prevalence estimates of PTSD among service members who served in Iraq and Afghanistan: possible explanations. J Trauma Stress 23(1):59–68, 2010

Rauch SA, Grunfeld TE, Yadin E, et al: Changes in reported physical health symptoms and social function with prolonged exposure therapy for chronic posttraumatic stress disorder. Depress Anxiety 26(8):732–738, 2009

Rheingold AA, Acierno R, Resnick HS: Trauma, posttraumatic stress disorder, and health risk behaviors, in Trauma and Health: Physical Health Consequences of Exposure to Extreme Stress. Edited by Schnurr PP, Green BL. Arlington, VA, American Psychological Association, 2004, pp 217–243

Samson AY, Bensen S, Beck A, et al: Posttraumatic stress disorder in primary care. J Fam Pract 48(3):222–227, 1999

Schnurr PP, Green BL: Understanding relationships among trauma, posttraumatic stress disorder, and health outcomes, in Trauma and Health: Physical Health Consequences of Exposure to Extreme Stress. Edited by Schnurr PP, Green BL. Arlington, VA, American Psychological Association, 2004, pp 247–275

Schnurr PP, Jankowski MK: Physical health and post-traumatic stress disorder: review and synthesis. Semin Clin Neuropsychiatry 4(4):295–304, 1999

Schnurr PP, Spiro A III: Combat exposure, posttraumatic stress disorder symptoms, and health behaviors as predictors of self-reported physical health in older veterans. J Nerv Ment Dis 187(6):353–359, 1999

Schnurr PP, Spiro A III, Aldwin CM, et al: Physical symptom trajectories following trauma exposure: longitudinal findings from the normative aging study. J Nerv Ment Dis 186(9):522–528, 1998

Schnurr PP, Ford JD, Friedman MJ, et al: Predictors and outcomes of posttraumatic stress disorder in World War II veterans exposed to mustard gas. J Consult Clin Psychol 68(2):258–268, 2000a

Schnurr PP, Spiro A III, Paris AH: Physician-diagnosed medical disorders in relation to PTSD symptoms in older male military veterans. Health Psychol 19(1):91–97, 2000b

Schnurr PP, Friedman MJ, Foy DW, et al: Randomized trial of trauma-focused group therapy for posttraumatic stress disorder: results from a department of veterans affairs cooperative study. Arch Gen Psychiatry 60(5):481–489, 2003

Schnurr PP, Green BL, Kaltman S: Trauma exposure and physical health, in Handbook of PTSD: Science and Practice. Edited by Friedman M. New York, Guilford, 2007, pp 406–424

Shemesh E, Yehuda R, Milo O, et al: Posttraumatic stress, nonadherence, and adverse outcome in survivors of a myocardial infarction. Psychosom Med 66(4):521–526, 2004

Sibai AM, Fletcher A, Armenian HK: Variations in the impact of long-term wartime stressors on mortality among the middle-aged and older population in Beirut, Lebanon, 1983–1993. Am J Epidemiol 154(2):128–137, 2001

Smith BN, Shipherd JC, Schuster JL, et al: Posttraumatic stress symptomatology as a mediator of the association between military sexual trauma and post-deployment physical health in women. J Trauma Dissociation 12(3):275–289, 2011

Stein MB, McQuaid JR, Pedrelli P, et al: Posttraumatic stress disorder in the primary care medical setting. Gen Hosp Psychiatry 22(4):261–269, 2000

Taft CT, Stern AS, King LA, et al: Modeling physical health and functional health status: the role of combat exposure, posttraumatic stress disorder, and personal resource attributes. J Trauma Stress 12(1):3–23, 1999

Taubman-Ben-Ari O, Rabinowitz J, Feldman D, et al: Post-traumatic stress disorder in primary-care settings: prevalence and physicians' detection. Psychol Med 31(3):555–560, 2001

Ullman SE, Siegel JM: Traumatic events and physical health in a community sample. J Trauma Stress 9(4):703–720, 1996

Uomoto JM, Williams RM: Post-acute polytrauma rehabilitation and integrated care of returning veterans: toward a holistic approach. Rehabil Psychol 54(3):259–269, 2009

Visintainer PF, Barone M, McGee H, et al: Proportionate mortality study of Vietnam-era veterans of Michigan. J Occup Environ Med 37(4):423–428, 1995

Wagner AW, Wolfe J, Rotnitsky A, et al: An investigation of the impact of posttraumatic stress disorder on physical health. J Trauma Stress 13(1):41–55, 2000

Walker EA, Gelfand AN, Katon WJ, et al: Adult health status of women with histories of childhood abuse and neglect. Am J Med 107(4):332–339, 1999

Weathers FW, Litz BT, Herman DS, et al: The PTSD checklist: reliability, validity, and diagnostic utility. Paper presented at the annual meeting of the International Society for Traumatic Stress Studies, San Antonio, TX, 1993

Wolfe J, Schnurr PP, Brown PJ, et al: Posttraumatic stress disorder and war-zone exposure as correlates of perceived health in female Vietnam War veterans. J Consult Clin Psychol 62(6):1235–1240, 1994

Yeager DE, Magruder KM, Knapp RG, et al: Performance characteristics of the posttraumatic stress disorder checklist and SPAN in Veterans Affairs primary care settings. Gen Hosp Psychiatry 29(4):294–301, 2007

Zatzick D, Rivara F, Jurkovich G, et al: Enhancing the population impact of collaborative care interventions: mixed method development and implementation of stepped care targeting posttraumatic stress disorder and related comorbidities after acute trauma. Gen Hosp Psychiatry 33(2):123–134, 2011

Zen AL, Whooley MA, Zhao S, et al: Post-traumatic stress disorder is associated with poor health behaviors: findings from the heart and soul study. Health Psychol 31(2):194–201, 2012

Chapter 6

Combat Stress Reactions and Psychiatric Disorders After Deployment

David E. Cabrera, Ph.D., LTC, USA, MSC
David M. Benedek, M.D.

THE UNITED STATES has long recognized the challenges its military members face on return from war (Leventman 1978; Wecter 1944). Concerns surrounding the ability of military members to successfully reintegrate into civilian society have resulted from the recognition that aggressive behavior that may be adaptive or necessary on the battlefield may persist on return and that exposure to the trauma of war may result in a variety of negative emotional and behavioral consequences. Although psychiatrists and other clinicians have long observed psychological changes on return from battle, medical science has struggled to develop a clear description of the symptoms, etiology, and course of war-related psychiatric disorders.

By the mid-1970s it became apparent that large numbers of soldiers returning from Vietnam were experiencing more protracted difficulties with readjustment. During this period clinicians and researchers began to develop criteria that have since evolved to define posttraumatic stress disorder (PTSD), first officially recognized in DSM-III (American Psychiatric Association 1980). As the definition of PTSD has evolved, so too has our recognition that the range of responses to the trauma of war cannot be circumscribed by a single diagnostic label. Just as may occur after exposures to the mass violence of natural or man-made disasters, war-related psychological symptoms occur across a full spectrum in terms of duration, characteristics, and severity.

Range of Postdeployment Response

At the individual level, the psychological response to combat experience is quite variable and ranges from transient and subclinical distress symptoms to well-characterized but nevertheless transient or self-limited psychiatric disorders to psychiatric disorders associated with longer-term impairment in social or occupational function. Across the spectrum of psychological responses to combat, PTSD has garnered much attention from the media and national leadership, and there has been considerable investment in research into the prevention and treatment of PTSD. However, other responses may cause significant (albeit transient) impairment in one's social or occupational function.

Symptom-inducing stressors include separation from loved ones or usual sources of support, austere living conditions, high operational tempo, extremes of climate, sleep deprivation, and—of course—exposure to mass violence resulting in the witnessing of death or the witnessing or experiencing of life-threatening or severe injury. The specific symptoms of a combat stress reaction or combat/operational stress reaction (COSR) may vary widely (ranging from symptoms of fear or worry to symptoms of anxiety, depression, or impaired reality testing) on the basis of the nature of traumatic exposure and a variety of population characteristics such as training and preparation for combat and cohesion and esprit de corps within the unit and individual factors such as coping skills, previous experience with combat, past medical or mental health history, and ongoing stressors occurring at the home (Gal and Jones 1995).

COSRs are, by military doctrine, distinct from psychiatric disorders and generally are treated according to the principles of immediacy, proximity (treatment near the point of injury identification or near the battlefront), simplicity (conservative measures focusing on support and restoration of nutrition, hygiene, and sleep), and expectancy (reassurance regarding the commonly observed and transient nature of COSRs). However, the line between COSRs and psychiatric diagnoses such as adjustment disorder or acute stress disorder has somewhat arbitrarily been drawn on the basis of duration of symptoms, with COSRs expected to resolve with implementation of the conservative treatment measures outlined above within 72 hours (see Tables 6–1 and 6–2).

Arguably, every service member is affected to some degree by the rigors of exposure to combat. The extent to which the changes brought about by

TABLE 6–1. Mild to moderate combat/operational stress reactions

Physical reactions	Emotional reactions	Behavioral reactions
Fatigue	Mild or moderate anxiety	Indecisiveness
Jumpiness	Mourning	Inattention
Sweating	Inability to concentrate	Carelessness
Difficulty sleeping	Nightmares	Hyperalertness
Rapid heartbeat	Self-doubt	Lack of motivation
Dizziness	Anger	Irritability
Nausea, vomiting, or diarrhea	Excessive concern with minor issues	Lack of initiative
		Tears, crying
Slow reaction times	Loss of confidence in self and unit	Inability to relax
Dry mouth		Argumentativeness
Muscular tension		

TABLE 6–2. Severe combat/operational stress reactions

Physical reactions	Emotional reactions	Behavioral reactions
Constant movement	Severe anxiety or panic	Disorientation
Severe startle response	Grief	Hallucinations
Shaking or trembling	Inability to concentrate	Paranoia or response to internal stimuli
Weakness and paralysis	Nightmares	
Impaired vision, hearing, and touch (loss of sensation)	Self-doubt	Carelessness
	Explosive anger or rage	Hyperalertness
	Excessive concern with minor issues	Lack of motivation
Total exhaustion		Irritability
Immobility	Loss of confidence in self and unit	Lack of initiative
Vacant stares		Constant tearfulness
Acute abdominal pain	Hopelessness	Inability to relax
Impaired speech or muteness		Argumentativeness
Staggering or swaying		
Heart palpitations		
Hyperventilation		
Insomnia or severe sleep disturbance		

combat experience affect one's life over the long term varies greatly. For many service members, the majority of initial symptoms (e.g., anxiety, fear, worry, insomnia) will resolve without the need for ongoing professional attention (Benedek and Rundell 2008). As such, providers must refrain from making a hasty diagnosis of PTSD in individuals presenting for assistance shortly after return home purely on the basis of a history of combat experience. They must ensure that a proper evaluation has been completed before a formal diagnosis is rendered in any medical record. Although there has been limited research regarding the prevalence of symptom embellishment or frank malingering, clinicians must also be aware that service members may present for evaluation in the context of ongoing legal or disciplinary proceedings or in disability evaluations involving potential financial compensation for both physical and psychological symptoms.

Other DSM-5 (American Psychiatric Association 2013) diagnoses that may emerge in the aftermath of combat deployments and in the context of reintegration into civilian life include adjustment disorders (e.g., with anxiety, with depressed mood, or mixed) and acute stress disorder. Although these conditions are also self-limited, other disorders that manifest after combat operations such as a major depressive disorder or PTSD may require more intensive or prolonged treatment. The assessment and management of these potentially more protracted and disabling illnesses are described in the section "Treatment of Postcombat Mental Disorders: Depression and PTSD." Assessment for substance use disorders, including abuse of and dependence on alcohol, illicit drugs, or prescribed medications (e.g., narcotic pain medications), is critical because these conditions, if not addressed, can affect the courses of and recovery from depression, PTSD, or physical injuries sustained in combat. Substance misuse and its treatment are addressed in Chapter 7, "Substance Use Disorders."

Subclinical Distress Reactions

Beyond the diagnostic entities noted above, responses to combat that are experienced after the return home may include the range of subsyndromal changes in behavior, which have been collectively and somewhat loosely termed *distress reactions*. Examples of these reactions are summarized in Table 6–3. Clinicians may be faced not only with managing these reactions but also, most importantly, with educating service members, spouses, or family members about these responses and helping service members and their families recognize when distress symptoms may evolve and require more directed clinical intervention.

TABLE 6–3.   Distress reactions after deployment

Reaction	Summary
Anger	Intensity and duration of modern combat combined with psychological burden provide fertile ground for anger in development.
	Anger serves a valuable role as a coping mechanism during the day-to-day mission requirements in the combat zone.
	Anger can serve as a protective mechanism during combat by providing the physical and psychological drive to sustain service members during patrols and firefights and while dealing with loss and injury of friends and peers.
	On return from deployment many are unable to "turn off" anger that served well in combat.
	At home anger may take the form of • Low tolerance for perceived "stupid actions" of others • Intense self-criticism for failure to perform to one's ability • An overall "intensity" that further isolates from civilian peers
Aggression	Aggression is the outward manifestation of the underlying anger issues above.
	The "burden" of anger may contribute to • Increased suicide rates • A nearly twofold increase in the number of misdemeanors • Traffic infractions • Driving under the influence or while intoxicated • Absent without leave behaviors • An increase in sexual assaults
	Problems have been resistant to education and treatment.

TABLE 6-3.   Distress reactions after deployment *(continued)*

Reaction	Summary
Sleep disturbances	Insomnia and nightmares are among the most common complaints of service members during combat and after returning.

Sleep difficulties are often transient and may resolve without formal treatment as the service member returns to routine responsibilities.

For some, persistent disruption in sleep duration and quality becomes debilitating.

Disturbances may require pharmacological or psychotherapeutic intervention.

Sleep disturbance varies in presentation and intensity but includes
- Nightmares
- Intrusive thoughts delaying sleep onset
- Easy awakening in response to "strange" sounds in one's home
- Difficulty falling asleep in "the deafening silence" of the home environment

Sleep difficulties can
- Exacerbate other COSRs in theater
- Impair social and familial interactions, occupational responsibilities, or other aspects of one's life on return

Management strategies may include
- Educational approaches such as a sleep hygiene regimen
- Psychotherapeutic interventions or pharmacological interventions to target sleep specifically or the symptoms of depression or PTSD

TABLE 6–3.   **Distress reactions after deployment** *(continued)*

Reaction	Summary
Emotional numbing	While in combat, many service members learn to blunt their emotional responses as a means to cope with the traumatic images, experiences, and losses associated with the deployment.
	This is an adaptive response to the rigors of combat and allows the service member to focus on the mission at hand and continue with his or her responsibilities.
	On return to one's family, this once adaptive response is often interpreted as a cold and distant remnant of the service member's personality that existed prior to the deployment.
	In its extreme form, emotional numbing can lower the service member's emotional baseline to a state that is nearly immune to the tears of a spouse or needs of a child.
	In this case, the service member has seen enough suffering and loss in combat that the needs of friends and family members seem irrelevant or complaining compared with the wartime experience in his or her mind.
	The sense of loss within the service member can be either direct loss, which includes a divorce while deployed, or indirect loss, which occurs on return from the deployment when various marital issues lead to separation or divorce.
	Indirect loss often heightens the individual's emotional numbing and continued distancing from the family members and/or the untreated intensity or anger that had been a protective factor while in combat.
	Clinical researchers have shown that this type of secondary trauma is analogous to PTSD symptoms and emphasize the importance of treatment of these subclinical behavioral changes.
	These secondary traumatic symptoms are widely believed to be underreported, underdiagnosed, and undertreated in many treatment settings.

TABLE 6–3.   Distress reactions after deployment *(continued)*

Reaction	Summary
Substance misuse	Individuals often attempt to "self-medicate" the effects of combat stress reactions long before they seek outside support. Alcohol is a readily available and potent means to attempt to drown out one's intrusive thoughts, guilt, anger, etc. Excessive use can lead to • Fights • Inability to function in one's job • DUIs • Other social and occupational complications Alternatives include marijuana, cocaine, "Spice," and amphetamines.
High-risk behaviors	Some service members feel incapable of tolerating "boredom" of civilian life. They may seek the physiological and psychological "high" that comes from the adrenaline rush of combat. This may become "addictive" and manifest as dangerous or illegal activities. In this case, the individual is more likely to engage in • High-speed driving • Extreme sports • Dangerous and/or illegal activities (e.g., provoking assaults)
Impulse control difficulties	Anger and impulsivity are common on redeployment. Some may express discomfort with or unwillingness to be in crowded public areas such as shopping malls, birthday parties, or clubs. Some may feel a need to carry a weapon to "feel safe" in these environments and may discharge weapons after misinterpreting environmental cues.

TABLE 6–3. Distress reactions after deployment *(continued)*

Reaction	Summary

Impulse control difficulties *(continued)*	Precipitants of impulsive behavior may include
	• Hyperstartle or hyperarousal during inappropriate situations in which other individuals are generally not alarmed
	• Memories of traumatic events experienced in combat
	• Hyperstartle reactions are manifested in many ways, commonly seen
	  • As a response to sudden loud noises
	  • When drifting off to sleep
	  • As a persistent sense of danger while in public situations such at restaurants and shopping malls
	  • During celebrations including fireworks
	  • As a response to sudden movements within the perimeter of one's perceived comfort zone (e.g., when a colleague steps into the individual's office without notice)

Social isolation or withdrawal	Withdrawal can manifest in both a physical and a psychological sense. Service members may utilize physical withdrawal as a coping response to the persistent sense of danger in public places that is often experienced with hyperstartle responses. Service members may choose to avoid gatherings in public places and withdraw to the perceived safety of their homes or other locations. In relationships with family members and close friends, service members may use distancing strategies such as rejection, anger, or avoidance to avert a continued sense of loss, abandonment, and rejection by others. In the subclinical arena, these behaviors are often the precursors to depression if not resolved or treated in a clinical context

Anger

The intensity and duration of modern combat operations combined with the psychological burden exacted on the individual provide fertile ground for anger in our combat veterans. As one of the primal emotions for our mammalian brains, anger serves a valuable role as a coping mechanism during the day-to-day mission requirements in the combat zone. It can serve as a protective mechanism during combat by providing the physical and psychological drive to sustain service members during patrols and firefights and while dealing with the loss and injury of friends or peers. On redeployment (return from deployment), many individuals find themselves unable to simply turn off the anger that served them well in combat, which can then manifest in difficulties in their home, job, and personal relationships. These issues can take the form of low tolerance for perceived "stupid actions" of others, intense self-criticism for failure to perform to one's ability, and an overall "intensity" that further isolates service members from the ability to fully reintegrate on return from combat.

Aggression

The outward manifestation of the underlying anger issues discussed in the previous section is aggression. After a decade of active warfare, the true long-term impact on service members has become glaringly obvious. Symptoms of this problem include a steadily rising rate of suicide, a nearly twofold increase in the number of misdemeanors committed by service members (e.g., traffic infractions, driving under the influence, absence without leave), and an increase in sexual assault. These problems have all been resistant to a dedicated effort of education and treatment, likely because they are symptoms of a much more pervasive epidemic of combat stress reactions.

Sleep Disturbance

Insomnia and nightmares are among the most common complaints of service members both in combat and after returning from deployment. Sleep difficulties are often transient and frequently resolve as the service member returns to the more routine responsibilities of "normal" life at home. For others, the common disruption in one's sleep quality can become debilitating if not corrected with professional assistance in the form of pharmacological or psychotherapeutic intervention. Sleep disturbances vary in presentation and intensity but are generally characterized by nightmares, intrusive thoughts, easy awakening in response to "strange" sounds in one's home, or difficulty in transitioning back to what is described as "the deafening silence" of one's home environment on redeployment. Sleep difficulties can exacerbate COSRs in the operational theater and may complicate social and familial interactions, occupational responsibilities, or other aspects of one's life on return. A recent study (Robson 2011) concluded that sleep disorders reported by troops may be a normal result of exposure to combat as opposed to symptoms of PTSD or mild traumatic brain injury (mTBI). For many service members, mild sleep disturbances will subside within days or weeks of redeployment. For symptoms that fail to subside or worsen over time, professional intervention is warranted. Treatment strategies may include educational approaches such as a sleep hygiene regimen, psychotherapeutic interventions, or pharmacological interventions to target sleep specifically or the symptoms of depression or PTSD, which often include sleep disturbance.

Impulse Control Difficulties

Another group of individuals is represented by the lingering anger and impulsivity that are seen in many returning combat troops. This group of individuals often experiences an inability or unwillingness to be in areas of large groups of individuals such as shopping malls, birthday parties, or clubs. In order to retain a sense of safety, an individual may carry a weapon into these environments and utilize the weapon as a means of perceived self-defense when in reality the individual's life is not in danger. He or she is simply experiencing the flashbacks or lingering effects of the trauma and loss experienced in combat. These lingering effects can manifest in many ways, including hyperstartle reactions, emotional numbing, substance misuse, and high-risk behaviors.

Hyperstartle Reaction

Hyperstartle reaction is characterized by the enhanced startle reaction of the individual during inappropriate situations in which other individuals are generally not alarmed. This response may also be accompanied by memories of traumatic events experienced in combat. Hyperstartle reactions can manifest in many ways but are commonly seen as a response to sudden loud noises, when drifting off to sleep, as a persistent sense of danger while in public situations such at restaurants and shopping malls, during celebrations including fireworks, and as a response to sudden movements within the perimeter of one's perceived comfort zone (e.g., when a colleague steps into the individual's office without notice).

Social Isolation and Withdrawal

Social isolation and withdrawal can manifest in both a physical and a psychological sense. Service members may utilize physical withdrawal as a coping response to the persistent sense of danger in public places that is often experienced with hyperstartle responses. Service members may choose to avoid gatherings in public places and withdraw to the perceived safety of their homes or other locations. In relationships with family members and close friends, service members may use distancing strategies such as rejection, anger, or avoidance to avert a continued sense of loss, abandonment, and rejection by others. In the subclinical arena, these behaviors are often the precursors to depression if not resolved or treated in a clinical context.

Emotional Numbing

While in combat, many service members learn to blunt their emotional responses as a means to cope with the traumatic images, experiences, and losses associated with the deployment. This is an adaptive response to the rigors of combat and allows the service member to focus on the mission at hand and continue with his or her responsibilities. On return to one's family, this once adaptive response is often interpreted as a cold and distant remnant of the service member's personality that existed prior to the deployment. In its extreme form, emotional numbing can lower the service member's emotional baseline to such an extent that he or she is nearly immune to the tears of a spouse or needs of a child. In this case, the service member has seen enough suffering and loss in combat that the needs of friends and family members seem irrelevant or complaining compared with the wartime experience in his or her mind. The sense of loss experienced by the service member can be either direct loss, which includes a divorce while deployed, or indirect loss, which occurs on return from the deployment when various marital issues lead to separation or divorce. The latter type of loss often heightens the individual's emotional numbing and continued distancing from the family members and/or the untreated intensity or anger that had been a protective factor while in combat. Clinical researchers have shown that this type of secondary trauma is analogous to PTSD symptoms and emphasize the importance of treatment of these subclinical behavioral changes. These secondary traumatic symptoms are widely believed to be underreported, underdiagnosed, and undertreated in many treatment settings (Coffey et al. 2003; Dansky et al. 1997; Ouimette and Brown 2003).

Substance Misuse

Although substance misuse is discussed in detail in Chapter 7, it is important to note that individuals often attempt to "self-medicate" the effects of combat stress reactions long before they seek outside support. Alcohol is a readily available and potent means to attempt to drown out one's intrusive thoughts, guilt, anger, etc. Excessive use can lead to fights, inability to function in one's job, DUIs, and other social and occupational complications. When alcohol is no longer sufficient to mask the psychological or physical pain, an individual may seek alternative drugs such as marijuana, cocaine, or Spice. This substance misuse perpetuates the cycle and ultimately leads to detrimental effects on the individual and his or her family. When anger issues are combined with drugs, additional types of criminal behavior become more prevalent. This type of behavior can include crimes against people such as robbery, assault, or suicide and other actions that go against the good order and discipline of the Armed Services.

High-Risk Behaviors

Some members of the military return from combat and feel incapable of tolerating the boredom of day-to-day living. They seek the physiological "high" that comes from the daily stress and adrenaline rush of combat. The adrenaline that kept these young men and women alert and alive in combat can become as addictive as any synthetic drug for some service members. In this case, the individual is more likely to perform "extreme" sports and actions, or participate in dangerous or illegal activities (e.g., driving at excessively high speeds, provoking assaults) that serve the individual's need to satiate the desired thrill effect. The fight or flight rush of adrenaline that served to protect this type of service member in combat now serves as an impediment to his or her reintegration.

Postdeployment Mental Disorders and Mild Traumatic Brain Injury

PTSD and the more transient acute stress disorder are distinguished from most other mental disorders in DSM-5 (American Psychiatric Association 2013) by the requirement of a traumatic environmental exposure as part of the diagnostic criteria. Given that military deployment may involve direct involvement in firefights and the witnessing of sudden and unanticipated death, serious injury, or destruction with or without serious physical injury to one's self, it is not surprising that these disorders are often diagnosed along with other medical and behavioral health issues in combat veterans. The DSM-5 criteria for PTSD are described in Box 6–1.

Box 6–1.   DSM-5 Criteria for Posttraumatic Stress Disorder

309.81 (F43.10)

Posttraumatic Stress Disorder

Note: The following criteria apply to adults, adolescents, and children older than 6 years. For children 6 years and younger, see corresponding criteria in DSM-5.

A. Exposure to actual or threatened death, serious injury, or sexual violence in one (or more) of the following ways:

1. Directly experiencing the traumatic event(s).

2. Witnessing, in person, the event(s) as it occurred to others.

3. Learning that the traumatic event(s) occurred to a close family member or close friend. In cases of actual or threatened death of a family member or friend, the event(s) must have been violent or accidental.

4. Experiencing repeated or extreme exposure to aversive details of the traumatic event(s) (e.g., first responders collecting human remains; police officers repeatedly exposed to details of child abuse).

    Note: Criterion A4 does not apply to exposure through electronic media, television, movies, or pictures, unless this exposure is work related.

B. Presence of one (or more) of the following intrusion symptoms associated with the traumatic event(s), beginning after the traumatic event(s) occurred:

1. Recurrent, involuntary, and intrusive distressing memories of the traumatic event(s).

    Note: In children older than 6 years, repetitive play may occur in which themes or aspects of the traumatic event(s) are expressed.

2. Recurrent distressing dreams in which the content and/or affect of the dream are related to the traumatic event(s).

    Note: In children, there may be frightening dreams without recognizable content.

3. Dissociative reactions (e.g., flashbacks) in which the individual feels or acts as if the traumatic event(s) were recurring. (Such reactions may occur on a continuum, with the most extreme expression being a complete loss of awareness of present surroundings.)

    Note: In children, trauma-specific reenactment may occur in play.

4. Intense or prolonged psychological distress at exposure to internal or external cues that symbolize or resemble an aspect of the traumatic event(s).

5. Marked physiological reactions to internal or external cues that symbolize or resemble an aspect of the traumatic event(s).

C. Persistent avoidance of stimuli associated with the traumatic event(s), beginning after the traumatic event(s) occurred, as evidenced by one or both of the following:

1. Avoidance of or efforts to avoid distressing memories, thoughts, or feelings about or closely associated with the traumatic event(s).

2. Avoidance of or efforts to avoid external reminders (people, places, conversations, activities, objects, situations) that arouse distressing memories, thoughts, or feelings about or closely associated with the traumatic event(s).

D. Negative alterations in cognitions and mood associated with the traumatic event(s), beginning or worsening after the traumatic event(s) occurred, as evidenced by two (or more) of the following:

1. Inability to remember an important aspect of the traumatic event(s) (typically due to dissociative amnesia and not to other factors such as head injury, alcohol, or drugs).

2. Persistent and exaggerated negative beliefs or expectations about oneself, others, or the world (e.g., "I am bad," "No one can be trusted," "The world is completely dangerous," "My whole nervous system is permanently ruined").

3. Persistent, distorted cognitions about the cause or consequences of the traumatic event(s) that lead the individual to blame himself/herself or others.

4. Persistent negative emotional state (e.g., fear, horror, anger, guilt, or shame).

5. Markedly diminished interest or participation in significant activities.

6. Feelings of detachment or estrangement from others.

7. Persistent inability to experience positive emotions (e.g., inability to experience happiness, satisfaction, or loving feelings).

E. Marked alterations in arousal and reactivity associated with the traumatic event(s), beginning or worsening after the traumatic event(s) occurred, as evidenced by two (or more) of the following:

1. Irritable behavior and angry outbursts (with little or no provocation) typically expressed as verbal or physical aggression toward people or objects.

2. Reckless or self-destructive behavior.

3. Hypervigilance.

4. Exaggerated startle response.

5. Problems with concentration.

6. Sleep disturbance (e.g., difficulty falling or staying asleep or restless sleep).

F. Duration of the disturbance (Criteria B, C, D, and E) is more than 1 month.

G. The disturbance causes clinically significant distress or impairment in social, occupational, or other important areas of functioning.

H. The disturbance is not attributable to the physiological effects of a substance (e.g., medication, alcohol) or another medical condition.

Specify whether:

With dissociative symptoms: The individual's symptoms meet the criteria for posttraumatic stress disorder, and in addition, in response to the stressor, the individual experiences persistent or recurrent symptoms of either of the following:

1. **Depersonalization:** Persistent or recurrent experiences of feeling detached from, and as if one were an outside observer of, one's mental processes or body (e.g., feeling as though one were in a dream; feeling a sense of unreality of self or body or of time moving slowly).

2. **Derealization:** Persistent or recurrent experiences of unreality of surroundings (e.g., the world around the individual is experienced as unreal, dreamlike, distant, or distorted).

Note: To use this subtype, the dissociative symptoms must not be attributable to the physiological effects of a substance (e.g., blackouts, behavior during alcohol intoxication) or another medical condition (e.g., complex partial seizures).

Specify if:

With delayed expression: If the full diagnostic criteria are not met until at least 6 months after the event (although the onset and expression of some symptoms may be immediate).

PTSD diagnoses often co-occur with other disorders that may have preceded the onset of PTSD or manifested as a concurrent result of exposures to the trauma of combat. Any comorbid diagnosis can co-occur with PTSD, although some are more prevalent in association with this diagnosis. Of particular relevance is the association between PTSD (a mental disorder) and mTBI (a neurological disorder resulting from concussive trauma to the brain). Both PTSD and mTBI are associated with changes in mood (e.g., irritability, anger), behavior (e.g., impulsivity, aggression), and cognition (e.g., difficulties with memory and concentration). Because the physical trauma that can result in mTBI (e.g., resulting from close proximity to an improvised explosive devise or other blast) can most certainly initiate both psychological and physiological stress responses and injury and because the exact neurological mechanisms of mTBI have not been identified, the extent to which symptoms of mTBI represent some components of the stress response of PTSD rather than a distinct pathophysiological response to blast or concussive trauma remains an area of ongoing investigation (Eshel 2007; Lew et al. 2005; U.S. Department of Defense 2006).

Importantly, although PTSD and TBI have been described as the "signature wounds" of the current conflicts in Iraq and Afghanistan, it should be noted that major depressive disorder is highly prevalent in both general and military populations, remains the most prevalent psychiatric diagnosis in the aftermath of such traumatic exposures as natural or man-made disaster, and may be frequently diagnosed in service members both during and after deployment (Fullerton et al. 2004; Ursano et al. 1995). Primary care clinicians and others caring for service members returning from deployment are most likely familiar with the diagnostic criteria for depression (i.e., at least 2 weeks of persistent sadness or irritability accompanied by tearfulness, diminished interest in usually pleasurable activities, decreased concentration and energy, decreased appetite, decreased libido, and inappropriate feelings of guilt that may or may not be accompanied by suicidal thoughts or impaired reality testing). However, while focusing increased attention on the assessment for potential TBI or PTSD, it is important not to overlook this illness as a substantial contributor to postdeployment adjustment difficulty or precipitant of care seeking. (See Chapter 9, "Traumatic Brain Injury," for more information on TBI.)

PTSD and Depression After Combat Deployment: Epidemiology, Assessment, and Treatment

Epidemiology

The numerous studies conducted to estimate the prevalence of PTSD in military personnel during the Iraq and Afghanistan wars have generally shown consistency in rates when similarly exposed populations are studied (e.g., when Army and Marine combat infantry units are compared with one another as opposed to populations of combat support units or units not directly involved in combat). In 2004, Hoge and colleagues found that 3 months after service members returned from high-intensity combat in Iraq, the prevalence of PTSD was 12.9% in soldiers and 12.2% in Marines (Hoge et al. 2004). The prevalence of PTSD in troops deployed to Afghanistan in that time frame (when combat there was less intense) was 6.2% (Terhakopian et al. 2008). However, a study of National Guard brigade combat teams after combat intensified demonstrated a rate of 15% at 3 months postdeployment, which rose to 17%–25% 12 months after return (Thomas et al. 2010). Although general population studies that do not focus specifically on combat units have found lower rates than in high-combat samples, predeployment rates have ranged from 3% to 6%—comparable to civilian rates reported in the National Comorbidity Study (Kessler et al. 2005)—whereas postdeployment rates have ranged from 6% to 20%. As a whole, these studies demonstrate variability in the time course of PTSD symptoms after combat but have consistently found combat intensity and frequency to be the best predictors of postdeployment PTSD.

Assessment and Management of Depression and PTSD for the Individual Patient: Diagnostic Assessment

The U.S. Department of Defense (DOD) has implemented the Post-Deployment Health Assessment/Post-Deployment Health Reassessment (PDHA/PDHRA) Program in an effort to enhance early identification of postdeployment distress reactions; symptoms of TBI; and mental disorders, including depression and PTSD. Although these programs may result in a referral for care, clinicians must be aware that other service members and veterans not identified by the PDHA/PDHRA may present for assistance in a variety of care settings and typically do not identify their complaints of pain or somatic equivalents of anxiety, fatigue, insomnia, or other behavioral changes as symptoms of psychiatric illness. Therefore, it is important that clinicians in both primary care and specialty settings screen their patients for current or prior military service, military deployment, and nature and degree of combat exposure. Although current practice guidelines for management of PTSD recommend screening for military service and combat exposure, it is not clear to what extent these practices have been implemented in civilian behavioral health or primary care treatment facilities. Although a variety of paper and pencil or computer-based screens exist for PTSD (e.g., the Primary Care PTSD Screen, the PTSD Brief Screen, the PTSD Checklist) and depression (the Beck Depression Inventory, the Patient Health Questionnaire-9), the use of any of these instruments as opposed to questions systematically incorporated into the clinician's intake evaluation history is debatable. What is clear is that clinicians must be aware that postdeployment distress reactions, depression, and PTSD result in a significant health burden, so incorporating processes for screening, followed by more thorough diagnostic interviews, will enhance the likelihood of rendering appropriate diagnoses and treatment across a very broad range of postdeployment complaints or concerns.

Treatment of Postcombat Mental Disorders: Depression and PTSD

Major depression, like adjustment disorders and substance use disorders as a consequence of deployment, have been less well studied than has been PTSD. Nonetheless, data indicate that these disorders also occur at higher than average rates in the aftermath of human-caused disasters involving mass violence, including combat (Galea et al. 2002; Kessler et al. 1999; Miguel-Tobal et al. 2006). Major depression, substance use, and adjustment disorders (with anxiety and/or depression) may be relatively common in the 6–12 months after return from deployment and may reflect the returning veteran's struggles with physical injuries and feelings surrounding participation in combat or reflect mental health challenges that existed prior to deployment. The occurrence of these psychiatric disorders may result from such secondary stressors as unemployment or marital discord (Epstein et al. 1998; Vlahov et al. 2002). Major depression and substance abuse (illicit drugs, alcohol, and/or tobacco) are frequently comorbid with PTSD (Davidson and Fairbank 1992; Shalev et al. 1990). Increased substance use that does not constitute abuse or dependence may also be seen and may affect the overall dynamics of postdeployment adjustment through its contribution to motor vehicle accidents, sexual behaviors, or family violence (Fullerton et al. 2004).

The recommendations of various PTSD treatment practice guidelines and consensus statements are summarized in Table 6–4. The American Psychiatric Association's *Practice Guideline for the Treatment of Patients With Acute Stress Disorder and Posttraumatic Stress Disorder* was published in October 2004 (American Psychiatric Association 2004b). Since that time, a number of well-designed randomized controlled trials of pharmacological and psychotherapeutic interventions for PTSD have been conducted in various populations exposed to trauma and have generally augmented the evidence supporting the use of exposure-based psychotherapies as well as selective serotonin reuptake inhibitors (SSRIs) and venlafaxine as first-line agents if medications are to be used (see Table 6–4).

In 2008, the Institute of Medicine (IOM) also reviewed and summarized the evidence supporting treatment for PTSD (Institute of Medicine 2007). The IOM recognized that there is evidence for psychopharmacological treatment of PTSD but believed the evidence base did not meet standards of large randomized controlled trials present in other areas of medicine. The IOM concluded that existing evidence was sufficient only to establish the efficacy of exposure-based psychotherapies in the treatment of PTSD.

The best evidence from recent studies (Management of Post-Traumatic Stress Working Group 2010) bolsters existing support not only for exposure-based psychotherapies but also for pharmacological intervention in many circumstances. Generally, these analyses support the use of some forms of cognitive-behavioral therapy (CBT) and also of pharmacological treatment (usually with selective serotonin reuptake inhibitors [SSRIs] and most recently with venlafaxine). Other antidepressants have received some support, but the efficacy of mood stabilizers, beta blockers, and antipsychotic medications has not been demonstrated.

Similar guidelines have been published summarizing a substantial evidence basis for the treatment of major depression, panic disorder, and substance abuse (American Psychiatric Association 2006). CBT is also a mainstay of depression treatment. Cognitive-behavioral approaches have also been demonstrated in substance abuse and insomnia. Antidepressant medications, particularly the SSRIs, have a substantial evidence basis for their efficacy across the range of mood and anxiety disorders, including PTSD (Craighead et al. 2013). The most recent of these guidelines have also noted that the antihypertensive medication prazosin, although not approved by the U.S. Food and Drug Administration for treatment of PTSD, has been shown to be effective for nightmares and insomnia in the aftermath of trauma exposure including combat-related trauma exposure (Raskind et al. 2003, 2007; Taylor et al. 2008).

Most recently, multidisciplinary experts within the Departments of Defense and Veterans Affairs have collaborated on a systematic review of exist-

TABLE 6–4. PTSD practice guidelines and consensus statements

Guideline	Year	Population	Recommendations
Management of Post-Traumatic Stress Working Group (2010)	2010	Adults (veterans)	Significant benefit: trauma-focused psychotherapy with components of exposure and/or cognitive restructuring; stress inoculation training; SSRIs, SNRIs Some benefit: patient education, imagery rehearsal therapy, psychodynamic therapy, hypnosis, relaxation, group therapy; mirtazapine, TCAs, MAOIs, nefazodone, prazocin (for sleep or nightmares) EMDR (eye movements not critical)
Institute of Medicine (2007)	2007	Adults	First-line treatment: exposure therapies Second-line treatment: EMDR, cognitive restructuring, coping skills, group therapy Insufficient evidence for efficacy of pharmacotherapy
Forbes et al. (2007)	2007	Adults	First line: trauma-focused psychological treatment Second line: SSRIs Third line: mirtazapine, TCAs, phenelzine for treatment-resistant PTSD
National Collaborating Centre for Mental Health (2005)	2005	Adults, children	First line: trauma-focused CBT or EMDR Second line: paroxetine, mirtazapine, amitriptyline, phenelzine, non-trauma-focused psychological interventions

TABLE 6–4.   PTSD practice guidelines and consensus statements *(continued)*

Guideline	Year	Population	Recommendations
Baldwin et al. (2005)	2005	Adults	First line: SSRIs (fluoxetine, paroxetine), amitriptyline, imipramine, phenelzine, mirtazapine, venlafaxine, lamotrigine Trauma-focused individual CBT and EMDR
Swinson et al. (2006)	2005	Adults, children	First line: some SSRIs (fluoxetine, paroxetine, sertraline), venlafaxine XR, CBT Second line: mirtazapine, fluvoxamine, moclobemide, phenelzine
American Psychiatric Association (2004a)	2004	Adults	First line: SSRIs, CBT, EMDR Second line: MAOIs, TCAs, stress inoculation, imagery rehearsal, prolonged exposure

Note.   CBT=cognitive-behavior therapy; EMDR=eye-movement desensitization and reprocessing; MAOIs=monoamine oxidase inhibitors; SNRIs=serotonin-norepinephrine reuptake inhibitors; SRIs=serotonin reuptake inhibitors; SSRIs=selective serotonin reuptake inhibitors; TCAs=tricyclic antidepressants.

ing evidence that has resulted in the development of the *VA/DoD Clinical Practice Guideline for Management of Post-traumatic Stress* (Management of Post-Traumatic Stress Working Group 2010). The guideline, like its predecessors, does not clearly prioritize either pharmacotherapy or psychosocial treatments as being preferential. It suggests that a decision regarding medication versus psychotherapy should be guided by patient choice. This review of existing evidence found SSRIs and serotonin-norepinephrine reuptake inhibitors (SNRIs) to be of "significant benefit," noting that risks and benefits of long-term medication should be discussed with patients before and during treatment and that single-medication dosing should be optimized before additional agents are started. The guideline also identified trauma-focused therapy, including components of exposure and/or cognitive restructuring (e.g., prolonged exposure therapy, cognitive reprocessing therapy), and stress inoculation—a set of coping skills for management of anxiety that includes deep muscle relaxation training, breathing control, positive thinking, thought stopping, and assertiveness—as having "significant benefit." The review noted that eye movement desensitization and reprocessing (EMDR) is an effective treatment, although eye movements are not critical to the effects of EMDR (American Psychiatric Association 2006).

As a group, the existing published guidelines for the treatment of depression and PTSD, which are based on extensive reviews of methodologically sound clinical trials, support cognitive-behavioral approaches and pharmacological treatments of both disorders. SSRIs and SNRIs appear to be effective first-line agents for both PTSD and depression. Unfortunately, specific postdeployment depression studies of these agents or other medications have not been conducted. Because emerging evidence suggests that combat-related PTSD response to existing medications may not be as robust as in civilian trauma (Benedek et al. 2009), caution must be exercised in generalizing predominantly civilian depression studies to military populations.

Conclusions

Although society has long observed (and struggled with) the emotional challenges faced by returning veterans as they reintegrate into civilian life, the past quarter-century has seen much progress in our ability to identify and classify trauma-related psychological responses associated with military combat. Predisposing, exacerbating, and mitigating factors have been identified, and the neurobiology underlying traumatic stress response has become increasingly clarified. A previous and perhaps naively optimistic belief that combat-related distress symptoms were generally transient and self-limited has been replaced with the recognition that psychological response to war exposures occurs across the full spectrum of duration and severity on the basis of characteristics of the exposure and the individual and the nature of the community to which he or she returns.

In the past decade, considerable research has emerged supporting psychotherapeutic and pharmacological approaches to the most prevalent psychiatric disorders occurring in the aftermath of combat, including PTSD and major depressive disorder. Moreover, the important contributions of potential co-occurring disorders to the overall course of these conditions have been clarified, and therapeutic approaches to these comorbidities have been refined. Finally, a heightened recognition of the prevalence of psychological and behavioral consequences to combat exposure has resulted in the implementation of a number of DOD-sponsored public health approaches to identification and prevention, the efficacy of which must still be established. The most recent evaluations of existing treatments for PTSD have suggested that pharmacotherapy for civilian therapy may not be as effective in combat-related PTSD. Although the relative efficacy of existing treatments for civilian versus combat-related depression has not been explored, the findings related to PTSD suggest that exposure to war trauma may provoke a different response than does exposure to physical or sexual assault, motor vehicle accident, or even natural disaster and that further effort must be devoted to the identification of pharmacological and psychotherapeutic treatments for combat-related psychiatric disorders.

SUMMARY POINTS

- The psychological response to combat experience is variable and ranges from transient and subclinical distress symptoms to well-characterized but nevertheless transient or self-limited psychiatric disorders to long-term psychiatric disorders.

- *Combat stress reaction* and *combat/operational stress reaction* are the terms used to describe the wide range of generally transient psychological symptoms that may emerge in response to the stressors of the combat environment.

- Subclinical distress reactions may include anger, aggression, sleep disturbance, impulse control difficulties, hyperstartle reactions, social isolation or withdrawal, emotional numbing, substance misuse, and high-risk behaviors.

- PTSD and depression are disorders that commonly occur in the aftermath of combat exposure and, when present, are best managed with use of established evidence-based treatments.

- Combat-related PTSD may provoke a different response than does exposure to physical or sexual assault, motor vehicle accident, or even natural disaster; therefore, unique pharmacological and psychotherapeutic treatments may be required.

References

American Psychiatric Association: Diagnostic and Statistical Manual of Mental Disorders, 3rd Edition. Washington, DC, American Psychiatric Association, 1980

American Psychiatric Association: Diagnostic and Statistical Manual of Mental Disorders, 5th Edition. Washington, DC, American Psychiatric Association, 2013

American Psychiatric Association: Practice Guideline for the Treatment of Patients with Acute Stress Disorder and Posttraumatic Stress Disorder. Arlington, VA, American Psychiatric Association, 2004a

American Psychiatric Association: Practice guideline for the treatment of patients with schizophrenia, 2nd Edition. Am J Psychiatry 161 (suppl 2):1–56, 2004b

American Psychiatric Association: American Psychiatric Association Practice Guidelines for the Treatment of Psychiatric Disorders: Compendium. Arlington, VA, American Psychiatric Association, 2006

American Psychiatric Association: Diagnostic and Statistical Manual of Mental Disorders, 5th Edition. Arlington, VA, American Psychiatric Association, 2013

Baldwin D, Anderson I, Nutt D, et al: Evidence based guidelines for the pharmacological treatment of anxiety disorders: recommendations from the British Association for Psychopharmacology. J Psychopharmacol 19:567–596, 2005

Benedek DM, Rundell JR: Military psychiatry, in Massachusetts General Hospital Comprehensive Textbook of Psychiatry. Edited by Stern TA, Rosenbaum JF, Fava M, et al. Philadelphia, PA, Moseby, 2008, pp 1207–1213

Benedek DM, Freidman MJ, Zatzick D, et al: Guideline watch (March 2009): Practice Guideline for the Treatment of Patients with Acute Stress Disorder and Posttraumatic Stress Disorder. Arlington, VA, American Psychiatric Association, 2009. Available at: http://www.psychiatryonline.com/content.aspx?aid=156498d. Accessed August 18, 2011. doi:10.1176/appi.books.9780890423479.156498

Coffey SF, Dansky BS, Brady KT: Exposure-based, trauma-focused therapy for comorbid posttraumatic stress disorder–substance use disorder, in Trauma and Substance Abuse: Causes, Consequences, and Treatment of Comorbid Disorders. Edited by Ouimette PC, Brown, PJ. Washington, DC, American Psychological Association, 2003, pp 27–146

Craighead WE, Craighead LW, Ritschel LA, et al: Behavior therapy and cognitive-behavioral therapy, in Handbook of Psychology, 2nd Edition, Vol 8: Clinical Psychology. Hoboken, NJ, Wiley, 2013, pp 291–319

Dansky BS, Roitzsch JC, Brady KT, et al: Posttraumatic stress disorder and substance abuse: use of research in a clinical setting. J Trauma Stress 10(1):141–148, 1997

Davidson JR, Fairbank JA: The epidemiology of posttraumatic stress disorder, in Posttraumatic Stress Disorder: DSM-IV and Beyond. Edited by Davidson JRT, Foa EB. Washington, DC, American Psychiatric Press, 1992, pp 147–169

Epstein RS, Fullerton CS, Ursano RJ: Posttraumatic stress disorder following an air disaster: a prospective study. Am J Psychiatry 155(7):934–938, 1998

Eshel D: IED blast related injuries: the silent killer. Defense Update, May 27, 2007. Available at: http://defense-update.com/analysis/analysis_270507_blast.htm. Accessed September 1, 2013.

Forbes D, Creamer M, Phelps A, et al: Australian guidelines for the treatment of adults with acute stress disorder and post-traumatic stress disorder. Aust NZ J Psychiatry 41:637–648, 2007

Fullerton CS, Ursano RJ, Wang L: Acute stress disorder, posttraumatic stress disorder, and depression in disaster or rescue workers. Am J Psychiatry 161(8):1370–1376, 2004

Gal R, Jones FD: A psychological model of combat stress, in War Psychiatry. Edited by Davis L. Falls Church, VA, Office of the Surgeon General, 1995

Galea S, Ahern J, Resnick H, et al: Psychological sequelae of the September 11 terrorist attacks in New York City. N Engl J Med 346(13):982–987, 2002

Hoge CW, Castro CA, Messer SC, et al: Combat duty in Iraq and Afghanistan, mental health problems, and barriers to care. N Engl J Med 351(1):13–22, 2004

Institute of Medicine: Treatment of PTSD: An Assessment of the Evidence. Washington, DC, National Academies Press, 2007

Kessler RC, Barber C, Birnbaum HG, et al: Depression in the workplace: effects on short-term disability. Health Aff (Millwood) 18(5):163–171, 1999

Kessler RC, Berglund P, Demler O, et al: Lifetime prevalence and age-of-onset distributions of DSM-IV disorders in the National Comorbidity Survey Replication. Arch Gen Psychiatry 62(6):593–602, 2005

Leventman S: Epilogue: social and historical perspectives on the Vietnam veteran, in Stress Disorders Among Vietnam Veterans: Theory, Research and Treatment. Edited by Figley CR. New York, Brunner, 1978, pp 292–295

Lew HL, Poole JH, Alvarez S, et al: Soldiers with occult traumatic brain injury. Am J Phys Med Rehabil 84(6):393–398, 2005

Management of Post-Traumatic Stress Working Group: VA/DoD Clinical Practice Guideline for Management of Post-traumatic Stress, U.S. Department of Veterans Affairs, 2010. Available at: http://www.healthquality.va.gov/ptsd/cpg_PTSD-FULL-201011612.pdf. Accessed September 1, 2013.

Miguel-Tobal JJ, Cano-Vindel A, Gonzalez-Ordi H, et al: PTSD and depression after the Madrid March 11 train bombings. J Trauma Stress 19(1):69–80, 2006

National Collaborating Centre for Mental Health: Posttraumatic Stress Disorder: The Management of PTSD in Adults and Children in Primary and Secondary Care. London, Gaskell, 2005

Ouimette PC, Brown PJ: Epilogue: future directions, in Trauma and Substance Abuse: Causes, Consequences, and Treatment of Comorbid Disorders. Edited by Ouimette PC, Brown, PJ. Washington, DC, American Psychological Association, 2003, pp 243–246

Raskind MA, Peskind ER, Kanter ED, et al: Reduction of nightmares and other PTSD symptoms in combat veterans by prazosin: a placebo-controlled study. Am J Psychiatry 160(2):371–373, 2003

Raskind MA, Peskind ER, Hoff DJ, et al: A parallel group placebo controlled study of prazosin for trauma nightmares and sleep disturbance in combat veterans with post-traumatic stress disorder. Biol Psychiatry 61(8):928–934, 2007

Robson S: Study: sleep disorders normal for post-combat troops. Stars and Stripes, June 10, 2011

Shalev A, Bleich A, Ursano RJ: Posttraumatic stress disorder: somatic comorbidity and effort tolerance. Psychosomatics 31(2):197–203, 1990

Swinson RP, Antony MM, Bleau PB, et al: Clinical practice guidelines: management of anxiety disorders. Can J Psychiatry 51 (suppl 2):1–92, 2006

Taylor FB, Martin P, Thompson C, et al: Prazosin effects on objective sleep measures and clinical symptoms in civilian trauma posttraumatic stress disorder: a placebo-controlled study. Biol Psychiatry 63(6):629–632, 2008

Terhakopian A, Sinaii N, Engel CC, et al: Estimating population prevalence of posttraumatic stress disorder: an example using the PTSD checklist. J Trauma Stress 21(3):290–300, 2008

Thomas JL, Wilk JE, Riviere LA, et al: Prevalence of mental health problems and functional impairment among active component and National Guard soldiers 3 and 12 months following combat in Iraq. Arch Gen Psychiatry 67(6):614–623, 2010

Ursano RJ, Fullerton CS, Kao TC, et al: Longitudinal assessment of posttraumatic stress disorder and depression after exposure to traumatic death. J Nerv Ment Dis 183(1):36–42, 1995

U.S. Department of Defense: Implementation and application of joint medical surveillance for deployments. DoD Instruction Number 6490.3. U.S. Department of Defense, 2006. Available at: http://www.dtic.mil/whs/directives/corres/pdf/649003p.pdf. Accessed September 1, 2013.

Vlahov D, Galea S, Resnick H, et al: Increased use of cigarettes, alcohol, and marijuana among Manhattan, New York, residents after the September 11th terrorist attacks. Am J Epidemiol 155(11):988–996, 2002

Wecter D: When Johnny Comes Marching Home. Cambridge, MA, Houghton Mifflin, 1944

Chapter 7

Substance Use Disorders

Patcho Santiago, M.D., M.P.H., CDR, USN, MC

SUBSTANCE-RELATED and addictive disorders in the military are relatively common. As in the civilian world, substance use problems can have significant negative impact on service members' and veterans' lives, careers, and mission as a whole. These disorders likely impact their own health and occupational outcomes as well as important social, family, and intimate relationships. Substance use disorders complicate the treatment of comorbid physical conditions and psychiatric disorders. The military has special prohibitions against illicit drug use—service members can lose their jobs. In addition, exposure to combat is associated with higher rates of substance use and misuse, and combat veterans report higher rates of substance abuse and dependence compared with civilian populations (Blume et al. 2010; Hoge et al. 2005, 2008). Clinicians must assess substance use as a potential postdeployment health outcome (Larson et al. 2012; Seal et al. 2007). In this chapter we review the epidemiology of and the regulations regarding service members and veterans with substance use disorder and review evaluation and treatment options. For updated DSM-5-related substance use categories (American Psychiatric Association [APA] 2013), see Table 7–1.

Epidemiology

Substance use disorders are chronic, relapsing mental disorders and are common in the military (Bray and Hourani 2007; McLellan et al. 2000). In

TABLE 7-1.   DSM-5 substance-related and addictive disorder categories

Substance-related disorders

A. Alcohol-related disorders

1. Alcohol use disorder[a, b]
   Specify current severity: mild, moderate, or severe

2. Alcohol intoxication
   Specifiers: with use disorder, mild; with use disorder, moderate or severe; without use disorder

3. Alcohol withdrawal[c, d]
   Specify if: with or without perceptual disturbances

4. Other alcohol-induced disorders

5. Unspecified alcohol-related disorder

B. Caffeine-related disorders

1. Caffeine intoxication

2. Caffeine withdrawal

3. Other caffeine-induced disorders

4. Unspecified caffeine-related disorder

C. Cannabis-related disorders

1. Cannabis use disorder[a, b]
   Specify current severity: mild, moderate, or severe

2. Cannabis intoxication[c]
   Specify if: with or without perceptual disturbances
   Specifiers: with use disorder, mild; with use disorder, moderate or severe; without use disorder

3. Cannabis withdrawal[d]

4. Other cannabis-induced disorders

5. Unspecified cannabis-induced disorder

D. Hallucinogen-related disorders

1. Phencyclidine use disorder[a, b]
   Specify current severity: mild, moderate, or severe

2. Other hallucinogen use disorder[a, b]
   Specify the particular hallucinogen
   Specify current severity: mild, moderate, or severe

3. Phencyclidine intoxication
   Specifiers: mild, moderate, severe

TABLE 7–1. **DSM-5 substance-related and addictive disorder categories** *(continued)*

4. Other hallucinogen intoxication
   Specify if: with or without perceptual disturbances
   Specifiers: with use disorder, mild; with use disorder, moderate or severe; without use disorder

5. Hallucinogen persisting perception disorder

6. Other phencyclidine-induced disorders

7. Other hallucinogen-induced disorders

8. Unspecified phencyclidine-induced disorder

9. Unspecified hallucinogen-related disorder

E. **Inhalant-related disorders**

1. Inhalant use disorder[a, b]
   Specify the particular inhalant
   Specify current severity: moderate or severe

2. Inhalant intoxication
   Specifiers: with use disorder, mild; with use disorder, moderate or severe; without use disorder

3. Other inhalant-induced disorders

4. Unspecified inhalant-related disorder

F. **Opioid-related disorders**

1. Opioid use disorder[a]
   Specify if: on maintenance therapy, in a controlled environment
   Specify current severity: mild, moderate, or severe

2. Opioid intoxication[c]
   a. Without perceptual disturbances
      i. *Specifiers:* with use disorder, moderate or severe; without use disorder
   b. With perceptual disturbances
      i. *Specifiers:* with use disorder, mild; with use disorder, moderate or severe; without use disorder

3. Opioid withdrawal[d]

4. Other opioid-induced disorders

5. Unspecified opioid-related disorder

TABLE 7-1.   **DSM-5 substance-related and addictive disorder categories** *(continued)*

G. Sedative-, hypnotic-, or anxiolytic-related disorders

 1. Sedative, hypnotic, or anxiolytic use disorder[a, b]
    Specify current severity: mild, moderate, or severe

 2. Sedative, hypnotic, or anxiolytic intoxication
    Specifiers: with use disorder, mild; with use disorder, moderate or severe; without use disorder

 3. Sedative, hypnotic, or anxiolytic withdrawal[c, d]
    Specify if: with or without perceptual disturbances

 4. Other sedative-, hypnotic-, or anxiolytic-induced disorders

 5. Unspecified sedative-, hypnotic-, or anxiolytic-induced disorder

H. Stimulant-related disorders

 1. Stimulant use disorder[a, b]
    Specify current severity: mild, moderate, or severe
    a. Amphetamine-type substance
    b. Cocaine
    c. Other or unspecified stimulant

 2. Stimulant intoxication[c]
    Specify the specific intoxicant
    a. Amphetamine or other stimulant
       Specify if: with or without perceptual disturbances
       Specifiers: with use disorder, mild; with use disorder, moderate or severe; without use disorder
    b. Cocaine
       Specify if: with or without perceptual disturbances
       Specifiers: with use disorder, mild; with use disorder, moderate or severe; without use disorder

 3. Stimulant withdrawal[d]
    Specify the specific substance causing the withdrawal syndrome
    a. Amphetamine or other stimulant
    b. Cocaine

 4. Other stimulant-induced disorders

 5. Unspecified stimulant-related disorder
    a. Amphetamine or other stimulant
    b. Cocaine

I. Tobacco-related disorders

 1. Tobacco use disorder[a]
    Specify if: on maintenance therapy, in a controlled environment
    Specify current severity: mild, moderate, or severe

TABLE 7–1.   DSM-5 substance-related and addictive disorder categories *(continued)*

   2. Tobacco withdrawal[d]

   3. Other tobacco-induced disorders

   4. Unspecified tobacco-related disorder

J. **Other (or unknown) substance–related disorders**

   1. Other (or unknown) substance use disorder[a, b]
       Specify current severity: mild, moderate, or severe

   2. Other (or unknown) substance intoxication
       Specifiers: with use disorder, mild; with use disorder, moderate or severe; without use disorder

   3. Other (or unknown) substance withdrawal[d]

   4. Other (or unknown) substance-induced disorders

   5. Unspecified other (or unknown) substance-related disorder

Non-substance-related disorders

   1. Gambling disorder[a]
       Specify if: episodic, persistent
       Specify current severity: mild, moderate, or severe

The following specifiers and note apply to substance-related and addictive disorders where indicated:
[a]*Specify* if: in early remission, in sustained remission.
[b]*Specify* if: in a controlled environment.
[c]*Specify* if: with perceptual disturbances.
[d]The ICD-10-CM code indicates the comorbid presence of a moderate or severe substance use disorder, which must be present in order to apply the code for substance withdrawal.

the 2008 U.S. Department of Defense Survey of Health Related Behaviors Among Active Duty Military Personnel, the prevalence of active duty service members using tobacco products was 31%, the prevalence of illicit drug use was 12%, the prevalence of prescription drug misuse was 11%, and the prevalence of heavy alcohol use was 20% (Bray et al. 2010). In 2010, substance use disorders were the seventh most common reason for hospitalization in military treatment facilities (Armed Forces Health Surveillance Center 2011). Another study found that 36% of returning service members were misusing alcohol after returning from deployment (Burnett-Zeigler et al. 2011). The Land Combat Study found that after deployment, the number of soldiers and Marines who responded affirmatively to the question "Have you used more alcohol more than you meant to?" jumped from 17% before deployment to 24%–35% after deployment to Iraq and Afghanistan (Hoge et al. 2004). The Millennium Cohort Study found that returnees from combat deployment engage in binge drinking at a rate of 54%, with a new onset rate of 26% (Jacobson et al. 2008), and that military deployments are associated with higher odds of smoking initiation and smoking recidivism, especially in service members with long or multiple deployments (Smith et al. 2008). The U.S. Department of Veterans Affairs (VA) reported that spending on substance use disorders increased from 2000 to 2007 (Wagner et al. 2011), and substance use is among the highest risk factors for homelessness among veterans (Edens et al. 2011).

In addition, misuse of substances in military and veteran populations reflects the use and misuse in the civilian population. Historically, as use of substances such as alcohol, marijuana, cocaine, and heroin increased in civilian communities, such use increased in military and veteran ones as well (Benjamin et al. 2007; Compton et al. 2007; Moore et al. 2004; Polich 1981; Wallace et al. 2009). Today, as synthetic cannabinoids (e.g., Spice), inhalants, prescription pain killers, methamphetamines, and even over-the-counter synthetic stimulants (e.g., "bath salts") make headlines as being used and misused by increasing numbers of people, their use in military and veteran populations is also observed (Barry et al. 2011; Johnson et al. 2011; Lacy and Ditzler 2007; Lacy et al. 2008; Prosser and Nelson 2012; Rosenbaum et al. 2012).

Tobacco use also deserves increased scrutiny in military and veteran populations. Traditional determinations of use over the patient's lifetime may hide an increase in tobacco use during and immediately following deployment because tobacco use is associated with stress mitigation and increased social contact in combat zones (Widome et al. 2011). Among veterans, nicotine dependence is diagnosed in 15% of patients receiving VA health care services, and tobacco use is disproportionately greater compared with civilian populations (Tsai et al. 2011).

Military Perspectives

Military Regulations on Substance Use

From a military perspective, alcohol, tobacco, and illicit drug use are important issues and can seriously undermine the mission readiness of operational units. As stated in Army Regulation 600–85, "Abuse of alcohol or use of illicit drugs by both military and civilian personnel is inconsistent with Army values, the Warrior Ethos, and standards of performance, discipline, and readiness necessary to accomplish the Army's mission" (U.S. Department of the Army 2009, p. 2). The Navy instruction is clear that

> Military members determined to be using drugs…or who are diagnosed as drug dependent, shall be disciplined as appropriate and processed for ad-

ministrative separation.... Additionally, military members who incur a subsequent alcohol incident after entering a prescribed treatment program (successful completion notwithstanding) precipitated by a prior alcohol incident, shall be disciplined as appropriate, and processed for administrative separation (U.S. Department of the Navy 2011, pp. 2–3).

At the same time, the military is actively engaged in supporting service members with substance use disorders. For example, Army Regulation AR 600–85 (U.S. Department of the Army 2009) requires leaders to promote a command climate that dissuades soldiers from misusing alcohol and drugs with public health prevention interventions and encourages treatment for soldiers with substance use disorders. The Air Force writes specifically, "The Air Force recognizes alcoholism as a primary, chronic disease that affects the entire family. Alcoholism is both preventable and treatable" (Green et al. 2009, p. 197). Service members who are found to have drug or alcohol use disorders are automatically directed by their command to treatment, regardless of whether or not they are likely to be retained on active duty.

Military Treatment Programs

Military drug and alcohol treatment is known by different acronyms, most commonly SARP, the Navy Substance Abuse Rehabilitation Program; ASAP, the Army Substance Abuse Program; and ADAPT, the Air Force Alcohol and Drug Abuse Prevention and Treatment program. It may be useful to ask the patient if he or she has ever attended or been referred to any one of these programs, even if the patient denies a history of alcohol or drug treatment, because he or she may still have been ordered to complete drug and alcohol education after, for example, an alcohol-related incident even if no diagnosis of substance use disorder was found by a provider. After the patient is in the care of a practitioner, care can be coordinated with the patient's command via identified officers known by various acronyms: the Navy command DAPA (Drug and Alcohol Program Advisor), the Air Force ADAPTPM (ADAPT Program Manager), and the Army command ADCO (Alcohol and Drug Control Officer).

Screening and Evaluation

Screening for substance misuse is a critical step for practitioners in all settings and at a minimum can help identify patients who are engaged in such potentially dangerous alcohol-related behaviors as drinking and driving or illicit drug use (Santiago et al. 2010). The National Institute on Alcohol Abuse and Alcoholism clinician's guide recommends that all patients be asked, "Do you sometimes drink beer, wine or other alcoholic beverages?" (U.S. Department of Health and Human Services 2005, p. 4). If the answer is "yes," the patient should complete the Alcohol Use Disorders Identification Test (AUDIT), a 5-minute screening questionnaire (Reinert and Allen 2002). High scores indicate the need to evaluate for alcohol use disorders because negative outcomes are markedly elevated for heavy drinkers in active duty populations (Mattiko et al. 2011). Even subthreshold scores can lead to appropriate alcohol education, which may be particularly important in a military population given the potential for normative attitudes toward excessive drinking (Ames et al. 2007; Benjamin et al. 2007; Poehlman et al. 2011).

Specific instruments to screen for substance dependence have not been validated in military populations, likely because of the career implications under a zero tolerance policy. However, clinicians may wish to examine some existing tools, such as the established Drug Abuse Screening Test (Skinner 1982) or the newer Substance Dependence Screening Questionnaire, which shows some promise to be both sensitive and specific (Vázquez et al. 2007). Additionally, the single-item screening question "How many times in the past year have you used an illegal drug or used a prescription medication for nonmedical reasons?" has been tested in primary care patients (Smith et al. 2010) and may be useful in military populations as well.

Further evaluation must examine more closely reported substance use because such use often is minimized by patients (Morral et al. 2000), and history of other mental disorders may warrant deeper examination of substance use because depression, posttraumatic stress disorder, and anxiety disorders are frequently comorbid with substance use disorders in this population (Skidmore and Roy 2011). The VA recommends in its referral algorithm (VA/DoD Clinical Practice Guideline Working Group 2009, p. 25) obtaining a comprehensive biopsychosocial assessment to "evaluate an individual's strengths, needs, abilities, and preferences, and to determine priorities so that an initial treatment plan can be developed" (Table 7–2).

Treatment

When first approaching a military or veteran patient about the prospect of addressing substance use disorders, a recommended process for clinicians is to establish the first treatment goal of the patient acknowledging and recognizing the problem. The clinician's goal is to increase the patient's motivation to take action. In taking a patient's chief complaint and showing how substance use relates to it, a provider can show a patient what else he or she could anticipate in the future with continued substance use. Regardless of how one attempts to develop a collaborative relationship and build trust, mutual commitment to outcomes is critical (Schuckit 2010). When the cli-

TABLE 7–2. **Elements of a comprehensive biopsychosocial assessment for substance use disorders**

History of the present episode, including precipitating factors, current symptoms, and pertinent present risks:

- Family history:
    - Family alcohol and drug use history, including past treatment episodes
    - Family social history, including profiles of parents (or guardians or other caretakers), home atmosphere, economic status, religious affiliation, cultural influences, leisure activities, monitoring and supervision, and relocations
    - Family medical and psychiatric history
- Developmental history, including pregnancy and delivery, developmental milestones, and temperament
- Comprehensive substance use history, including onset and pattern of progression, past sequelae, and past treatment episodes (including all substances, e.g., alcohol, illicit drugs, tobacco, caffeine, over-the-counter medications, prescription medications, inhalants)
- Nearly all daily nicotine users are nicotine dependent. Identification and treatment of comorbid nicotine dependence may improve recovery rates of other substance use disorders. For patients using nicotine, offer and recommend tobacco use cessation treatment.
- Recent pattern of substance use based on self-report and urine drug screening
- Personal and social history (including housing issues, religious or spiritual affiliation, cultural influences)
- School history
- Military history
- Marital history
- Peer relationships and friendships
- Leisure activities
- Sexual activity
- Physical or sexual abuse
- Legal and nonjudicial punishment history, including past behaviors and their relation to substance use, arrests, adjudications, and details of current status
- Psychiatric history, including symptoms and their relation to substance use, current and past diagnoses, treatments, and providers
- Medical history, including pertinent medical problems and treatment, surgeries, head injuries, present medications, and allergies
- Review of systems, including present and past medical and psychological symptoms

TABLE 7–2.   Elements of a comprehensive biopsychosocial assessment for substance use disorders *(continued)*

Laboratory tests for infectious diseases (HIV, hepatitis C, sexually transmitted disease) and consequences of substance use (e.g., liver function tests)

Mental status examination

Survey of assets, vulnerabilities, and supports

Patient's perspective on current problems, treatment goals, and preferences

Source. Adapted from VA/DoD Clinical Practice Guideline Working Group 2009.

nician develops a positive therapeutic alliance, buy-in about diagnosis and agreement on need for change can overcome concerns that treatment for substance use can derail a military career or negatively affect what benefits a service member receives. Instead, treatment can be seen as enhancing the patient's career and life in total, and the patient can see that readjusting to life without substance misuse can lead to many more opportunities.

Psychotherapy and Web-Based Interventions

There are many psychosocial programs and interventions incorporating individual and group psychotherapies in various structures targeting all sorts of populations that are tested in studies large and small. Military and veteran programs available to any individual patient will vary greatly, and some effort may be needed to locate appropriate psychosocial interventions for patients. Additionally, because of the complexity of learning psychotherapy, we will not attempt to cover either all the available programs or how to conduct psychotherapy. However, it is useful to describe both motivational interviewing and cognitive-behavioral therapy (CBT) because patients are likely to be engaged in programs utilizing these proven techniques, and familiarity with their core concepts will help providers guide their patients' next actions in their own treatment.

The central tenet of CBT is that thoughts, feelings, and behaviors are all intertwined and drive one another rather than an individual being driven by external events in his or her life. The aspect under the most direct conscious control is thoughts, and by having a patient examine his or her own thoughts and how they drive emotion and action, a patient can potentially change how he or she feels and behaves (Craighead et al. 2013). In the context of substance dependence, there are many triggers that promote ongoing substance use, but by examining automatic thoughts in their experience, patients can work to change those automatic thoughts to more accurately reflect a balanced view of the world around them. For example, if a person focuses on the negative aspects of interpersonal interaction, say, with a boss who offers constructive criticism in the workplace, the opportunity for professional growth is overshadowed by thoughts of not having met expectations. This could lead to feelings of failure, which could be a trigger for someone to resume maladaptive behaviors such as binge drinking. By using CBT, practitioners strive to help patients develop the skills to interrupt the automatic thoughts as they occur and to circumvent the development of negative feelings and, consequently, negative behaviors. In veteran populations especially, this psychotherapy has proved useful (Brown et al. 1997; Burling et al. 1994; McCarthy and O'Sullivan 2010).

Motivational interviewing begins with the idea that the motivation for change must begin with the patient rather than being imposed on the patient (Rollnick 2004). Unlike CBT, which is often manualized and can require homework with specific goals and skill sets to develop, motivational interviewing is more stylistic. Its central tenets are to express empathy and minimize resistance. A practitioner's directions for the patient have less to do with telling patients what to do (i.e., telling them to stop using drugs and alcohol) and more about having the patients observe their internal conflict and the contradictions in their behaviors via talking therapy. Then, through introspection of the discrepancy between what the patient wants from his life and what he currently makes his life out to be, he can overcome his ambivalence and make real changes in his behavior (Rollnick 2004).

Online interventions are also available and are varied in their scope, target audience, and availability given their often experimental nature. Results of systematic review are mixed (White et al. 2010), but if a patient is very interested in self-help techniques using these online tools, practitioners should be aware that they may be attractive to patients less likely to engage in traditional substance dependence programs, such as those in the military who are concerned about the impact on their careers, National Guard and Reservists who may have limited access to treatment programs after leaving active duty, and veterans who are not yet motivated for formal treatment (Pemberton et al. 2011). Nonetheless, the Department of Defense and the VA both provide a wealth of information regarding substance use disorder treatment that exists for service members and veterans. On the VA Web site, practitioners can find a substance use disorder program locator (http://www2.va.gov/directory/guide/SUD_flsh.asp?isFlash=1) and smoking and tobacco use cessation program information (http://www.publichealth.va.gov/smoking/) to guide potential patients to local services. Also very useful is the VA's Make the Connection (http://www.maketheconnection.net), where veterans can share their concerns and read the stories of other veterans who have addressed their own mental health challenges. Often, encountering someone with a similar background who has undergone mental health treatment is the most effective means of reducing the stigma associated with seeking behavioral health services (Byrne 1999). For active duty military, access to care is most often coordinated through representatives from their own commands, but each of the service branches has a Web site that also helps guide patients to treatment. For service members who were wounded in a combat zone, case management is available through Wounded Warrior programs (Hudak et al. 2009). Finding meetings for Alcoholics Anonymous or Narcotics Anonymous can be facilitated by visiting http://www.aa.org or http://www.na.org.

Medications

There are a number of medications approved for the treatment of drug, alcohol, and nicotine dependence, although the literature shows wide variation in reports of their efficacy (De Sousa 2010; Lin 2013; Mann 2004; Miller et al. 2011; Stead and Lancaster 2012). None of the medications is automatically disqualifying for ongoing active duty service, but those that are considered "psychotropic" by instruction (e.g., bupropion) would require the patient to be stable on the medication for 3 months before being able to deploy. Regulations attempt to identify "medical conditions usually precluding contingency deployment" and include "chronic medical conditions that require ongoing treatment with antipsychotics, lithium or anticonvulsants" (U.S. Department of Defense 2010, pp. 10–12). Although it appears that the intent of this regulation is to limit service members with psychotic or manic symptoms from deployment, a patient with alcohol dependence but in remission and stable on topiramate would appear to require at least a waiver given the instruction. Regardless, the patient's medical needs should come first, and a discussion with the patient about how substance use treatment would impact deployment readiness should include the information that untreated substance use disorders would preclude deployment because of the likelihood of impaired duty performance while under the routine stressors of a deployed environment (U.S. Department of Defense 2010). Other considerations when deploying a service member on these medications are the safety and feasibility of having the patient deploy with a 180-day supply of the medication, the likelihood that the patient can obtain a refill if required, and the potential for harm to the patient or others should he or she be unable to obtain a refill in the austere conditions possible while deployed (Benedek et al. 2007).

Alcohol Use

Acamprosate

Acamprosate is U.S. Food and Drug Administration approved for the treatment of alcohol dependence and may modulate glutamate neurotransmission at metabotropic 5 glutamate receptors in the nucleus accumbens, which is thought to be responsible for reinforcing drinking behaviors (Harris et al. 2002). The most common side effects include nausea, diarrhea, flatulence, and headache, and although dose dependent, these side effects often resolve with time. In most studies, acamprosate generally shows a modest treatment effect with efficacy similar to naltrexone, and when it is used in combination with naltrexone (see section "Naltrexone") and/or psychosocial interventions, efficacy is improved (Boothby and Doering 2005). However, acamprosate failed as a solo agent in the maintenance of alcohol abstinence in two large double-blind U.S. studies, leaving clinicians to wonder if most of the positive effect comes from concurrent psychotherapeutic interventions (Johnson 2008).

Acamprosate is manufactured as 333-mg delayed-released tablets and prescribed at 666 mg (two tablets) orally three times a day except in cases of renal dysfunction. When the creatinine clearance is between 30 and 50 mL/min, the manufacturer recommends one tablet three times daily, and when the creatinine clearance is below 30 mL/min, acamprosate is contraindicated. Although it is recommended to start after withdrawal ends and abstinence begins, there are no clear guidelines for how long to continue the medication. After a year of monthly checkups, if sobriety has been maintained and a firm plan for ongoing abstinence is in place, consider withdrawing the medication at that time. Often, the medication is continued even during relapse, although repeated relapse is often associated with ongoing nonadherence to any medication regimen (Wright and Myrick 2006).

Naltrexone

Naltrexone is a μ-opioid receptor antagonist with moderate efficacy in the treatment of alcohol dependence, and its mechanism of action is likely related to cortico-mesolimbic dopamine system modulation with decreased dopamine reward. Naltrexone has been shown to reduce the number of heavy drinking days and help to maintain abstinence (Ray et al. 2010) even in a VA population with comorbid depression or anxiety (Krystal et al. 2008).

Oral naltrexone is prescribed at 50 mg/day for alcohol dependence. (It is often started at 25 mg/day for opiate dependence and then increased to 50 mg daily if there are no signs of withdrawal.) For alcohol dependence, outpatient treatment with a scheduled taper of a benzodiazepine can be utilized to promote a period of alcohol abstinence before naltrexone is started. Common side effects include nausea and fatigue. Treatment to promote alcohol abstinence usually continues for at least 2 months. Liver function tests should be monitored regularly because naltrexone has a black box warning for hepatotoxicity; it is more often of concern in patients taking higher than approved doses (i.e., 100 mg/day) (Adi et al. 2007; Garbutt 2010; Soyka and Rösner 2008). Depot naltrexone is also available.

Disulfiram

There is a dearth of literature regarding the use of disulfiram in military populations, with the last publication in 1975 (Rock and Donley 1975), except for a case report of fulminant hepatic failure in a soldier taking disulfiram (Mendenhall 2004). It has been used since 1948 as adjunctive treatment for alcohol dependence through its mechanism of inhibiting aldehyde dehydrogenase in the liver. After alcohol consumption, serum acetaldehye levels rise and lead to vomiting, diaphoresis, dizziness, nausea, headache, and anxiety. Possible side effects include dermatitis, muscle weakness, fatigue, depression, and decreased libido. Hepatotoxicity is rare and more likely in those with previous hepatic disease (Wright and Moore 1990). One VA study pointed to continued heavy drinking as the true cause of liver toxicity and not disulfiram, which had poor medication adherence in their study population (Iber et al. 1987). Disulfiram is typically dosed between 250 and 500 mg orally per day and requires a patient with significant motivation to change his or her drinking behaviors as well as substantial investment with other treatment interventions such as Alcoholics Anonymous and individual and group psychotherapy (Jørgensen et al. 2011; Krampe and Ehrenreich 2010).

Topiramate

Topiramate is a GABAergic anticonvulsant that has been shown to be effective in the treatment of alcohol dependence to maintain remission and may even have better performance than naltrexone (Baltieri et al. 2008; Flórez et al. 2011; Kenna et al. 2009; Paparrigopoulos et al. 2011). It acts at the nonbenzodiazepine site on the γ-aminobutyric acid (GABA) type A receptor and is associated with improvement in obesity, liver disease, and elevated cholesterol that alcoholics often experience (Ait-Daoud et al. 2006; Shinn and Greenfield 2010). Topiramate is started at 25 mg/day orally and increased every week for 8 weeks to a dose of 150 mg twice a day. Side effects include poor concentration and memory, psychomotor retardation, paresthesia, anorexia, and taste changes, although it is generally well tolerated. If patients cannot tolerate a higher dose, the medication may still be effective at doses as low as 50 mg twice a day and can continue for 1 year to promote ongoing abstinence (Johnson 2008). Topiramate also has been shown to be useful in the maintenance of abstinence in methamphetamine use disorder (Elkashef et al. 2012) and may be useful in the treatment of cocaine use disorder, although sample sizes in those studies have been small (Shinn and Greenfield 2010).

Nicotine Use

Nicotine Replacement Therapies

Nicotine replacement using gum, transdermal patch, nasal spray, inhaler, and sublingual tablets has been shown to have mild to moderate efficacy in promoting nicotine abstinence. Although rates of smoking cessation improve by 50%–70%, even without additional psychotherapeutic or psychosocial interventions, overall quit rates hover around 7% in most studies, with few individuals successfully quitting tobacco at their first attempt (Stead et al. 2012). Of note, combined use of the nicotine patch and gum may improve smoking cessation rates, although such a tactic is not common (Kornitzer et al. 1995). Practitioners should note that military and VA patients seldom have to pay out of pocket for treatment and that tobacco control managers are often present at military bases and VA hospitals (Hamlett-Berry et al. 2009; Jahnke et al. 2010; VA/DoD Clinical Practice Guideline Working Group 2004).

Bupropion (Zyban)

Bupropion is an atypical antidepressant, likely a norepinephrine-dopamine reuptake inhibitor, that is often used to promote smoking cessation. Compared with placebo, some studies found it doubles smoking cessation rates. The sustained release preparation is generally started at 150 mg/day for 3–7 days and then increased to 150 mg daily for 3 months or longer. It is generally safe and well tolerated, with the most common side effects being dry mouth, insomnia, and headache (Hurt et al. 1997). Like varenicline (described in the next section), it carries a black box warning for serious behavioral symptoms, including suicidal ideation, suicide attempt, hostility, depression, and agitation. However, the data are not sufficient to conclude true elevated risk of self-harm using bupropion, and other plausible mechanisms for the association between smoking cessation and suicide exist (Hughes 2008). In addition, bupropion has shown some efficacy in reducing methamphetamine use among mild abusers (Elkashef et al. 2008; Karila et al. 2010).

Varenicline (Chantix)

Varenicline is a partial nicotinic acetylcholine receptor agonist found to effectively promote smoking cessation (Cahill et al. 2012). It is thought to stimulate enough dopamine release to reduce nicotine craving and withdrawal while blocking the further release of dopamine by preventing nicotine binding (Mihalak et al. 2006). It is typically started at 0.5 mg/day for 3 days and then increased to 0.5 mg twice daily for another 3–4 days and then 1 mg twice daily. Dosing is reduced to 0.5 mg/day or twice daily for patients with renal dysfunction (Gonzales et al. 2006). Although common side effects, including nausea, headache, insomnia, and disturbing dreams are tolerable, there is a black box warning regarding suicidal ideation and hostility.

Conclusions

The negative consequences of substance-related and addictive disorders on our service members and veterans affect all aspects of their lives, from their social relationships to their work performance to their physical and mental health. Early identification and intervention can reduce the morbidity and mortality associated with substance use disorders and other comorbid mental disorders. Early engagement and retention of patients in treatment can greatly improve outcomes, from reduction in relapse to increase in quality of life.

SUMMARY POINTS

- Substance use problems can have significant negative impact on service members' and veterans' lives, careers, and mission as a whole.
- Screening for substance misuse is a critical step for practitioners in all settings and can help identify patients who are engaged in potentially dangerous alcohol or illicit drug use.
- Motivational interviewing and cognitive-behavioral therapy are proven techniques that can be effectively utilized in substance use treatment programs.
- Certain medications may have a role in supporting comprehensive substance use treatment plans, including acamprosate, naltrexone, disulfiram, topiramate, nicotine replacement therapies, bupropion, and varenicline.

References

Adi Y, Juarez-Garcia A, Wang D, et al: Oral naltrexone as a treatment for relapse prevention in formerly opioid-dependent drug users: a systematic review and economic evaluation. Health Technol Assess 11(6):iii–iv, 1–85, 2007

Ait-Daoud N, Malcolm RJ Jr, Johnson BA: An overview of medications for the treatment of alcohol withdrawal and alcohol dependence with an emphasis on the use of older and newer anticonvulsants. Addict Behav 31(9):1628–1649, 2006

American Psychiatric Association: Diagnostic and Statistical Manual of Mental Disorders, 5th Edition. Arlington, VA, American Psychiatric Association, 2013

Ames GM, Cunradi CB, Moore RS, et al: Military culture and drinking behavior among U.S. Navy careerists. J Stud Alcohol Drugs 68(3):336–344, 2007

Armed Forces Health Surveillance Center: Hospitalizations among members of the active component, U.S. Armed Forces, 2010. MSMR 18(4):8–15, 2011

Baltieri DA, Daró FR, Ribeiro PL, et al: Comparing topiramate with naltrexone in the treatment of alcohol dependence. Addiction 103(12):2035–2044, 2008

Barry DT, Goulet JL, Kerns RK, et al: Nonmedical use of prescription opioids and pain in veterans with and without HIV. Pain 152(5):1133–1138, 2011

Benedek DM, Schneider BJ, Bradley JC: Psychiatric medications for deployment: an update. Mil Med 172(7):681–685, 2007

Benjamin KL, Bell NS, Hollander IE: A historical look at alcohol abuse trends in Army and civilian populations, 1980–1995. Mil Med 172(9):950–955, 2007

Blume AW, Schmaling KB, Russell ML: Stress and alcohol use among soldiers assessed at mobilization and demobilization. Mil Med 175(6):400–404, 2010

Boothby LA, Doering PL: Acamprosate for the treatment of alcohol dependence. Clin Ther 27(6):695–714, 2005

Bray RM, Hourani LL: Substance use trends among active duty military personnel: findings from the United States Department of Defense Health Related Behavior Surveys, 1980–2005. Addiction 102(7):1092–1101, 2007

Bray RM, Pemberton MR, Lane ME, et al: Substance use and mental health trends among U.S. military active duty personnel: key findings from the 2008 DoD Health Behavior Survey. Mil Med 175(6):390–399, 2010

Brown RA, Evans DM, Miller IW, et al: Cognitive-behavioral treatment for depression in alcoholism. J Consult Clin Psychol 65(5):715–726, 1997

Burling TA, Seidner AL, Salvio MA, et al: A cognitive-behavioral therapeutic community for substance dependent and homeless veterans: treatment outcome. Addict Behav 19(6):621–629, 1994

Burnett-Zeigler I, Ilgen M, Valenstein M, et al: Prevalence and correlates of alcohol misuse among returning Afghanistan and Iraq veterans. Addict Behav 36(8):801–806, 2011

Byrne P: Stigma of mental illness: changing minds, changing behaviour. Br J Psychiatry 174:1–2, 1999

Cahill K, Stead LF, Lancaster T: Nicotine receptor partial agonists for smoking cessation. Cochrane Database of Systematic Reviews 2012, Issue 4. Art. No.: CD006103. DOI: 10.1002/14651858.CD006103.pub6

Craighead WE, Craighead LW, Ritschel LA, et al: Behavior therapy and cognitive-behavioral therapy, in Handbook of Psychology, 2nd Edition, Vol 8: Clinical Psychology. Hoboken, NJ, Wiley, 2013, pp 291–319

Compton WM, Thomas YF, Stinson FS, et al: Prevalence, correlates, disability, and comorbidity of DSM-IV drug abuse and dependence in the United States: results from the national epidemiologic survey on alcohol and related conditions. Arch Gen Psychiatry 64(5):566–576, 2007

De Sousa A: The pharmacotherapy of alcohol dependence: a state of the art review. Mens Sana Monogr 8(1):69–82, 2010 doi:10.4103/0973-1229.58820

Edens EL, Kasprow W, Tsai J, et al: Association of substance use and VA service-connected disability benefits with risk of homelessness among veterans. Am J Addict 20(5):412–419, 2011

Elkashef AM, Rawson RA, Anderson AL, et al: Bupropion for the treatment of methamphetamine dependence. Neuropsychopharmacology 33(5):1162–1170, 2008

Elkashef A, Kahn R, Yu E, et al: Topiramate for the treatment of methamphetamine addiction: a multi-center placebo-controlled trial. Addiction 107(7):1297–1306, 2012 [abstract corrected in Addiction 197(9):1718, 2012]

Flórez G, Saiz PA, García-Portilla P, et al: Topiramate for the treatment of alcohol dependence: comparison with naltrexone. Eur Addict Res 17(1):29–36, 2011

Garbutt JC: Efficacy and tolerability of naltrexone in the management of alcohol dependence. Curr Pharm Des 16(19):2091–2097, 2010

Gonzales D, Rennard SI, Nides M, et al: Varenicline, an alpha4beta2 nicotinic ace-tylcholine receptor partial agonist, vs sustained-release bupropion and placebo for smoking cessation: a randomized controlled trial. JAMA 296(1):47–55, 2006

Green KW, Oakley RD, Herrera CM (eds): The military commander and the law. U.S. Air Force, 2009. Available at: http://www.afjag.af.mil/shared/media/document/AFD-091026-025.pdf. Accessed April 3, 2012.

Hamlett-Berry K, Davison J, Kivlahan DR, et al: Evidence-based national initia-tives to address tobacco use as a public health priority in the Veterans Health Administration. Mil Med 174(1):29–34, 2009

Harris BR, Prendergast MA, Gibson DA, et al: Acamprosate inhibits the binding and neurotoxic effects of trans-ACPD, suggesting a novel site of action at metabotropic glutamate receptors. Alcohol Clin Exp Res 26(12):1779–1793, 2002

Hoge CW, Castro CA, Messer SC, et al: Combat duty in Iraq and Afghanistan, mental health problems, and barriers to care. N Engl J Med 351(1):13–22, 2004

Hoge CW, Toboni HE, Messer SC, et al: The occupational burden of mental dis-orders in the U.S. military: psychiatric hospitalizations, involuntary separa-tions, and disability. Am J Psychiatry 162(3):585–591, 2005

Hoge CW, Castro CA, Messer CS, et al: Combat duty in Iraq and Afghanistan, mental health problems and barriers to care. US Army Med Dep J (Jul–Sep)7–17, 2008

Hudak RP, Morrison C, Carstensen M, et al: The U.S. Army Wounded Warrior Program (AW2): a case study in designing a nonmedical case management pro-gram for severely wounded, injured, and ill service members and their families. Mil Med 174(6):566–571, 2009

Hughes JR: Smoking and suicide: a brief overview. Drug Alcohol Depend 98(3):169–178, 2008

Hurt RD, Sachs DP, Glover ED, et al: A comparison of sustained-release bupropion and placebo for smoking cessation. N Engl J Med 337(17):1195–1202, 1997

Iber FL, Lee K, Lacoursiere R, Fuller R: Liver toxicity encountered in the Veterans Administration trial of disulfiram in alcoholics. Alcohol Clin Exp Res 11(3):301–304, 1987

Jacobson IG, Ryan MA, Hooper TI, et al: Alcohol use and alcohol-related problems before and after military combat deployment. JAMA 300(6):663–675, 2008

Jahnke SA, Haddock CK, Poston WS, et al: A qualitative analysis of the tobacco control climate in the U.S. military. Nicotine Tob Res 12(2):88–95, 2010

Johnson BA: Update on neuropharmacological treatments for alcoholism: scientific basis and clinical findings. Biochem Pharmacol 75(1):34–56, 2008

Johnson LA, Johnson RL, Alfonzo C: Spice: a legal marijuana equivalent. Mil Med 176(6):718–720, 2011

Jørgensen CH, Pedersen B, Tønnesen H: The efficacy of disulfiram for the treat-ment of alcohol use disorder. Alcohol Clin Exp Res 35(10):1749–1758, 2011 doi:10.1111/j.1530-0277.2011.01523.x

Karila L, Weinstein A, Aubin HJ, et al: Pharmacological approaches to metham-phetamine dependence: a focused review. Br J Clin Pharmacol 69(6):578–592, 2010

Kenna GA, Lomastro TL, Schiesl A, et al: Review of topiramate: an antiepileptic for the treatment of alcohol dependence. Curr Drug Abuse Rev 2(2):135–142, 2009

Kornitzer M, Boutsen M, Dramaix M, et al: Combined use of nicotine patch and gum in smoking cessation: a placebo-controlled clinical trial. Prev Med 24(1):41–47, 1995

Krampe H, Ehrenreich H: Supervised disulfiram as adjunct to psychotherapy in alcoholism treatment. Curr Pharm Des 16(19):2076–2090, 2010

Krystal JH, Gueorguieva R, Cramer J, et al: Naltrexone is associated with reduced drinking by alcohol dependent patients receiving antidepressants for mood and anxiety symptoms: results from VA Cooperative Study No. 425, "Naltrexone in the treatment of alcoholism." Alcohol Clin Exp Res 32(1):85–91, 2008

Lacy BW, Ditzler TF: Inhalant abuse in the military: an unrecognized threat. Mil Med 172(4):388–392, 2007

Lacy BW, Ditzler TF, Wilson RS, et al: Regional methamphetamine use among U.S. Army personnel stationed in the continental United States and Hawaii: a six-year retrospective study (2000–2005). Mil Med 173(4):353–358, 2008

Larson MJ, Wooten NR, Adams RS, et al: Military combat deployments and substance use: review and future directions. J Soc Work Pract Addict 12(1):6–27, 2012

Lin SK: Pharmacological means of reducing human drug dependence: a selective and narrative review of the clinical literature. Br J Clin Pharmacol May 23, 2013 [Epub ahead of print] doi:10.1111/bcp.12163

Mann K: Pharmacotherapy of alcohol dependence: a review of the clinical data. CNS Drugs 18(8):485–504, 2004

Mattiko MJ, Olmsted KL, Brown JM, et al: Alcohol use and negative consequences among active duty military personnel. Addict Behav 36(6):608–614, 2011

McCarthy PM, O'Sullivan D: Efficacy of a brief cognitive behavioral therapy program to reduce excessive drinking behavior among new recruits entering the Irish Navy: a pilot evaluation. Mil Med 175(11):841–846, 2010

McLellan AT, Lewis DC, O'Brien CP, et al: Drug dependence, a chronic medical illness: implications for treatment, insurance, and outcomes evaluation. JAMA 284(13):1689–1695, 2000

Mendenhall M: Disulfiram-induced fulminant hepatic failure in an active duty soldier. Mil Med 169(8):671–672, 2004

Mihalak KB, Carroll FI, Luetje CW: Varenicline is a partial agonist at alpha4beta2 and a full agonist at alpha7 neuronal nicotinic receptors. Mol Pharmacol 70(3):801–805, 2006

Miller PM, Book SW, Stewart SH: Medical treatment of alcohol dependence: a systematic review. Int J Psychiatry Med 42(3):227–266, 2011

Moore RS, Cunradi CB, Ames GM: Did substance use change after September 11th? An analysis of a military cohort. Mil Med 169(10):829–832, 2004

Morral AR, McCaffrey D, Iguchi MY: Hardcore drug users claim to be occasional users: drug use frequency underreporting. Drug Alcohol Depend 57(3):193–202, 2000

Paparrigopoulos T, Tzavellas E, Karaiskos D, et al: Treatment of alcohol dependence with low-dose topiramate: an open-label controlled study. BMC Psychiatry 11:41, 2011

Pemberton MR, Williams J, Herman-Stahl M, et al: Evaluation of two Web-based alcohol interventions in the U.S. military. J Stud Alcohol Drugs 72(3):480–489, 2011

Poehlman JA, Schwerin MJ, Pemberton MR, et al: Socio-cultural factors that foster use and abuse of alcohol among a sample of enlisted personnel at four Navy and Marine Corps installations. Mil Med 176(4):397–401, 2011

Polich JM: Epidemiology of alcohol abuse in military and civilian populations. Am J Public Health 71(10):1125–1132, 1981

Prosser JM, Nelson LS: The toxicology of bath salts: a review of synthetic cathinones. J Med Toxicol 8(1):33–42, 2012

Ray LA, Chin PF, Miotto K: Naltrexone for the treatment of alcoholism: clinical findings, mechanisms of action, and pharmacogenetics. CNS Neurol Disord Drug Targets 9(1):13–22, 2010

Reinert DF, Allen JP: The Alcohol Use Disorders Identification Test (AUDIT): a review of recent research. Alcohol Clin Exp Res 26(2):272–279, 2002

Rock NL, Donley PJ: Treatment program for military personnel with alcohol problems, part II: the program. Int J Addict 10(3):467–480, 1975

Rollnick SJA: Motivational interviewing, in The Essential Handbook of Treatment and Prevention of Alcohol Problems. Edited by Heather N, Stockwell T. West Sussex, UK, Wiley, 2004, pp 105–115

Rosenbaum CD, Carreiro SP, Babu KM: Here today, gone tomorrow…and back again? A review of herbal marijuana alternatives (K2, Spice), synthetic cathinones (bath salts), kratom, Salvia divinorum, methoxetamine, and piperazines. J Med Toxicol 8(1):15–32, 2012

Santiago PN, Wilk JE, Milliken CS, et al: Screening for alcohol misuse and alcohol-related behaviors among combat veterans. Psychiatr Serv 61(6):575–581, 2010

Schuckit MA: Drug and Alcohol Abuse: A Clinical Guide to Diagnosis and Treatment. New York, Springer, 2010

Seal KH, Bertenthal D, Miner CR, et al: Bringing the war back home: mental health disorders among 103,788 US veterans returning from Iraq and Afghanistan seen at Department of Veterans Affairs facilities. Arch Intern Med 167(5):476–482, 2007

Shinn AK, Greenfield SF: Topiramate in the treatment of substance-related disorders: a critical review of the literature. J Clin Psychiatry 71(5):634–648, 2010

Skidmore WC, Roy M: Practical considerations for addressing substance use disorders in veterans and service members. Soc Work Health Care 50(1):85–107, 2011

Skinner HA: The drug abuse screening test. Addict Behav 7(4):363–371, 1982

Smith B, Ryan MA, Wingard DL, et al: Cigarette smoking and military deployment: a prospective evaluation. Am J Prev Med 35(6):539–546, 2008

Smith PC, Schmidt SM, Allensworth-Davies D, et al: A single-question screening test for drug use in primary care. Arch Intern Med 170(13):1155–1160, 2010

Soyka M, Rösner S: Opioid antagonists for pharmacological treatment of alcohol dependence: a critical review. Curr Drug Abuse Rev 1(3):280–291, 2008

Stead L, Lancaster T: Combined pharmacotherapy and behavioural interventions for smoking cessation. J Evid Based Med 5(4):242, 2012 doi:10.1111/jebm.12012

Stead LF, Perera R, Bullen C, et al: Nicotine replacement therapy for smoking cessation. Cochrane Database of Systematic Reviews 2012, Issue 11. Art. No.: CD000146. DOI: 10.1002/14651858.CD000146.pub4

Tsai J, Edens EL, Rosenheck RA: Nicotine dependence and its risk factors among users of veterans health services, 2008–2009. Prev Chronic Dis 8(6):1–12, 2011

U.S. Department of Defense: Deployment-limiting medical conditions for service members and DoD civilian employees. Instruction No. 6490.07. U.S. Department of Defense, 2010. Available at: http://www.dtic.mil/whs/directives/corres/pdf/649007p.pdf. Accessed February 23, 2012.

U.S. Department of Health and Human Services: Helping patients who drink too much: a clinician's guide. Bethesda, MD, National Institute on Alcohol Abuse and Alcoholism, 2005. Available at: http://pubs.niaaa.nih.gov/publications/Practitioner/CliniciansGuide2005/guide.pdf. Accessed March 1, 2012.

U.S. Department of the Army: The Army Substance Abuse Program Headquarters Rapid Action Revision (RAR). Army Regulation 600–85. Washington, DC, U.S. Department of the Army, 2009. Available at: www.army.mil/usapa/epubs/pdf/r600_85.pdf. Accessed February 23, 2012.

U.S. Department of the Navy: Military substance abuse prevention and control. SECNAV Instruction 5300.28E. Washington, DC, U.S. Department of the Navy, 2011. Available at: http://doni.daps.dla.mil/Directives/05000%20General%20Management%20Security%20and%20Safety%20Services/05-300%20Manpower%20Personnel%20Support/5300.28E.pdf. Accessed February 23, 2012.

VA/DoD Clinical Practice Guideline Working Group: Management of tobacco use. Office of Quality and Performance Publication 10Q-CPG/TUC-04. Washington, DC, Veterans Health Administration, Department of Veterans Affairs and Health Affairs, U.S. Department of Defense, 2004

VA/DoD Clinical Practice Guideline Working Group: Management of substance use disorder (SUD). Washington, DC, Veterans Health Administration, U.S. Department of Veterans Affairs, 2009

Vázquez FL, Blanco V, López M: Performance of a new substance dependence screening questionnaire (SDSQ) in a non-clinical population. Addict Behav 32(5):1082–1087, 2007

Wagner TH, Sinnott P, Siroka AM: Mental health and substance use disorder spending in the Department of Veterans Affairs, fiscal years 2000–2007. Psychiatr Serv 62(4):389–395, 2011

Wallace AE, Sheehan EP, Young-Xu Y: Women, alcohol, and the military: cultural changes and reductions in later alcohol problems among female veterans. J Womens Health (Larchmt) 18(9):1347–1353, 2009

White A, Kavanagh D, Stallman H, et al: Online alcohol interventions: a systematic review. J Med Internet Res 12(5):e62, 2010

Widome R, Joseph AM, Polusny MA, et al: Talking to Iraq and Afghanistan war veterans about tobacco use. Nicotine Tob Res 13(7):623–626, 2011

Wright C, Moore RD: Disulfiram treatment of alcoholism. Am J Med 88(6):647–655, 1990

Wright TM, Myrick H: Acamprosate: a new tool in the battle against alcohol dependence. Neuropsychiatr Dis Treat 2(4):445–453, 2006

Chapter 8

Care of Combat-Injured Service Members

Harold Wain, Ph.D.
Robert M. Perito Jr., M.D.

COMBAT INJURY has a profound effect on military service members, impacting their psychological and physical functioning as well as their interpersonal lives. During the acute phase of medical care, treatment is often complicated by delirium, pain, and sleep deprivation as well as iatrogenic issues such as drug interactions and nosocomial infections. Further complications may arise as a result of traumatic brain injuries (TBIs) and can present unique challenges for clinicians and patients. In this chapter we review the physical and psychological sequelae of severe combat injury and the unique challenges of working with patients who have been injured in a combat theater, as well as the important psychotherapeutic and psychopharmacological approaches that serve to support recovery in the short term and over time.

Combat Injuries

Since the start of the wars in Iraq and Afghanistan, more than 47,000 men and women have been injured in theater (http://icasualties.org, accessed December 30, 2012). Advances in medical practices have increased the rates of injury survival (Gawande 2004), resulting in many more survivors of severe and complex injuries requiring months to years of medical treatment. The most common causes of physical injuries are related to blasts and improvised explosive devices (Ramsamy et al. 2008; Beckett et al. 2012). Injuries include TBIs, amputations, genital injuries, musculoskeletal injuries, spinal cord and nerve injuries, multi-organ trauma, and burns, as well as facial, ocular, and other disfiguring injuries. Clinicians must anticipate the potential for significant psychological consequences from these injuries and the events surrounding them.

Psychological Consequences of Combat Injury

Morgan et al. (2001) stated that nearly all survivors exposed to traumatic events briefly exhibit one or more stress-related symptoms. In many instances these symptoms dissipate within a reasonable period of time. O'Donnell et al. (2004) reported that 20%–40% of patients followed 1 year after trauma met criteria for a psychiatric disorder. Koren et al. (2005) reported rates of posttraumatic stress disorder (PTSD) 15 months postinjury that were more than five times higher (16.7% versus 2.5%) in their combat-injured Israeli soldier population when compared with similarly combat-exposed noninjured soldiers. Given high rates of reported PTSD in noninjured combat veterans (Hoge et al. 2004), it is reasonable to conclude that injury increases the risk of psychiatric disorders above the exposure to combat alone, making it an imperative to monitor the injured as an at-risk population.

Factors Impacting Recovery

Social and Family Relationships

Access to resources and psychological support from clinicians, family members, and the greater community (both military and civilian) are essential to facilitating injury recovery. Frierson and Lippmann (1987) described social isolation as a common occurrence after amputation that can complicate recovery and needs to be actively monitored and addressed as part of routine clinical care. In the same vein, social discomfort and body image anxiety may need to be worked through with appropriate support and therapy (Horgan and MacLachlan 2004). It is not uncommon for severely injured service members to believe that their injury has left them less than human, in which case they may avoid social settings or lose opportunities for community support. In the case of comorbid PTSD, patients may be further burdened by social isolation and avoidance that can limit interpersonal connectedness and negatively impact treatment outcomes, especially as they move from the hospital to the community setting.

Delirium, Pain, and Sleep Deprivation

The acute phase following injury and the early course of recovery are often marked by circumstances that can adversely impact recovery and must be targeted for treatment, specifically, delirium, pain, and sleep deprivation. Pain is a multifaceted experience with emotional, cognitive, autonomic, and neuroendocrine aspects. Increased sympathetic outflow associated with pain may play a role in increasing or perpetuating neurophysiological changes associated with extremes of stress. The problem of controlling pain in patients suffering from catastrophic injuries leads to aggressive efforts beginning soon after injury. Unmanaged pain has been shown to contribute to the development or worsening of posttraumatic outcomes, and therefore behavioral health clinicians must ensure that medical-surgical colleagues are adequately addressing pain management.

Similarly, sleep can be highly compromised in the acute care and intensive care settings, often worsened by pain, delirium, or environmental stimuli. Posttraumatic symptoms can further disrupt sleep. Clinicians must recognize that prolonged and serious disruptions to sleep can undermine patient recovery and may often go unnoticed by medical-surgical treatment teams. Effective sleep management likely requires a combination of environmental strategies as well as pharmacotherapy. The psychopharmacology of delirium, pain, and sleep is further described in the section "Pharmacological Intervention."

Psychological Defenses in Response to Trauma

Recognizing the important role that psychological defenses play in helping injured service members maintain a state of equilibrium is an indispensable part of any evaluation and informs treatment approaches. Misdirected interventions that rapidly break down psychological defenses can create distress that complicates treatment. Some of the more common defense mechanisms in the combat injured include dissociation, regression, intellectualization, rationalization, and denial. Avoidance may also be a problematic coping strategy and may correlate with increased rates of PTSD. Dissociation may occur during or subsequent to trauma and serves to distance the service member from the impact of the trauma but may ultimately lead to poorer outcome. Regression occurs when a person temporarily reverts to an earlier stage of psychological development in the face of significant stress. As the psyche attempts to cope with the medical and psychological trauma, premorbid maladaptive personality traits may become more prominent and be impediments in recovery. However, the diagnosis of a personality disorder is inappropriate in the initial phases of recovery.

Interventions That Facilitate Recovery

In a study examining PTSD and depression symptoms in combat-injured soldiers, 80% of soldiers who met disorder threshold criteria 7 months after injury met criteria for neither disorder at initial assessment (Grieger et al. 2006). These findings, in conjunction with previously cited literature, suggest the importance of careful clinical attention to the injured population. Wain (1979, 1993) and colleagues (Wain et al. 2002, 2006) have written previously about successful strategies when working with this population that emphasize a preventive approach to care. Critical to these efforts is developing the therapeutic alliance, addressing stigma, and using empathic exposure strategies as well as other traditional approaches such as hypnosis and cognitive-behavioral strategies (see Table 8–1).

Developing the Alliance

The development of a therapeutic relationship with the injured patient is essential to both short-term and long-term clinical effectiveness. As a positive therapeutic alliance develops, the patient becomes more open to discussing complex issues, fears, and concerns about the future. This occurs only by "meeting the patients where they are" and utilizing a flexible and personalized evaluation and treatment approach. Patience is advised rather than rushing to gather data and making a diagnosis. In addition, it is best to focus initially on patient assets and strengths; reinforcing these characteristics facilitates the development of the therapeutic alliance and the beginning of treatment. To further support the therapeutic alliance, behavioral health clinicians can act as patient advocates and serve as liaisons with families and medical and support staff, addressing immediate needs in a timely manner.

Addressing Stigma

In an effort to decrease the stigma associated with mental illness, the preventive medical psychiatry (PMP) approach was developed to address the psychological needs of trauma victims, provide support to the individuals and their families, assess psychiatric status, provide early intervention when needed without stigmatization of the patient. As an adjunct to the program, support is also provided to the medical and surgical staff and support personnel. The major components of the PMP approach are as follows: making mental health a routine

TABLE 8–1. Intervention strategies with combat injured

Therapeutic alliance

Empathic exposure

Reinforcing ego strengths

Supportive therapy

Hypnosis-relaxation

Pharmacology

Cognitive reframing

Enhancing the patient's engagement in medical treatment

Reducing psychological distress

Increasing ability to cope with pain

Improving coping skills

Increasing autonomy and self-efficacy

Facilitating adaptation to injuries

Supporting the patient's ability to engage social supports

Facilitating the resolution of external conflicts

Bolstering self-esteem

part of trauma care, utilizing a biopsychosocial approach, developing a strong therapeutic alliance with the patient and family, normalization of the experience and the psychological response to the trauma, education, pharmacology, hypnosis, providing empathic exposure therapy, treating any psychiatric symptoms, reinforcing resilience, education, and promoting positive coping behaviors (Wain 1979, 1993; Wain et al. 2002, 2006). Traditional psychotherapeutic and psychodynamic concepts are also employed.

Use of Empathic Exposure

Empathic exposure allows for the normalization of the event and consolidation of the experience in the patient's memory and may help the service member integrate the past trauma into a normal stream of consciousness. Providers are taught to offer rapid caring empathic responses to patients as they recall their injury and associated trauma. As they continue to relate their trauma and become more aware of their experience, empathic reinforcing statements are made about their psychological assets, and positive behaviors displayed during the patient's narrative of traumatic events. Comments that identify and reinforce positive assets that emerge during the patient's narrative are interjected: "Where did you learn to do that?" or "How did you have the presence of mind to put on the tourniquet?" Nonthreatening techniques are employed and confrontational approaches are avoided. Acceptance, respect, empathy, warmth, advice, praise, affirmation, and a sense of hope are qualities and characteristics the clinician is encouraged to display while working with these patients. It is critical that providers are viewed as genuine in their concern and support of the patient while offering empathic validation and encouraging patients to elaborate on reactions relevant to the trauma.

Hypnosis

Hypnosis is a helpful tool that can capitalize on the healthy human capacity for dissociation. Components of hypnosis include absorption in a task, focused attention, decreased vigilance, openness to suggestion, dissociation, trance logic, rapid assimilation of data, and time distortion, all of which can be helpful to the combat-injured service member (Wain 1993). Hypnotic techniques (hypnoanalgesia, relaxation, imagery, and reframing) that guide constructive thought processes help individuals to cope with pain, insomnia, and injuries. These techniques allow patients to master or distance themselves from their treatment, feel safe, rapidly learn new coping techniques, and become productively engaged in the healing process (Beshai 2004; Patterson and Jensen 2003; Spiegel and Spiegel 1980; Wain 1979). In general, hypnotic techniques used judiciously as part of the psychotherapeutic approach to trauma can also help reintegrate compartmentalized experiences into the normal stream of consciousness.

Cognitive-Behavioral Techniques

Cognitive-behavioral therapy (CBT) provides powerful tools, and many CBT techniques translate well into the supportive framework. CBT interventions are generally aimed at identifying patterns of distortion and helping patients to assert healthier patterns of automatic thoughts. Because many combat-injured service members have complex and conflicting thoughts related to the experiences that led to their injuries, CBT can be very useful. These interventions can assist in changing the conceptual framework within which the patients understand themselves and their experiences, and this may allow for a healthier interpretation of their experience and a reduction in distress (Craighead et al. 2013).

Psychopharmacological Intervention

Medication management is a critical element in the effective treatment of combat-injured service members. Successful prescribing requires a broad biopsychosocial understanding of the case while recognizing appropriate targets for medication effect. Injuries and their sequelae are often complex and extensive, and multiple providers are typically involved in their care. Polypharmacy is commonplace and can become counterproductive and potentially dangerous at times. Collaborating within the larger medical care team, the behavioral health prescriber must review all prescribed medications, monitor for pharmacokinetic and pharmacodynamic medication interactions, evaluate for side effects, and streamline the psychotropic regimen where possible. All clinicians must be mindful of the abuse potential of many medications prescribed to the combat-injured population, especially over time.

Pain Management

Pain is a multifaceted experience that includes physical, emotional, cognitive, autonomic, and neuroendocrine aspects. Increased sympathetic outflow associated with pain may play a role in increasing or perpetuating neurophysiologic changes associated with extremes of stress. The effective management of pain can be challenging but is critical to combat injury recovery. One retrospective study identified a possible correlation between administration of morphine in the immediate period following injury and lower rates of screening positive for PTSD (Holbrook et al. 2010). Similarly, ketamine administration during debridement in patients in a military burn treatment center was associated with a lower relative risk of screening positive for PTSD (McGhee et al. 2008).

Opioids

In polytrauma patients, very high doses of opioids are often used for extended periods, and as a result, some of the subtler pharmacodynamic effects may become significant. Though these effects are better studied in animal models, it is not uncommon to see idiosyncratic reactions to opioids, such as hyperalgesia, and in extreme cases agitation and psychosis (Chen et al. 2009; Chu et al. 2008; King et al. 2005; Silverman 2009; van Dorp et al. 2009). More frequently, myoclonic jerks can be observed in patients on high-dose opioids, especially in the sleep-wake transition, and are particularly troublesome for patients with multiple injuries where limb movement causes pain. This can be remedied by reduction of the opioid. When that is not practicable, the movements can often be treated with $\alpha_2\delta$ ligands or benzodiazepines (Jiménez-Jiménez et al. 2004).

Opiates have drug-drug interactions impacting serotonin levels that are worthy of note. For example, tramadol hydrochloride is a significant serotonin and norepinephrine reuptake inhibitor and can interact with other pro-serotonergic medications. Tramadol is a prodrug whose active metabolite O-desmethyltramadol has activity at the µ-opioid receptor. It can have both pharmacodynamic and pharmacokinetic interactions with psychotropic medications. Duloxetine, a CYP450 2D6 inhibitor, can slow metabolism of the tramadol to the active form, resulting in decreased efficacy, and the increase in serotonin from tramadol and duloxetine can lead to serotonin-related side effects and, in worst case, to serotonin syndrome (Meyer and Maurer 2011; Smith 2009). Synthetic opioids (but not opiates or semisynthetics) are weak serotonin uptake inhibitors (Ables and Nagubilli 2010; Dvir and Smallwood 2008; Rastogi et al. 2011) and at higher doses, in overdose, or in combination with other pro-serotonergic medications can lead to excessive serotonergic activity.

Antidepressants in Pain Treatment

Antidepressant medications are often started by primary care providers, pain specialists, physiatrists, and orthopedic surgeons. Although tricyclic antidepressants (TCAs), duloxetine, venlafaxine, and perhaps milnacipran may be effective in ameliorating pain, evidence demonstrates comparatively little benefit from serotonin-specific reuptake inhibitors (Barkin and Fawcett 2000; Bellingham and Peng 2010; McCleane 2008; Saarto and Wiffen 2007; Smith and Nicholson 2007; Verdu et al. 2008). There is evidence for use of TCAs and serotonin-norepinephrine reuptake inhibitors in treatment of chronic neuropathic pain, but evidence for treatment of acute pain and pain due to traumatic nerve injury is lacking.

In the setting of polytrauma, where patients are often receiving serial surgeries, which may include repeated incision and debridement, revision of amputations, or skin grafts, clinicians must consider the impact that serotonin-blocking agents may have on platelet function. Studies have demonstrated an increased risk (relative risk as high as 3.7; Movig et al. 2003) of receiving a transfusion while on a serotonin uptake–blocking medication in the perisurgical period for orthopedic surgeries (Looper 2007; Movig et al. 2003). Risk increases significantly with coadministration of nonsteroidal anti-inflammatory drugs or COX-2 inhibitors. When used alone, medications that block serotonin uptake appear to be safe in general; however, other medications such as enoxaparin or warfarin are used as prophylaxis against venous thrombosis or in treatment of pulmonary embolism as part of standard practice in polytrauma patients, and platelet counts may be low because of consumption in clotting.

Other important effects of antidepressants, particularly while patients are acutely ill, are the potential of syndrome of inappropriate antidiuretic hormone secretion leading to hyponatremia and medication interactions leading to serotonin syndrome (see the section "Opioids") (Jacob and Spinler 2006; Looper 2007; Mago et al. 2008). Because all antidepressant medications bear the U.S. Food and Drug Administration's black box warning for increased suicidality in patients under 24 years old, young service members and their families should be warned about this potential risk.

The $\alpha_2\delta$ Ligands

Another area of overlap between psychotropics and augmenting agents for the treatment of pain are the $\alpha_2\delta$ ligands, including pregabalin and gabapentin. Frequently, these medications are used to address neuropathic and central pain, including phantom pain (Kroenke et al. 2009). Although gabapentin appears to have only mild efficacy in treating anxiety, pregabalin has robust effects. Studies demonstrate efficacy in the treatment of generalized anxiety disorder, and in Europe, the medication is used in treatment of generalized anxiety disorder and social phobia (Feltner et al. 2008; Mula et al. 2007; Rickels et al. 2005; Van Ameringen et al. 2004; Wensel et al. 2012). In patients demonstrating anxiety who are suffering with neuropathic pain, it may be worthwhile switching to or initiating treatment with pregabalin. Anecdotally, pregabalin does not appear to help in acute anxiety states such as a panic attack or flashback. It may, however, lower the background level of anxiety.

Benzodiazepines

Benzodiazepines are frequently started by providers outside of the behavioral health field to address patient distress, anxiety, sleep, or other problems. In the case of severe orthopedic injuries or polytrauma, diazepam and other benzodiazepines may be used as muscle relaxants and are also frequently used for the treatment of neuropathic pain and phantom limb pain (Bartusch et al. 1996; Malchow and Black 2008; Tremont-Lukats et al. 2000). These medications can have unintended effects. One of the primary drawbacks of the use of benzodiazepines in hospitalized combat-injured patients is their potential to precipitate or exacerbate delirium in the setting of significant medical compromise, TBI, and polypharmacy. Although rare, disinhibition may produce paradoxical agitation or emotional dysregulation, particularly in patients with brain injury (Hall and Zisook 1981; Nielsen et al. 2011).

Pharmacological Interventions for Sleep Problems

Sleep problems are common among hospitalized patients as well as warriors returning from combat, who fly across multiple time zones to U.S. hospitals. Although hospital procedures and the stimulating hospital environment (intensive care units) can initially contribute to sleep disruption, the discomfort from patients' injuries often continues to make sleep difficult. Sleep disruption may occur as part of delirium, TBI, or combat-related stress disorders or as a result of the persistent hyperaroused state many service members experience as part of their adaptation to living in a combat zone or dealing with combat-related stress disorders.

Sedative-Hypnotics

There are several good medications to address problems related to sleep. For uncomplicated insomnia (not related to delirium or caused by awakening from nightmares) benzodiazepine-like sedative-hypnotics are good choices. With its rapid onset and short half-life, zolpidem is a well-tolerated and attractive option to address early insomnia, and a controlled release formulation of zolpidem is available. Eszopiclone has a slightly longer half-life and may be helpful in cases where mid sleep cycle awakening is a problem or if treatment with zolpidem does not help the patient sleep for a sufficient period of time. Drawbacks of this class of medications include tolerance and potential for addiction. These medications may also cause parasomnias or promote dissociative experiences and can worsen nightmares, making them a poor choice for a patient with nightmares, acute stress disorder, or PTSD (Monti and Pandi-Perumal 2007; Toner et al. 2000).

Sedating Antidepressants

The antidepressants trazodone and mirtazapine may be attractive sleep-enhancing agents in the combat-injured population. There is little potential for addiction, and patients may be less likely to develop habituation. The medications are less likely to precipitate delirium, and there is no association with increased nightmares or dissociative experiences. The most common problem with both of these medications is the "hangover effect" of excessive morning somnolence and weight gain associated with mirtazapine. Mirtazapine can prove difficult to manage for patients whose physical activity may be limited by confinement to bed or a wheelchair. Fluctuation in weight can create significant setbacks or delay progress in those phases of rehabilitation in which the fitting of a prosthetic and effort required to ambulate are key factors.

Psychopharmacology for Nightmares

Presently, there are two medication strategies to address nightmares: second-generation antipsychotic agents (SGAs) and prazosin, an α_1 adrenergic receptor antagonist. The choice of which type of medication to use is dictated by the clinical situation and other ongoing medical problems.

Prazosin has been shown to reduce combat-related nightmares in most studies, demonstrating effects at bedtime doses between 3 and 12 mg (Daly et al. 2005; Taylor et al. 2008; Thompson et al. 2008). Titrating the medication dose over several days reduces risk of orthostasis. In general, prazosin is better tolerated than SGAs, and in a retrospective study comparing prazosin with quetiapine it was found to have significantly lower rates of discontinuation due to side effects (Byers et al. 2010).

In low bedtime doses (from 25 to 200 mg) quetiapine works well to treat nightmares, in our experience. It may also be a good choice in patients whose nightmares are related to delirium, patients who are vulnerable to developing delirium (Ahearn et al. 2011; Ipser and Stein 2012; Rowe 2007), or patients whose nightmares are related to side effects of other medications, such as opioids. However, in general, because of the deleterious side effects, SGAs should be considered a short-term intervention and may be better suited to the inpatient setting.

Other Medications for Sleep

Antihistamines may be useful medications to assist with sleep, but they have several drawbacks. Patients on multiple medications often develop problematic anticholinergic side effects. Urinary hesitancy or urinary retention, especially in patients with urogenital injury or urethral stricture from traumatic catheterization, can lead to serious problems. Constipation is always an issue with the use of opioids and can be worsened by the addition of medications with high anticholinergic activity.

Delirium

Delirium is common in the early phase of injury recovery, particularly in the ICU (Burns et al. 2004). Although delirium is easily identified when it manifests with psychomotor agitation, it may be missed when it is of the "quiet" or mixed motoric subtypes (Maldonado 2008; Meagher et al. 2008). Delirium is the manifestation of end organ (brain) dysfunction and indicates an ongoing underlying medical process. Often, proximate causes will be apparent, as in the case of infection with increased white blood count and fever. In other cases, however, the underlying cause may be less clear, as with medication interactions, and in polytrauma patients, delirium is likely to be multifactorial. Delirium is independently associated with poorer outcomes (e.g., increased mortality, increased hospital stay, increased time on a ventilator, cognitive deficits) (Ely et al. 2004; Lin et al. 2004; Pandharipande et al. 2005; Rockwood et al. 1999; Thomason and Ely 2004; van Zyl and Seitz 2006). Delirium can be extremely distressing for patients and their families. For patients the experiences of distorted reality associated with this state can be traumatic events in their own right (Breitbart et al. 2002; Griffiths and Jones 2007). The definitive treatment for delirium requires identifying and correcting the underlying medical cause. Antipsychotic medications are the mainstay of the medical management of delirium. The specific antipsychotic agent should be selected to address acuity of symptoms with consideration given to its side effect profile (Eisendrath and Shim 2006).

First-Generation Antipsychotics

In acute states of agitation driven by delirium, especially where the patient is at risk for harming himself or herself or staff, intravenous (IV) formulations may be required. Substantial evidence exists for the use of haloperidol in the treatment of delirium (Bienvenu et al. 2012; Milbrandt et al. 2005; Wang et al. 2012). However, the U.S. Food and Drug Administration has issued a statement regarding the risk associated with the use of IV haloperidol, and this route of administration should be carefully considered (Meyer-Massetti et al. 2010). All antipsychotics should be used with caution in medically compromised patients, and adverse cardiac effects (including torsades de pointes), along with other side effects of antipsychotics, are cause for concern among medically ill patients.

Second-Generation Antipsychotics

If IV access is not available and the patient requires medication as needed to deal with acute agitation, several immediate-release SGAs are available at this time for intramuscular administration, including aripiprazole, olanzapine, and ziprasidone. In less acute situations, delirium can often be managed with oral SGAs, usually at low to moderate doses (Chaput and Bryson 2012; Steiner 2011). Selection of a useful SGA can be guided by effects and side effects of the specific agent. Some of the SGAs come in rapidly dissolving forms such as Zyprexa Zydis, Risperdal M-Tab, and Abilify Discmelt. These formulations may be associated with more rapid onset because they are already in solution when they reach the stomach. They are also difficult to spit out and impossible to "cheek."

Benzodiazepines

In delirium, benzodiazepines, benzo-like sedative-hypnotics, and medications with high anticholinergic side effects should be avoided whenever possible because of their propensity to disinhibit behavior or impair cognition. Benzodiazepines can play a role in treating agitation associated with delirium when used in conjunction with antipsychotics, though this strategy should be employed with some caution. The exception to this rule is delirium associated with withdrawal from pro-GABAergic substances such as alcohol, benzodiazepines, barbiturates, or γ-hydroxybutyrate (GHB), for which benzodiazepines are the treatment of choice (Clegg and Young 2011; Hughes et al. 2012).

Pharmacological Intervention With Traumatic Brain Injury

Prescribing physicians must be aware of the unique challenges of using medications in TBI and anoxic brain injury patients. For example, studies have shown that in animal models of TBI, administration of haloperidol is associated with delayed recovery of function. The theoretical explanation for this effect is that dopamine is essential for neuronal recovery (Arciniegas et al. 2008; Hoffman et al. 2008; Kline et al. 2008). Although definitive research is lacking with human subjects, these findings suggest that high-potency antipsychotics, particularly first-generation antipsychotics, should be used sparingly in patients recovering from brain injury (Arciniegas et al. 2008; Elovic et al. 2008). When an antipsychotic medication is necessary, an SGA may be a better choice. Other medications should also be prescribed cautiously. Benzodiazepines and benzo-like sedative-hypnotics should be used with care in patients with brain injury because of the potential for delayed recovery or cognitive and motor impairment and the possibility of paradoxical disinhibition (Flanagan et al. 2007). An additional effect of brain injury is fatigue, and TBI patients often tire quickly, simply from hospital routine, making it difficult for them to engage in physical and occupational therapy. Stimulant medications such as methylphenidate or amphetamine-based psychostimulants or wake-promoting agents such as modafinil or armodafinil can help alleviate this problem (Chew and Zafonte 2009; Liepert 2008; Shoumitro and Crownshaw 2004). These medications should be avoided in patients who are delirious or psychotic because they can exacerbate symptoms of psychosis.

Ongoing Care

Combat-injured service members and veterans are confronted with many challenges as they transition from the hospital to the outpatient setting. After discharge, they are faced with returning home, moving to new communities, engaging new health care providers, and/or reestablishing existing relationships with growing awareness of the challenges their injuries impose. In circumstances where combat stress disorders, including PTSD, are present, patients may face greater challenges in dealing with symptoms as they move into a world that is more chaotic and stimulating than the safety of the hospital setting. Anger may evolve and lead to unanticipated conflicts in the marital relationship, with other family members, or with good friends. In an attempt to soothe themselves, patients and family members may resort to alcohol and drugs. Systems of care can best address these potential complications by developing positive and proactive engagement of mental health services with patients and families early in the hospitalization.

Conclusions

Combat injuries result in multifaceted physical and psychological sequelae, requiring complex and coordinated medical, surgical, and psychiatric care. Mental health services are best provided as an integrated part of the multidisciplinary, multiservice package of care and include psychoeducation, empathic exposure, cognitive reframing, and hypnosis or relaxation techniques as well as pharmacotherapy. The goal of the preventive medical psychiatry (PMP) approach is to actively engage all combat-injured patients simply as a matter or course, thus reducing stigma while developing a therapeutic alliance with and providing empathic exposure therapy to injured service members. Pharmacotherapy is used in conjunction with a variety of adjunctive treatments, and frequent contact with families, the treatment team, nursing staff, and command is maintained. Because combat-injured patients have complex medical-surgical problems, greater attention must be paid to polypharmacy and adverse effects. Complex medical and psychological sequelae are likely to require ongoing care, highlighting the importance of active and positive engagement with mental health as well as careful attention to transitions in care (see Chapter 4, "Military Health Care System and the U.S. Department of Veterans Affairs").

SUMMARY POINTS

- Combat injury has a profound effect on military service members, impacting their psychological and physical functioning as well as their interpersonal lives.
- Injury likely increases the risk of psychiatric disorders above the exposure to combat alone, making it imperative to monitor the injured as an at-risk population.
- Access to resources and psychological support from clinicians, family members, and the greater community (both military and civilian) are essential to facilitating injury recovery.
- The development of a therapeutic relationship with the injured patient is essential to both short-term and long-term clinical effectiveness.
- Effective psychopharmacology is a critical contributor to treatment outcomes in combat-injured service members.
- Unmanaged pain has been shown to contribute to the development or worsening of posttraumatic outcomes and therefore must be adequately addressed by medical-surgical teams.

References

Ables AZ, Nagubilli R: Prevention, recognition, and management of serotonin syndrome. Am Fam Physician 81(9):1139–1142, 2010

Ahearn EP, Juergens T, Cordes T, et al: A review of atypical antipsychotic medications for posttraumatic stress disorder. Int Clin Psychopharmacol 26(4):193–200, 2011

Arciniegas DB, Silver JM, McAllister TW: Stimulants and acetylcholinesterase inhibitors for the treatment of cognitive impairment after traumatic brain injury. Psychopharm Review 43(12):91–97, 2008

Barkin RL, Fawcett J: The management challenges of chronic pain: the role of antidepressants. Am J Ther 7(1):31–47, 2000

Bartusch SL, Sanders BJ, D'Alessio JG, et al: Clonazepam for the treatment of lancinating phantom limb pain. Clin J Pain 12(1):59–62, 1996

Beckett A, Pelletier P, Mamczak C, et al: Multidisciplinary trauma team care in Kandahar, Afghanistan: current injury patterns and care practices. Injury 43(12):2072–2077, 2012

Bellingham GA, Peng PWH: Duloxetine: a review of its pharmacology and use in chronic pain management. Reg Anesth Pain Med 35(3):294–303, 2010

Beshai JA: Toward a phenomenology of trance logic in posttraumatic stress disorder. Psychol Rep 94(2):649–654, 2004

Bienvenu OJ, Neufeld KJ, Needham DM: Treatment of four psychiatric emergencies in the intensive care unit. Crit Care Med 40(9):2662–2670, 2012

Breitbart W, Gibson C, Tremblay A: The delirium experience: delirium recall and delirium-related distress in hospitalized patients with cancer, their spouses/caregivers, and their nurses. Psychosomatics 43(3):183–194, 2002

Burns A, Gallagley A, Byrne J: Delirium. J Neurol Neurosurg Psychiatry 75(3):362–367, 2004

Byers MG, Allison KM, Wendel CS, et al: Prazosin versus quetiapine for nighttime posttraumatic stress disorder symptoms in veterans: an assessment of long-term comparative effectiveness and safety. J Clin Psychopharmacol 30(3):225–229, 2010

Chaput AJ, Bryson GL: Postoperative delirium: risk factors and management: continuing professional development. Can J Anaesth 59(3):304–320, 2012

Chen L, Malarick C, Seefeld L, et al: Altered quantitative sensory testing outcome in subjects with opioid therapy. Pain 143:65–70, 2009

Chew E, Zafonte RD: Pharmacological management of neurobehavioral disorders following traumatic brain injury: a state-of-the-art review. J Rehabil Res Dev 46(6):851–879, 2009

Chu LF, Angst MS, Clark D: Opioid-induced hyperalgesia in humans: molecular mechanisms and clinical considerations. Clin J Pain 24(6):479–496, 2008

Clegg A, Young JB: Which medications to avoid in people at risk of delirium: a systematic review. Age Ageing 40(1):23–29, 2011

Craighead WE, Craighead LW, Ritschel LA, et al: Behavior therapy and cognitive-behavioral therapy, in Handbook of Psychology, 2nd Edition, Vol 8: Clinical Psychology. Hoboken, NJ, Wiley, 2013, pp 291–319

Daly CM, Doyle ME, Radkind M, et al: Clinical case series: the use of prazosin for combat-related recurrent nightmares among Operation Iraqi Freedom combat veterans. Mil Med 170(6):513–515, 2005

Dvir Y, Smallwood P: Serotonin syndrome: a complex but easily avoidable condition. Gen Hosp Psychiatry 30(3):284–287, 2008

Eisendrath SJ, Shim JJ: Management of psychiatric problems in critically ill patients. Am J Med 119(1):22–29, 2006

Elovic EP, Jasey NN Jr, Eisenberg ME: The use of atypical antipsychotics after traumatic brain injury. J Head Trauma Rehabil 23(2):132–135, 2008

Ely EW, Shintani A, Truman B, et al: Delirium as a predictor of mortality in mechanically ventilated patients in the intensive care unit. JAMA 291(14):1753–1762, 2004

Feltner D, Wittchen HU, Kavoussi R, et al: Long-term efficacy of pregabalin in generalized anxiety disorder. Int Clin Psychopharmacol 23(1):18–28, 2008

Flanagan SR, Greenwald B, Wieber S: Pharmacological treatment of insomnia for individuals with brain injury. J Head Trauma Rehabil 22(1):67–70, 2007

Frierson RL, Lippmann SB: Psychiatric consultation for acute amputees. Report of a ten-year experience. Psychosomatics 28(4):183–189, 1987

Gawande A: Casualties of war—military care for the wounded from Iraq and Afghanistan. N Engl J Med 351(24):2471–2475, 2004 doi:10.1056/NEJMp048317

Grieger TA, Cozza SJ, Ursano RJ, et al: Posttraumatic stress disorder and depression in battle-injured soldiers. Am J Psychiatry 163:1777–1783, 2006

Griffiths RD, Jones C: Delirium, cognitive dysfunction and posttraumatic stress disorder. Curr Opin Anaesthesiol 20(2):124–129, 2007

Hall RCW, Zisook S: Paradoxical reactions to benzodiazepines. Br J Clin Pharmacol 11:99S–104S, 1981

Hoffman AN, Cheng JP, Zafonte RD, et al: Administration of haloperidol and risperidone after neurobehavioral testing hinders the recovery of traumatic brain injury-induced deficits. Life Sci 83(17–18):602–607, 2008

Hoge CW, Castro CA, Messer SC, et al: Combat duty in Iraq and Afghanistan, mental health problems, and barriers to care. N Engl J Med 351(1):13–22, 2004

Holbrook TL, Galarneau MR, Dye JL, et al: Morphine use after combat injury in Iraq and post-traumatic stress disorder. N Engl J Med 362(2):110–117, 2010

Horgan O, MacLachlan M: Psychosocial adjustment to lower-limb amputation: a review. Disabil Rehabil 26(14–15):837–850, 2004

Hughes CG, Patel MB, Pandharipande PP: Pathophysiology of acute brain dysfunction: what's the cause of all this confusion? Curr Opin Crit Care 18(5):518–526, 2012

Ipser JC, Stein DJ: Evidence-based pharmacotherapy of post-traumatic stress disorder (PTSD). Int J Neuropsychopharmacol 15(6):825–840, 2012

Jacob S, Spinler SA: Hyponatremia associated with selective serotonin-reuptake inhibitors in older adults. Ann Pharmacother 40(9):1618–1622, 2006

Jiménez-Jiménez FJ, Puertas I, de Toledo-Heras M: Drug-induced myoclonus: frequency, mechanisms and management. CNS Drugs 18(2):93–104, 2004

King T, Ossipov MH, Vanderah TW, et al: Is paradoxical pain induced by sustained opioid exposure an underlying mechanism of opioid antinociceptive tolerance? Neurosignals 14(4):194–205, 2005

Kline AE, Hoffman AN, Cheng JP, et al: Chronic administration of antipsychotics impede behavioral recovery after experimental traumatic brain injury. Neurosci Lett 448(3):263–267, 2008

Koren D, Norman D, Cohen A, et al: Increased PTSD risk with combat-related injury: a matched comparison study of injured and uninjured soldiers experiencing the same combat events. Am J Psychiatry 162(2):276–282, 2005

Kroenke K, Krebs EE, Bair MJ: Pharmacotherapy of chronic pain: a synthesis of recommendations from systematic reviews. Gen Hosp Psychiatry 31(3):206–219, 2009

Liepert J: Pharmacotherapy in restorative neurology. Curr Opin Neurol 21:639–643, 2008

Lin SM, Liu CY, Wang CH, et al: The impact of delirium on the survival of mechanically ventilated patients. Crit Care Med 32(11):2254–2259, 2004

Looper KJ: Potential medical and surgical complications of serotonergic antidepressant medications. Psychosomatics 48(1):1–9, 2007

Mago R, Mahajan R, Thase ME: Medically serious adverse effects of newer antidepressants. Curr Psychiatry Rep 10(3):249–257, 2008

Malchow RJ, Black IH: The evolution of pain management in the critically ill trauma patient: emerging concepts from the global war on terrorism. Crit Care Med 36(7) (suppl):S346–S357, 2008

Maldonado JR: Delirium in the acute care setting: characteristics, diagnosis and treatment. Crit Care Clin 24(4):657–722, vii, 2008

McCleane G: Antidepressants as analgesics. CNS Drugs 22(2):139–156, 2008

McGhee LL, Maani CV, Garza TH, et al: The correlation between ketamine and posttraumatic stress disorder in burned service members. J Trauma 64:S195–S199, 2008

Meagher D, Moran M, Raju B, et al: A new data-based motor subtype schema for delirium. J Neuropsychiatry Clin Neurosci 20(2):185–193, 2008

Meyer MR, Maurer HH: Absorption, distribution, metabolism and excretion pharmacogenomics of drugs of abuse. Pharmacogenomics 12(2):215–233, 2011

Meyer-Massetti C, Cheng CM, Sharpe BA, et al: The FDA extended warning for intravenous haloperidol and torsades de pointes: how should institutions respond? J Hosp Med 5(4):E8–E16, 2010

Milbrandt EB, Kersten A, Kong L, et al: Haloperidol use is associated with lower hospital mortality in mechanically ventilated patients. Crit Care Med 33(1):226–229, discussion 263–265, 2005

Monti JM, Pandi-Perumal SR: Eszopiclone: its use in the treatment of insomnia. Neuropsychiatr Dis Treat 3(4):441–453, 2007

Morgan CA III, Hazlett G, Wang S, et al: Symptoms of dissociation in humans experiencing acute, uncontrollable stress: a prospective investigation. Am J Psychiatry 158(8):1239–1247, 2001

Movig KLL, Janssen MWHE, de Waal Malefijt J, et al: Relationship of serotonergic antidepressants and need for blood transfusion in orthopedic surgical patients. Arch Intern Med 163(19):2354–2358, 2003

Mula M, Pini S, Cassano GB: The role of anticonvulsant drugs in anxiety disorders: a critical review of the evidence. J Clin Psychopharmacol 27(3):263–272, 2007

Nielsen J, Graff C, Kanters JK, et al: Assessing QT interval prolongation and its associated risks with antipsychotics. CNS Drugs 25(6):473–490, 2011

O'Donnell ML, Creamer M, Pattison P: Posttraumatic stress disorder and depression following trauma: understanding comorbidity. Am J Psychiatry 161(8):1390–1396, 2004

Pandharipande P, Jackson J, Ely EW: Delirium: acute cognitive dysfunction in the critically ill. Curr Opin Crit Care 11(4):360–368, 2005

Patterson DR, Jensen MP: Hypnosis and clinical pain. Psychol Bull 129(4):495–521, 2003

Ramsamy A, Harrison SE, Clasper JC: Injuries from roadside improvised explosive devices. J Trauma Injury Infect Crit Care 65(4):910–914, 2008

Rastogi R, Swarm RA, Patel TA: Case scenario: opioid association with serotonin syndrome: implications to the practitioners. Anesthesiology 115(6):1291–1298, 2011

Rickels K, Pollack MH, Feltner DE, et al: Pregabalin for treatment of generalized anxiety disorder: a 4-week, multicenter, double-blind, placebo-controlled trial of pregabalin and alprazolam. Arch Gen Psychiatry 62(9):1022–1030, 2005

Rockwood K, Cosway S, Carver D, et al: The risk of dementia and death after delirium. Age Ageing 28(6):551–556, 1999

Rowe DL: Off-label prescription of quetiapine in psychiatric disorders. Expert Rev Neurother 7(7):841–852, 2007

Saarto T, Wiffen PJ. Antidepressants for neuropathic pain. Cochrane Database of Systematic Reviews 2007, Issue 4. Art. No.: CD005454. DOI: 10.1002/14651858.CD005454.pub2

Shoumitro D, Crownshaw T: The role of pharmacotherapy in the management of behavior disorders in traumatic brain injury patients. Brain Injury 18(1):1–31, 2004

Silverman SM: Opioid induced hyperalgesia: clinical implications for the pain practitioner. Pain Physician 12(3):679–684, 2009

Smith HS: Opioid metabolism. Mayo Clin Proc 84(7):613–624, 2009

Smith T, Nicholson RA: Review of duloxetine in the management of diabetic peripheral neuropathic pain. Vasc Health Risk Manag 3(6):833–844, 2007

Spiegel D, Spiegel H: Hypnosis in psychosomatic medicine. Psychosomatics 21(1):35–41, 1980

Steiner LA: Postoperative delirium, part 2: detection, prevention and treatment. Eur J Anaesthesiol 28(10):723–732, 2011

Taylor HR, Freeman MK, Cates ME: Prazosin for treatment of nightmares related to posttraumatic stress disorder. Am J Health Syst Pharm 65(8):716–722, 2008

Thomason JW, Ely EW: Delirium in the intensive care unit is bad: what is the confusion? Crit Care Med 32(11):2352–2354, 2004

Thompson CE, Taylor FB, McFall ME, et al: Nonnightmare distressed awakenings in veterans with posttraumatic stress disorder: response to prazosin. J Trauma Stress 21(4):417–420, 2008

Toner LC, Tsambiras BM, Catalano G, et al: Central nervous system side effects associated with zolpidem treatment. Clin Neuropharmacol 23(1):54–58, 2000

Tremont-Lukats IW, Megeff C, Backonja MM: Anticonvulsants for neuropathic pain syndromes: mechanisms of action and place in therapy. Drugs 60(5):1029–1052, 2000

Van Ameringen M, Mancini C, Pipe B, et al: Antiepileptic drugs in the treatment of anxiety disorders: role in therapy. Drugs 64(19):2199–2220, 2004

van Dorp ELA, Kest B, Kowalczyk WJ, et al: Morphine-6beta-glucuronide rapidly increases pain sensitivity independently of opioid receptor activity in mice and humans. Anesthesiology 110(6):1356–1363, 2009

van Zyl LT, Seitz DP: Delirium concisely: condition is associated with increased morbidity, mortality, and length of hospitalization. Geriatrics 61(3):18–21, 2006

Verdu B, Decosterd I, Buclin T, et al: Antidepressants for the treatment of chronic pain. Drugs 68(18):2611–2632, 2008

Wain HJ: Hypnosis on a consultation-liaison service. Psychosomatics 20(10):678–689, 1979

Wain HJ: Medical hypnosis, in Medical Psychiatric Practice, Vol 2. Edited by Stou-
demire A, Fogel BS. Washington, DC, American Psychiatric Press, 1993, pp
36–66

Wain HJ, Grammer GG, Stasinos JJ, et al: Meeting the patients where they are:
consultation-liaison response to trauma victims of the Pentagon attack. Mil
Med 167(9) (suppl):19–21, 2002

Wain HJ, Grammer G, Stasinos J: Psychiatric intervention for medical surgical patients following traumatic injuries, in Mental Health Interventions in Terrorism and Natural Disaster. Edited by Ritchie EC, Friedman MJ, Watson PJ, et
al. New York: Guilford, 2006, pp 278–298

Wang W, Li HL, Wang DX, et al: Haloperidol prophylaxis decreases delirium incidence in elderly patients after noncardiac surgery: a randomized controlled
trial. Crit Care Med 40(3):731–739, 2012

Wensel TM, Powe KW, Cates ME: Pregabalin for the treatment of generalized
anxiety disorder. Ann Pharmacother 46(3):424–429, 2012

Chapter 9

Traumatic Brain Injury

Kimberly S. Meyer, APRN
Jamie B. Grimes, M.D.

TRAUMATIC BRAIN INJURY (TBI) is a leading cause of disability and death from injury in the United States, affecting all ages, ethnicities, and incomes (Coronado et al. 2009). TBI has also been referred to as the signature injury of current military conflicts in Iraq and Afghanistan (Jones et al. 2007). The Centers for Disease Control and Prevention (CDC) estimate that TBI affects more than 1.7 million Americans annually (Faul et al. 2010). Mortality across all TBI severities is approximately 3%; however, morbidity is more difficult to ascertain.

TBI is generally defined as a blow or jolt to the head that results in temporary or permanent cerebral dysfunction (Centers for Disease Control and Prevention 2010). This cerebral dysfunction may manifest as alterations of consciousness (AOC; feeling dazed or confused, seeing stars), loss of consciousness (LOC), or, in more severe cases, focal neurological findings.

Current conflicts in the Middle East have resulted in increased awareness of TBI in the military health care system. TBI surveillance within the U.S. Department of Defense (DOD) was initiated in 2000, and through the first quarter of 2012, 244,217 unique cases of TBI were identified in the U.S. Armed Forces population, with 77% mild TBI or concussion (Defense and Veterans Brain Injury Center 2011). These numbers include both deployment and nondeployment TBI-diagnosed injuries.

Epidemiology

In military combatants, blast injury is the most common cause of war injuries (Warden 2006) and the primary cause of TBI. Blast injury results from several mechanisms:

- Primary injury occurs as a result of rapid pressure shifts that predominantly impact areas of the body with air-fluid interfaces, including the brain and spinal cord.
- Secondary injury results from projectiles set in motion by blast energy.
- Tertiary injury results from impact with another object.
- Quaternary injury results from other mechanisms, including toxic inhalation, burns, radiation, or shock from severe blood loss.

Injury may also result from "blast plus" additional mechanisms of brain injury. This type of injury may occur when a blast causes a vehicle crash, resulting in a combination of blast and blunt TBI or other similar mechanisms.

Classification and Severity of Injury

TBI is a broad injury category encompassing a range of severities. Historically, TBI severity has been determined utilizing the Glasgow Coma Scale (GCS) score (Table 9–1), which incorporates eye opening, verbal responses, and motor responses. Although useful in severe injury, this categorization has limited application in patients sustaining less severe injury. Consequently, other parameters, including the duration of AOC or LOC and imaging findings, are also included in the determination of severity (Table 9–2). Interview questions should help identify gaps in time or memory, which are indicative of AOC. Broad questions, such as "Tell me about the accident," often fail to identify brief disruptions in time. Specific questions such as "What is the first thing you remember?" may be of more utility. It is important to note that delayed interviews following injury can be less likely to provide useful information on memory gaps because during the delay time period, friends or battle buddies may recount the incident to the injured, thereby reducing lapses or gaps in memory when the injured person is ultimately interviewed. Injuries that violate the skull and dura mater are considered penetrating brain injury regardless of classification by other parameters.

Appropriate assignment of injury severity is critical because this predicts necessary resources and, to a lesser degree, prognosis. Patients with mild

TABLE 9–1.   Glasgow Coma Scale

Scoring
(Use best response)

Response	Description	Score
Eye opening	Spontaneously	4
	To voice	3
	To pain	2
	None	1
Verbal response	Oriented	5
	Confused	4
	Inappropriate words	3
	Incomprehensible sounds	2
	None	1
Motor response	Follows commands	6
	Localizes to pain	5
	Withdraws	4
	Abnormal flexion	3
	Abnormal extension	2
	None	1
	Total score: ___	

TABLE 9–2.   TBI severity classification

Severity	GCS	AOC	LOC	PTA	Imaging
Mild	13–15	≤24 hours	0–30 minutes	≤24 hours	Negative
Moderate	9–12	>24 hours	>30 minutes <24 hours	>24 hours <7 days	Negative or positive
Severe	3–8	>24 hours	≥24 hours	≥7 days	Generally positive

Note. AOC=alteration of consciousness; GCS=Glasgow Coma Scale; LOC=loss of consciousness; PTA=posttraumatic amnesia.

TBI (mTBI), also called concussion, rarely require more than observation and a brief period of symptom management by a primary care provider. DOD criteria for mTBI follow the recommendations of the American College of Rehabilitation Medicine (1993), which include a traumatic event that results in temporary brain dysfunction that may include AOC, LOC for less than 30 minutes, or memory disturbance. In addition, DOD mTBI classification requires standardized structural neuroimaging to be normal (Management of Concussion/mTBI Working Group 2009). With single events, full recovery within days to weeks can be expected. Patients with a history of multiple concussions may suffer more severe symptomatology and require longer periods of recovery (Guskiewicz et al. 2003; Slobounov et al. 2007), but recovery is still anticipated. As in civilian populations, the majority of military-related TBI is classified as mild (Figure 9–1).

Moderate TBI often requires hospitalization, serial imaging, and, in many cases, acute rehabilitation. Cognitive deficits and other physical disabilities may persist in this population (Sandhaug et al. 2010). Evidence-based recommendations are scant for this subgroup of TBI.

Severe and penetrating TBI is resource intensive and is usually managed at designated trauma centers. Invasive monitoring of intracranial pressure, mechanical ventilation, and enteral feeding are often required (Brain Trauma Foundation 2007). Acute complications including infection, intracranial hypertension, and neuroworsening are common. Penetrating injury in particular may result in cerebral vasospasm, which can further worsen neurological function. Recovery following these injuries is less predictable, and long-term risks for other neurological conditions such as seizures (Bombardier et al. 2006; Wang et al. 2008) and hydrocephalus (Bauer et al. 2011) are increased. The yearly economic cost of TBI in the United States, including rehabilitation and medical costs as well as indirect economic costs, is estimated to be $60 billion (Finkelstein et al. 2006). According to the CDC, survivors of severe brain injury can require 5–10 years of intensive rehabilitative therapy, with the possibility of a single individual recovering from severe TBI having a lifetime cost of up to $4 million dollars.

Symptomatology

Problems following TBI can be categorized as neurological signs or symptoms. Neurological signs include seizures, focal neurological findings such as pupillary changes, or posturing. These signs are more likely to be seen in patients with moderate or severe TBI, with rare reports in mTBI. Self-reported symptoms are often vague and can be seen in numerous other medical conditions. Symptoms are frequently clustered into somatic, cognitive, or neuropsychiatric categories (see Table 9–3).

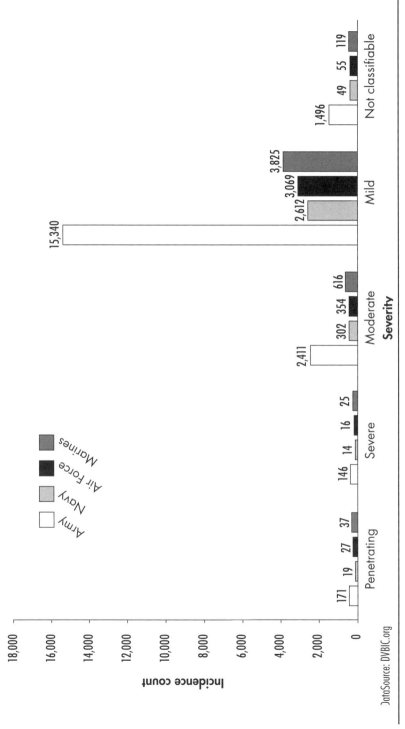

FIGURE 9–1. **TBI numbers by severity, all Armed Forces, 2010 (*N*=30,703).**

Source. Data are from DVBIC.org.

TABLE 9-3.   Categories of symptoms

Somatic	Cognitive	Neuropsychiatric
Headache	Memory problems	Anxiety
Dizziness or balance difficulties	Impaired attention	Irritability
Fatigue	Decreased concentration	Depression
Photophobia	Slowed processing speed	Emotional lability
Visual disturbances	Speech dysfluency	
Phonophobia or tinnitus		

Symptoms may occur in isolation or in combination. Following uncomplicated mTBI, symptoms are self-limiting over a short duration of time. Certain populations are known to have more pervasive symptoms. This is especially seen in children and in adults with prior TBI (Guskiewicz and Valovich McLeod 2011).

Assessment

Concussion and mTBI Strategies

Because the vast majority of TBI is concussive injury, in the remainder of this chapter we focus on the evaluation and management of this population. Resources for nondeployment care include the *VA/DoD Clinical Practice Guideline for Management of Concussion/Mild Traumatic Brain Injury (mTBI)*, which was published in 2009 and was ranked recently as one of the best assessment tools on the basis of cumulative assessments of multiple key domains for mTBI (Berrigan et al. 2011). On June 21, 2010, Directive Type Memorandum (DTM) 09-033 was signed, requiring implementation in combat zones of several medical algorithms for mTBI, including the use of the Military Acute Concussion Evaluation (MACE; Defense and Veterans Brain Injury Center 2010) at the time of the injury as well as four medical management algorithms: Combat Medic/Corpsman, Initial Provider, Comprehensive Concussion Evaluation, and Recurrent Concussion Assessment (three or more mTBIs documented in 12 months). Both the MACE and mTBI algorithms were updated in 2012 to expand short-term memory word lists for the MACE and to enhance clinical guidance for algorithms; the release date of both was July 2012.

A clinical interview is required to confirm the presence of either AOC or LOC following a traumatic insult to the head. The presence of AOC or

LOC establishes the diagnosis of concussion. Several tools are available to determine signs and symptoms that are temporally related to the concussive event, including such symptom inventories as the Rivermead Post-Concussion Symptoms Questionnaire (King et al. 1995) and the Neurobehavioral Symptom Inventory (Cicerone and Kalmar 1995). These and other surveys can be used during the initial concussion evaluation to identify symptoms and their severity and can then be used at subsequent evaluations to track symptoms over time.

Clinical evaluations begin with a complete neurological examination. During the interview, in addition to noting general orientation, the evaluator considers speech patterns, including word finding, fluency, and evidence of dysarthria. Pupillary function and motor strength are tested. Subtle evidence of upper extremity motor weakness can be elicited when checking for pronator drift. Gross balance can be assessed using the Romberg test, which can be made more sensitive with the Sharpened Romberg Test. The Balance Error Scoring System (BESS) can be used to further assess balance on both flat and unstable surfaces. A cranial nerve exam should be conducted, especially for patients with visual complaints.

Imaging in the acute setting is rarely necessary in concussion. In patients with a GCS of 15, only 5%–7% are likely to have positive findings on computed tomography (CT), with only 0.5% requiring neurosurgical intervention (Haydel et al. 2000; Smits et al. 2005). The New Orleans Criteria was the first successfully validated clinical decision rule for selective use of CT in minor head injury (Haydel et al. 2000). According to these criteria, patients who present with alcohol or drug intoxication; are greater than 60 years of age; experience seizure, worsening headache, persistent vomiting, or physical evidence of trauma above the clavicles; or are on anticoagulation medications should undergo acute imaging (Haydel et al. 2000). Magnetic resonance imaging (MRI) is considered more sensitive than CT in patients with mTBI (Levin et al. 1987), although findings do not generally alter the preestablished treatment plan. Additional imaging techniques, including functional MRI, diffusion tensor imaging, and positron emission tomography, show promise in identifying structural abnormalities in the setting of TBI but to date remain investigational.

Subjective memory and cognitive complaints are not uncommon following mTBI (Terrio et al. 2009). These complaints are generally short lived, resolving within several weeks following injury. Patients with persistent difficulties may benefit from formal neuropsychological testing. In most cases of mTBI, memory is not affected. Instead, deficits in attention, processing speed, and verbal learning are frequently identified (Cooper et al. 2010; Kashluba et al. 2008).

Treatment

Immediately following injury, treatment focuses on symptom management. In many cases, mitigation of the most offensive symptom will result in improvement of other related symptoms. For example, severe headaches may impair sleep and subsequently result in fatigue, irritability, and inability to manage emotions. After the headache is controlled, the other symptoms resolve or become more manageable. For this reason, it is advisable to identify the most troublesome symptoms and treat accordingly. This approach also minimizes the need for polypharmacy. When considering pharmacotherapy, one should be aware of the side effect profile and potential effect on cognitive function. Patients with persistent symptoms may benefit from more thorough screening for coexisting conditions.

Pharmacological Strategies for Management of TBI-Related Symptoms

In soldiers sustaining concussion during deployment, headache was the predominant complaint following injury (Terrio et al. 2009). According to DOD TBI management algorithms, aggressive early management of headaches using acetaminophen is encouraged. Acetaminophen has been shown to decrease headache severity (Pfaffenrath et al. 2009) without affecting platelet functionality or the coagulation cascade and is therefore the initial agent of choice in patients with minor intracranial pathology or in the absence of imaging. Patients with negative imaging findings may benefit from nonsteroidal anti-inflammatory medications such as ibuprofen or naproxen sodium. Abortive medications such as these should be used only for a short duration because prolonged use can precipitate analgesic rebound headaches. In patients with persistent headache, efforts to differentiate headache type should facilitate appropriate preventive pharmacological intervention. In blunt trauma, headaches are commonly described as tension type or cervicogenic in nature. However, patients with blast injury are more likely to report migrainous components (Lew et al. 2006).

Several drug classes have been shown to improve pain levels in patients with headaches. Antiepileptic drugs are useful in the management of chronic headaches associated with TBI. In a retrospective study of divalproex sodium, specifically in posttraumatic headache, 60% of participants reported mild to moderate improvement in headache status, with many converting from daily to episodic headaches (Packard 2000). Use of this medication is limited in combat settings secondary to the need for routine monitoring of serum drug levels and liver function tests. Other antiepileptic drugs, including lamotrigine, topiramate, and gabapentin, are shown to be efficacious in the management of migraine or chronic daily headaches (Gupta et al. 2007; Silberstein et al. 2007). Their use is often translated to posttraumatic headache. Calcium channel blockers, nonselective beta blockers (propranolol), and some antidepressants can be considered for patients whose headaches have migrainous features, whereas antidepressants and muscle relaxers are options for those with tension-type headaches (Lew et al. 2006).

Sleep disturbances are also common complaints following traumatic brain injury (Ouellet et al. 2006). Initial interventions should include sleep hygiene practices (e.g., avoidance of caffeine and nicotine, regular sleep schedule) and behavioral changes (Thaxton and Myers 2002). Some patients, however, will require pharmacological intervention. Some antidepressants, particularly trazodone and mirtazapine, can successfully facilitate sleep improvement. Nonbenzodiazepine sedative-hypnotic agents (zolpidem, zaleplon, eszopiclone) can be used for short-term management of insomnia. Careful monitoring is recommended because of the potentially dangerous side effects (e.g., sleepwalking) and development of tolerance. Benzodiazepines and antihistamines are not recommended for sleep management in patients with TBI secondary to adverse effects (e.g., hangover effects, cognitive worsening, dizziness) (Flanagan et al. 2007). Persistent sleep disturbance or fatigue may be indicative of other conditions such as depression or anxiety; therefore, further clinical screening may be indicated.

Dizziness and balance disturbances are also common somatic symptoms following mTBI. Screening using the BESS can be performed in the office (Davis et al. 2009). The BESS requires observation of closed-eye standing in various feet positions on both flat and unstable (foam) ground. Although the BESS is a useful screening tool currently employed in deployment settings, it does not provide details regarding the etiology of a given balance disturbance. Dynamic posturography is necessary to characterize dizziness after TBI (Hoffer et al. 2004, 2010). Vestibular dysfunction varies by traumatic mechanism. Patients with blast injury are more likely to demonstrate deficits in the vestibular ocular reflex (Hoffer et al. 2009). Vestibular rehabilitation and habituation exercises are the mainstay of treatment for dizziness and balance disturbances following TBI. Outcomes of this therapy vary by dizziness subtype: posttraumatic spatial disorientation, positional vertigo, and vestibular migraines (Hoffer et al. 2004). Medications such as meclizine, certain antimigraine medications, and quetiapine have been shown to adversely affect recovery and should be avoided whenever possible (Donaldson et al. 2010).

Substance abuse is known to be a contributing factor to TBI in the civilian population (O'Phelan et al. 2008). However, following TBI, substance use or abuse is sometimes seen in patients without preexisting tendencies, perhaps because of decreased inhibition or as an attempt to alleviate symptoms (Graham and Cardon 2008). The incidence of substance abuse following TBI is variable; therefore, screening and appropriate intervention are indicated (Graham and Cardon 2008; Vungkhanching et al. 2007). The use of certain antiepileptic medications appears to lessen emotional lability and alcohol use that is sometimes seen following TBI (Beresford et al. 2005).

Co-occurring TBI and Posttraumatic Stress Disorder

For service members, battlefield blast exposure resulting in concussion can occur in a setting of abject chaos; a deliberate life-threatening attack; and other injuries, including catastrophic and/or lethal wounds to self or battle mates. Posttraumatic stress disorder (PTSD) following civilian TBI is reported at rates from 10% to 30% (Bombardier et al. 2006). However, rates may be as high as 50% in service members with TBI (Brenner et al. 2010), which may contribute to increased symptom reporting (Kennedy et al. 2010). A recent collaboration between the U.S. Department of Veterans Affairs (VA) and the DOD resulted in a consensus paper regarding the treatment of mTBI and comorbid PTSD (National Center for Posttraumatic Stress Disorder 2011).

Integration of Care for Patients With TBI and Other Co-occurring Disorders

TBI commonly occurs with other conditions, both physical and psychological. Clinical practice guidelines exist for conditions such as mTBI, PTSD, and pain. However, these conditions seldom occur in isolation, and there is little to guide the management of these conditions when they coexist. Although care can be challenging, it is recommended that collaborative, interdisciplinary treatment plans guide the care for patients with multiple conditions. Keys to effective care include the use of consistent messages across providers and specific attention to minimize polypharmacy.

Pain associated with other traumatic injuries may also impact recovery from postconcussive symptoms. Pain is often managed with a variety of medications, including narcotics, antidepressants, and antiepileptics. However, alternative modalities such as transcutaneous electrical nerve stimulation, application of heat and cold, and other techniques may beneficial.

Concussion may also coexist with depression. Risk factors for developing depression after TBI include preexisting depressive symptoms and premorbid personality traits (Rogers and Read 2007). Increasing evidence suggests that women are at greater risk than men (Bay et al. 2009). It is unclear whether baseline traits or neuropathological consequences of TBI play a stronger role in the development of posttraumatic depression (Rogers and Read 2007). The Patient Health Questionnaire-9 (PHQ-9) has been shown to be a valid tool for depression screening in patients with TBI (Fann et al. 2005).

Interdisciplinary Approach to mTBI in Deployed Setting

An interdisciplinary team approach including occupational therapy and physical therapy for concussion can be implemented acutely but is especially helpful for a cohesive treatment approach if the concussed individual is not responding to initial treatment after a reasonable period of time. Uniquely in the acute setting of deployment arenas, occupational therapists along with occupational therapy techs have established a systematic approach at mTBI/concussion care centers. These centers ensure mandatory rest and provide education regarding expectation of recovery. Simultaneously, appropriate symptom management strategies are instituted, thereby facilitating the resolution of postconcussion symptoms. This team approach guides the service member in a standardized, gradual return to physical activity while being monitored for exacerbation of concussion symptoms in a manner similar to the civilian sports paradigm of graduated return to play.

Physical therapy can be an important discipline for assessing for and improving weakness, dizziness or vestibulopathy, dyscoordination, and co-occurring musculoskeletal complaints, including cervicogenic neck pain and tension-type headaches. Physical therapy, like occupational therapy, can oversee graduated return to physical activity and monitor for worsening symptoms after concussion sustained in a combat zone.

Spectrum of mTBI Rehabilitation

Patients with complicated mTBI (persistent or unusual symptoms) require individualized plans of care. Traditionally, cognitive rehabilitation in the setting of mTBI has been controversial. However, increasing evidence supports the use of interventions to improve attention, memory, communication skills, and executive functioning (Cicerone et al. 2011). Such methods as cueing, use of mnemonic techniques, and memory notebooks or calendars play a role in the recovery or development of compensatory strategies for cognitive impairment (Helmick and Members of Consensus Conference 2010). Additionally, assistive devices, including cellular telephones and personal digital assistants, may be beneficial in cognitive rehabilitation. Group therapy has been shown to improve problem-solving skills in patients with TBI by facilitating compensatory mechanisms (Rath et al. 2003).

Persistent balance deficits warrant detailed vestibular assessment for need of rehabilitation. Computerized posturography helps quantify postural instability and can guide vestibular rehabilitation (Pickett et al. 2007). Differences in visual-ocular reflexes and vestibular-spinal reflexes are seen in blast and blunt TBI (Hoffer et al. 2009), with those associated with blast injury resulting in variable recovery (Hoffer et al. 2010). Habituation exercises are the mainstay of vestibular rehabilitation, although a subset of patients with benign paroxysmal positional vertigo secondary to TBI may benefit from canalith repositioning maneuvers (Ahn et al. 2011). In many instances, this immediately improves the feeling of dizziness. The use of medications such as diazepam and meclizine is reserved for brief, acute use in severe cases of vestibular dysfunction because continued use can delay recovery.

Patients with mild to moderate TBI may complain of vague visual disturbances (e.g., blurry vision, difficulty reading). Standard vision testing is often within normal limits, but binocular testing can demonstrate accommodation or convergence insufficiency (Goodrich et al. 2007). Results of vision therapy are variable. Retraining of the eyes can be done in conjunction with occupational therapy or through the use of computerized programs to refocus the eyes (Ripley et al. 2010). In some cases, prism glasses may be prescribed to lessen the acute effects of visual disturbances.

Fitness for driving should also be assessed in selected cases of TBI. Both personality traits and cognitive ability impact one's ability to safely operate a motor vehicle (Sommer et al. 2010). Evaluation of fitness for driving is especially important in combat veterans who may be used to aggressive or erratic driving behaviors while deployed and who have cognitive impairments affecting attention and processing speeds. Driving simulators are effective means for both evaluating and remediating driving skills (Kraft et al. 2010).

Role of Complementary Medicine in TBI Care

Patients with refractory postconcussive symptoms may seek complementary therapies as adjuncts to traditional medical therapy. Some evidence suggests that acupuncture may decrease headache days and severity of headache in some chronic headache disorders (Vickers et al. 2004). Onabotulinum toxin A (Botox) has been used in a variety of headache conditions with variable results. One of the benefits of Botox is the long duration of action, up to 90 days (Pakalnis and Couch 2008). Neurofeedback, guided by quantitative electroencephalography, is sometimes used in the management of cognitive difficulties associated with TBI (Thornton and Carmody 2009). Biofeedback has also been used to improve balance.

Similar brain structures are thought to be involved in both mTBI and PTSD. In military cohorts, approximately 26% of service members screen positive for both TBI and PTSD (Brenner et al. 2010). Studies of lifetime prevalence of major depression in World War II veterans with TBI compared with veterans without TBI showed increased rate of depression (Holsinger et al. 2002). Incomplete treatment of one condition may result in inadequate recovery from the other condition. When determining treatment plans, both conditions should be considered, and treatments that can exacerbate complaints of one condition should be avoided whenever possible. The VA Workgroup on Co-occurring Conditions concluded that best practice should include prolonged exposure therapy and cognitive-behavioral therapy (National Center for Posttraumatic Stress Disorder 2011). Medications proven efficacious in PTSD treatment such as sertraline and paroxetine may also have benefit in treating mTBI (Arciniegas et al. 2000; Asnis et al. 2004; Fann et al. 2000).

Current State of TBI Care Within the Departments of Defense and Veterans Affairs

TBI care within the DOD begins on the battlefield. Aggressive event-based mandatory screening measures help identify service members at risk for TBI, and mandatory medical assessments help standardize the assessment and reporting of TBI in the durable medical record. The diagnosis is confirmed by licensed providers through clinical interview and review of MACE findings. Education, including the expectation of recovery, is paramount. Service members with symptoms but without neurological deficits are managed locally in a primary care model. In 2011, 11 concussion care clinics were established in the combat arenas. Establishment of these centers occurred in close coordination with combat operational stress centers and chaplains, thereby ensuring that treatment for both concussion and acute stress reaction or PTSD symptoms are managed in an interdisciplinary fashion. As previously described in the section "Interdisciplinary Approach to mTBI in Deployed

Setting," these facilities are run predominantly by occupational therapists, who focus on supervised rest, graded recovery, and return to duty and reintegration. All concussion care centers enter clinical assessments, treatments, and progress into the electronic military medical record to ensure accessibility across the continuum of care, from the deployment arena to stateside medical facilities. Complicated cases of mTBI are referred to neurologists at concussion specialty care centers, located at combat support hospitals. These facilities provide the highest level of concussion care in theater, including multidisciplinary specialty evaluations (e.g., ear, nose, and throat and optometry) and imaging (CT and MRI). Comprehensive recommendations are made for either ongoing in-theater care or stateside evacuation.

When the patient is stateside, medical management of persistent postconcussive symptoms continues, utilizing a primary care model. Service branches have established TBI centers with designated resources to facilitate multidiscipline care targeted to service members with persistent or uncontrolled symptoms. The Defense and Veterans Brain Injury Center (DVBIC), the primary TBI operational component of the Defense Centers of Excellence for Psychological Health and Traumatic Brain Injury, supports 18 clinical sites at military treatment facilities, VA facilities, and civilian rehabilitation sites (Figure 9–2). DVBIC has robust care, educational platforms, and care coordination programs that assist service members and their local case managers with identifying TBI-specific resources in the service member's home locale.

Patients with moderate, severe, or penetrating injury or mTBI with polytrauma are treated at one of the five VA polytrauma rehabilitation centers. These are comprehensive rehabilitation facilities offering a full range of state-of-the art equipment and neurorehabilitation. More recently, coma stimulation programs for patients in a minimally conscious state have been established. Veterans entering the VA medical system who have not been screened or diagnosed with TBI undergo mandatory TBI screening to determine if there are unmet needs.

Future of TBI

Investigators are in search of objective means to diagnose TBI, especially its mildest forms. Serum and cerebrospinal fluid biomarkers, including glial fibrillary acidic protein, S-100, and others are currently being evaluated. One study found that when elevated, these markers have been associated with poor neurological outcomes (Vos et al. 2010). The use of these and similar markers has been limited by concerns about sensitivity and specificity for TBI.

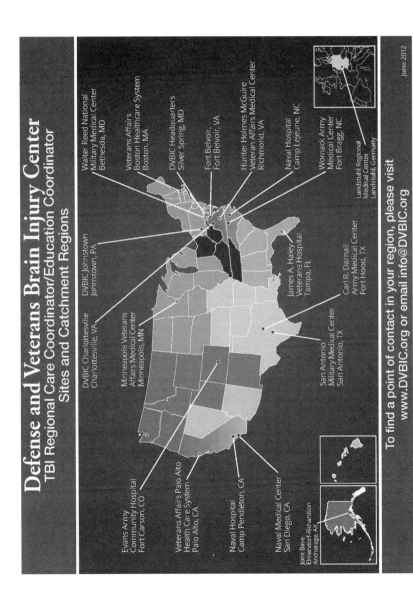

FIGURE 9–2. DVBIC clinical sites.

Several advanced imaging techniques show promise. Diffusion tensor imaging is sensitive to injury to the white matter tracts deep within the brain. Sponheim et al. (2011) demonstrated in a small sample that blast-related concussion was associated with disruptions in the anterior white matter tract. Similar results occurred in another military sample of blast injury (Mac Donald et al. 2011). Numerous larger studies evaluating the utility of various imaging modalities in the care of TBI are under way, including an institutional review board–approved clinical neuroimaging study in theater examining MRI findings in acute blast TBI in Afghanistan. Other more esoteric diagnostic methods are also being investigated.

Congressional funding for TBI research and care are ongoing, with $56 million allocated for fiscal year 2011. Many of these monies are disbursed through Congressionally Directed Medical Research Programs (CDMRP). CDMRP has funded a longitudinal study of traumatic brain injury that aims to determine the natural history of TBI. Other funded studies include the use of neurocognitive assessment batteries preinjury and postinjury, drugs with potential for neuroprotection, protective gear that can mitigate effects of blast injury, multimodal imaging of TBIs, and eye movement abnormalities associated with TBI.

Pharmacological studies are ongoing in the civilian setting. The National Institutes of Health is sponsoring a Phase III multicenter treatment trial, including San Antonio Military Medical Center, of progesterone as a neuroprotectant in moderate to severe TBI. Other funded trials evaluating the utility of antidepressants in the management of certain psychiatric and behavioral symptoms following TBI are under way at other centers. A collaborative workgroup, the Concussion Definition Consortium, which includes participants from the CDC, Brain Trauma Foundation, DOD, and academia, has convened to scientifically evaluate all mTBI literature. Although work is ongoing, the final product of this workgroup will be a universal definition of concussion and mTBI as well as an agreed-on set of diagnostic criteria.

Conclusions

TBI remains a significant problem in both the civilian and military medical systems. Although recovery from uncomplicated, isolated concussions is expected, less is known about the recovery and prognosis of patients sustaining multiple concussions. Ongoing efforts aimed at mitigation of blast-related injury, objective measures of diagnosis and recovery, and efficacious treatment modalities remain under investigation.

SUMMARY POINTS

- In military combatants, blast injury is the most common cause of war injuries and the primary cause of traumatic brain injury (TBI).
- TBI is a broad injury category encompassing a range of severities including mild, moderate, and severe TBI.
- TBI assessment requires a clinical interview and neurological evaluation and may also include imaging and neuropsychological testing.
- TBI treatment focuses on symptom management using pharmacotherapy and neurorehabilitative care.
- Given comorbidity of TBI with PTSD and pain, collaborative and interdisciplinary treatment plans are often required.

References

Ahn SK, Jeon SY, Kim JP, et al: Clinical characteristics and treatment of benign paroxysmal positional vertigo after traumatic brain injury. J Trauma 70(2):442–446, 2011

American College of Rehabilitation Medicine: Definition of mild traumatic brain injury. J Head Trauma Rehabil 8(3):86–87, 1993

Arciniegas DB, Topkoff J, Silver JM: Neuropsychiatric aspects of traumatic brain injury. Curr Treat Options Neurol 2(2):169–186, 2000

Asnis GM, Kohn SR, Henderson M, et al: SSRIs versus non-SSRIs in post-traumatic stress disorder: an update with recommendations. Drugs 64(4):383–404, 2004

Bauer DF, McGwin G Jr, Melton SM, et al: Risk factors for conversion to permanent ventricular shunt in patients receiving therapeutic ventriculostomy for traumatic brain injury. Neurosurgery 68(1):85–88, 2011

Bay E, Sikorskii A, Saint-Arnault D: Sex differences in depressive symptoms and their correlates after mild-to-moderate traumatic brain injury. J Neurosci Nurs 41(6):298–309, quiz 310–311, 2009

Beresford TP, Arciniegas D, Clapp L, et al: Reduction of affective lability and alcohol use following traumatic brain injury: a clinical pilot study of anti-convulsant medications. Brain Inj 19(4):309–313, 2005

Berrigan L, Marshall S, McCullagh S, et al: Quality of clinical practice guidelines for persons who have sustained mild traumatic brain injury. Brain Inj 25(7–8):742–751, 2011

Bombardier CH, Fann JR, Temkin N, et al: Posttraumatic stress disorder symptoms during the first six months after traumatic brain injury. J Neuropsychiatry Clin Neurosci 18(4):501–508, 2006

Brain Trauma Foundation: Guidelines for the management of severe traumatic brain injury 3rd edition. J Neurotrauma 24 (suppl 1):S1–S106, 2007

Brenner LA, Ivins BJ, Schwab K, et al: Traumatic brain injury and post-traumatic stress disorder symptom reporting among troops returning from Iraq. J Head Trauma Rehabil 25(5):307–312, 2010

Centers for Disease Control and Prevention: Injury prevention and control: traumatic brain injury, Centers for Disease Control and Prevention, 2010. Available at: http://www.cdc.gov/TraumaticBrainInjury/index.html. Accessed August 12, 2012.

Cicerone KD, Kalmar K: Persistent postconcussion syndrome: the structure of subjective complaints after mild traumatic brain injury. J Head Trauma Rehabil 10(3):1–17, 1995

Cicerone KD, Langenbahn DM, Braden C, et al: Evidence-based cognitive rehabilitation: updated review of the literature from 2003 through 2008. Arch Phys Med Rehabil 92(4):519–530, 2011

Cooper DB, Mercado-Couch JM, Critchfield E, et al: Factors influencing cognitive functioning following mild traumatic brain injury in OIF/OEF burn patients. NeuroRehabilitation 26(3):233–238, 2010

Coronado VG, Thurman DJ, Greenspan A, et al: Epidemiology, in Neurotrauma and Critical Care of the Brain. Edited by Jallo J, Loftus CM. New York, Thieme, 2009, pp 3–22

Davis GA, Iverson GL, Guskiewicz KM, et al: Contributions of neuroimaging, balance testing, electrophysiology and blood markers to the assessment of sport-related concussion. Br J Sports Med 43 (suppl 1):i36–i45, 2009

Defense and Veterans Brain Injury Center: Military Acute Concussion Evaluation (MACE) Pocket Cards. Defense and Veterans Brain Injury Center, 2010. Available at: http://www.dvbic.org/material/military-acute-concussion-evaluation-mace-pocket-cards. Accessed September 24, 2013.

Defense and Veterans Brain Injury Center: DoD worldwide numbers for TBI. Defense and Veterans Brain Injury Center, 2011. Available at: http://www.dvbic.org/dod-worldwide-numbers-tbi. Accessed September 24, 2013.

Donaldson CJ, Hoffer ME, Balough BJ, et al: Prognostic assessments of medical therapy and vestibular testing in post-traumatic migraine-associated dizziness patients. Otolaryngol Head Neck Surg 143(6):820–825, 2010

Fann JR, Uomoto JM, Katon WJ: Sertraline in the treatment of major depression following mild traumatic brain injury. J Neuropsychiatry Clin Neurosci 12(2):226–232, 2000

Fann JR, Bombardier CH, Dikmen S, et al: Validity of the Patient Health Questionnaire-9 in assessing depression following traumatic brain injury. J Head Trauma Rehabil 20(6):501–511, 2005

Faul M, Xu L, Wald MM, et al: Traumatic brain injury in the United States: emergency department visits, hospitalizations and deaths 2002–2006. Atlanta, GA, National Center for Injury Prevention and Control, Centers for Disease Control and Prevention, 2010

Finkelstein EA, Corso PS, Miller TR: The Incidence and Economic Burden of Injuries in the United States, New York, Oxford University Press, 2006

Flanagan SR, Greenwald B, Wieber S: Pharmacological treatment of insomnia for individuals with brain injury. J Head Trauma Rehabil 22(1):67–70, 2007

Goodrich GL, Kirby J, Cockerham G, et al: Visual function in patients of a polytrauma rehabilitation center: a descriptive study. J Rehabil Res Dev 44(7):929–936, 2007

Graham DP, Cardon AL: An update on substance use and treatment following traumatic brain injury. Ann NY Acad Sci 1141:148–162, 2008

Gupta P, Singh S, Goyal V, et al: Low-dose topiramate versus lamotrigine in migraine prophylaxis (the Lotolamp study). Headache 47(3):402–412, 2007

Guskiewicz KM, Valovich McLeod TC: Pediatric sports-related concussion. PM R 3(4):353–364, quiz 364, 2011

Guskiewicz KM, McCrea M, Marshall SW, et al: Cumulative effects associated with recurrent concussion in collegiate football players: the NCAA Concussion Study. JAMA 290(19):2549–2555, 2003

Haydel MJ, Preston CA, Mills TJ, et al: Indications for computed tomography in patients with minor head injury. N Engl J Med 343(2):100–105, 2000

Helmick KM, Members of Consensus Conference: Cognitive rehabilitation for military personnel with mild traumatic brain injury and chronic post-concussional disorder: results of April 2009 consensus conference. NeuroRehabilitation 26(3):239–255, 2010

Hoffer ME, Gottshall KR, Moore R, et al: Characterizing and treating dizziness after mild head trauma. Otol Neurotol 25(2):135–138, 2004

Hoffer ME, Donaldson C, Gottshall KR, et al: Blunt and blast head trauma: different entities. Int Tinnitus J 15(2):115–118, 2009

Hoffer ME, Balaban C, Gottshall K, et al: Blast exposure: vestibular consequences and associated characteristics. Otol Neurotol 31(2):232–236, 2010

Holsinger T, Steffens DC, Phillips C, et al: Head injury in early adulthood and the lifetime risk of depression. Arch Gen Psychiatry 59(1):17–22, 2002

Jones E, Fear NT, Wessely S: Shell shock and mild traumatic brain injury: a historical review. Am J Psychiatry 164(11):1641–1645, 2007

Kashluba S, Hanks RA, Casey JE, et al: Neuropsychologic and functional outcome after complicated mild traumatic brain injury. Arch Phys Med Rehabil 89(5):904–911, 2008

Kennedy JE, Leal FO, Lewis JD, et al: Posttraumatic stress symptoms in OIF/OEF service members with blast-related and non-blast-related mild TBI. NeuroRehabilitation 26(3):223–231, 2010

King NS, Crawford S, Wenden FJ, et al: The Rivermead Post Concussion Symptoms Questionnaire: a measure of symptoms commonly experienced after head injury and its reliability. J Neurol 242(9):587–592, 1995

Kraft M, Amick MM, Barth JT, et al: A review of driving simulator parameters relevant to Operation Enduring Freedom/Operation Iraqi Freedom veteran populations. Am J Phys Med Rehabil 89(4):336–344, 2010

Levin HS, Amparo E, Eisenberg HM, et al: Magnetic resonance imaging and computerized tomography in relation to the neurobehavioral sequelae of mild and moderate head injuries. J Neurosurg 66(5):706–713, 1987

Lew HL, Lin PH, Fuh JL, et al: Characteristics and treatment of headache after traumatic brain injury: a focused review. Am J Phys Med Rehabil 85(7):619–627, 2006

Mac Donald CL, Johnson AM, Cooper D, et al: Detection of blast-related traumatic brain injury in U.S. military personnel. N Engl J Med 364(22):2091–2100, 2011

Management of Concussion/mTBI Working Group: Va/DoD clinical practice guideline: management of concussion/mTBI, U.S. Department of Veterans Affairs, 2009. Available at: http://www.healthquality.va.gov/management_of_concussion_mtbi.asp. Accessed September 24, 2013.

National Center for Posttraumatic Stress Disorder: Report of (VA) consensus conference: practice recommendations for treatment of veterans with comorbid TBI, pain, and PTSD. U.S. Department of Veterans Affairs, 2011. Available at: http://www.mirecc.va.gov/docs/visn6/Report_Consensus_Conf_Practice_ Recommend_TBI_PTSD_Pain.pdf. Accessed September 24, 2013.

O'Phelan K, McArthur DL, Chang CW, et al: The impact of substance abuse on mortality in patients with severe traumatic brain injury. J Trauma 65(3):674–677, 2008

Ouellet MC, Beaulieu-Bonneau S, Morin CM: Insomnia in patients with traumatic brain injury: frequency, characteristics, and risk factors. J Head Trauma Rehabil 21(3):199–212, 2006

Packard RC: Treatment of chronic daily posttraumatic headache with divalproex sodium. Headache 40(9):736–739, 2000

Pakalnis A, Couch J: Headache therapy with botulinum toxin: form over substance. Arch Neurol 65(1):149–151, 2008

Pfaffenrath V, Diener HC, Pageler L, et al: OTC analgesics in headache treatment: open-label phase vs randomized double-blind phase of a large clinical trial. Headache 49(5):638–645, 2009

Pickett TC, Radfar-Baublitz LS, McDonald SD, et al: Objectively assessing balance deficits after TBI: Role of computerized posturography. J Rehabil Res Dev 44(7):983–990, 2007

Rath JF, Simon, D., Langenbahn DM, et al: Group treatment of problem-solving deficits in outpatients with traumatic brain injury: a randomised outcome study. Neuropsychol Rehabil 13(4)461–488, 2003

Ripley DL, Politzer T, Berryman A, et al: The vision clinic: an interdisciplinary method for assessment and treatment of visual problems after traumatic brain injury. NeuroRehabilitation 27(3):231–235, 2010

Rogers JM, Read CA: Psychiatric comorbidity following traumatic brain injury. Brain Inj 21(13–14):1321–1333, 2007

Sandhaug M, Andelic N, Vatne A, et al: Functional level during sub-acute rehabilitation after traumatic brain injury: course and predictors of outcome. Brain Inj 24(5):740–747, 2010

Silberstein SD, Lipton RB, Dodick DW, et al: Efficacy and safety of topiramate for the treatment of chronic migraine: a randomized, double-blind, placebo-controlled trial of quality of life. Headache 47(2):170–180, 2007

Slobounov S, Slobounov E, Sebastianelli W, et al: Differential rate of recovery in athletes after first and second concussion episodes. Neurosurgery 61(2):338–344, 2007

Smits M, Dippel DW, de Haan GG, et al: External validation of the Canadian CT Head Rule and the New Orleans Criteria for CT scanning in patients with minor head injury. JAMA 294(12):1519–1525, 2005

Sommer M, Heidinger Ch, Arendasy M, et al: Cognitive and personality determinants of post-injury driving fitness. Arch Clin Neuropsychol 25(2):99–117, 2010

Sponheim SR, McGuire KA, Kang SS, et al: Evidence of disrupted functional connectivity in the brain after combat-related blast injury. Neuroimage 54 (suppl 1):S21–S29, 2011

Terrio H, Brenner LA, Ivins BJ, et al: Traumatic brain injury screening: preliminary findings in a US Army brigade combat team. J Head Trauma Rehabil 24(1):14–23, 2009

Thaxton L, Myers MA: Sleep disturbances and their management in patients with brain injury. J Head Trauma Rehabil 17(4):335–348, 2002

Thornton KE, Carmody DP: Traumatic brain injury rehabilitation: QEEG biofeedback treatment protocols. Appl Psychophysiol Biofeedback 34(1):59–68, 2009

Vickers AJ, Rees RW, Zollman CE, et al: Acupuncture of chronic headache disorders in primary care: randomised controlled trial and economic analysis. Health Technol Assess 8(48):iii, 1–35, 2004

Vos PE, Jacobs B, Andriessen TM, et al: GFAP and S100B are biomarkers of traumatic brain injury: an observational cohort study. Neurology 75(20):1786–1793, 2010

Vungkhanching M, Heinemann AW, Langley MJ, et al: Feasibility of a skills-based substance abuse prevention program following traumatic brain injury. J Head Trauma Rehabil 22(3):167–176, 2007

Wang HC, Chang WN, Chang HW, et al: Factors predictive of outcome in post-traumatic seizures. J Trauma 64(4):883–888, 2008

Warden DW: Military TBI during the Iraq and Afghanistan wars. J Head Trauma Rehabil 21(5):398–402, 2006

Chapter 10

Suicidal Thoughts and Behaviors in Military Service Members and Veterans

James A. Naifeh, M.D.
Daniel W. Cox, Ph.D.
Matthew N. Goldenberg, M.D.
Matthew K. Nock, Ph.D.

The Problem of Suicidal Behaviors

There are inherent risks of injury and death associated with military service, particularly during times of war. The risks to life and limb associated with combat—from enemy fire, accidents, or other war-related events—are widely understood, expected, and even accepted. Less understood and, perhaps, less expected and accepted are self-inflicted injuries and deaths. Institutional and public concern over suicides and suicidal behavior among U.S. military service members and veterans dates back to at least the Civil War (Lande 2011). Over the course of the conflicts in Iraq and Afghanistan, the rate of suicide in the military surpassed that of the general public for the first time in decades. As a result, there has been widespread attention paid to the mental health issues of service members and veterans and increased scrutiny of the mental health care provided to them as well as intensified efforts aimed at suicide prevention (Kuehn 2009).

Classification of Self-Injurious Thoughts and Behaviors

It is important for both clinicians and researchers to distinguish between the various types of self-injurious thoughts and behaviors (SITB), which have different base rates, risk and protective factors, courses, and treatment outcomes (Brown et al. 2005; Kessler et al. 2005; Linehan et al. 1991; Nock and Kazdin 2002; Nock and Kessler 2006). Among clinicians, a lack of clarity and consistency in terminology hampers efforts to communicate about a patient's history and adequately assess patient risk. Among researchers, a lack of clarity and consistency presents challenges to the reliability and validity of the constructs under examination and complicates efforts to synthesize published literature.

Suicide ideation refers to thoughts about ending one's own life and should generally be considered distinct from passive thoughts about death or dying. Service members and veterans who have been exposed to life-threatening situations and death during combat deployments may experience thoughts about their own mortality or death in general. Such thoughts should not be classified as suicidal unless the content involves self-injury and/or a desire to die. A *suicide plan* refers to the development of a strategy by which one intends to die (e.g., date, time, place, and method). *Suicide attempt* refers to engagement in a potentially self-injurious behavior with intent to die. Given the numerous variations of suicidal SITB that may not cleanly fit into one of these categories, researchers have proposed additional distinctions, including *preparatory acts, aborted suicide attempts,* and *interrupted suicide attempts* (Barber et al. 1998; Marzuk et al. 1997b; Posner et al. 2007).

Not all self-injurious acts are necessarily suicidal. Whereas suicidal SITB involve at least some intent to die, nonsuicidal SITB are focused on the deliberate destruction of one's own body tissue without intent to die (Nock et al. 2008b). Superficial cutting or burning of the skin or hitting oneself are examples of such behaviors. The term *suicide gesture,* first used in reference to soldiers who intentionally injured themselves to escape active military duty (Fisch 1954; Tucker and Gorman 1967), has been used to describe self-injurious behaviors in which an individual seeks to give the appearance of having made a suicide attempt but where there is no actual intent to die. Some people have argued that the term is pejorative and should not be used (Silverman et al. 2007).

Epidemiology of Suicidal Thoughts and Behaviors in the General Population

Suicide is the tenth leading cause of death in the United States, occurring at an annual rate of 11.8 per 100,000 people and accounting for 1.4% of all deaths (National Center for Injury Prevention and Control 2005). Epidemiological data suggest that the lifetime prevalence of suicide ideation in the general population is 5.6%–14.3%. History of developing a suicide plan is reported by 3.9% of the general population, and 1.9%–8.7% report having made one or more suicide attempts (Nock et al. 2008a). Retrospective data suggest that 34% of persons reporting a history of suicide ideation will also make a suicide plan, and the majority (72%) who develop a plan will ultimately make an attempt. Notably, suicide attempts also are reported by 26% of ideators who deny ever making a plan. These transitions—between ideation, plan, and attempt—are most likely to occur within the first year after onset of suicide ideation (Kessler et al. 1999). Among suicide ideators who have not developed a plan or made an attempt, the risk of these transitions occurring decreases over time (Borges et al. 2008).

Epidemiology of Suicidal Thoughts and Behaviors in Military and Veteran Populations

Historically, service members in the U.S. military have experienced a lower suicide rate than civilians of the same age and sex in the general population. This discrepancy may have been due to the military's ability to screen out individuals with preenlistment mental health problems or criminality, both of which are related to increased risk for suicide (Boardman et al. 1999; Harris and Barraclough 1997; Hill et al. 2006). Other military-specific factors, such as universal access to health care, steady employment, and community support, may also have contributed to the military's historically lower rates. However, following the commencement of Operation Iraqi Freedom, the rate of suicide in the U.S. Army began to increase (Hill et al. 2006; Nelson 2004), rising from 9.0 suicides per 100,000 in 2001 to 21.7 per 100,000 in 2009. In 2008, the U.S. Army suicide rate surpassed the matched general population rate for the first time (Kuehn 2009). A similar pattern emerged in the Marine Corps, with the 2001 rate of 16.7 per 100,000 climbing to 22.3 per 100,000 in 2009. Air Force and Navy suicide rates also increased in recent years but remained lower than those of the Army and Marines (Department of Defense Task Force on the Prevention of Suicide by Members of the Armed Forces 2010).

Because of the methodological challenges of conducting suicide research on veterans, the data on this population are less clear (Kaplan et al. 2007). A recent study of all veterans receiving care from the U.S. Department of Veterans Affairs (VA) from 2000 to 2007 found that the suicide rate was significantly higher than that of the age- and gender-adjusted rates in the general U.S. population (Blow et al. 2012). However, because most studies of suicide among veterans have utilized VA health care data, the findings may not be representative of veterans who do not use VA services.

Understanding Suicidal Behaviors

Vulnerability-Stress Model

There is a large and growing body of research on the various factors that affect suicide risk. A *vulnerability-stress model*, variations of which dominate current approaches to suicide research, can facilitate the understanding of how wide-ranging risk factors contribute to suicidal behaviors. Within this conceptual framework, predisposing factors (*vulnerabilities*) interact with environmental events (*stressors*) to trigger suicidal behaviors. Factors identified serve as promising targets for future research with current and former service members.

Vulnerability Factors

Mental Disorders

Research indicates that mental disorders are among the most consistent risk factors for suicidal behavior in the civilian population (Kessler et al. 2005), with the greatest risk conveyed by mood, substance use, impulse control, psychotic, and personality disorders (Hawton et al. 2003; Kessler et al. 1999; Petronis et al. 1990). Although a history of major depression is one of the strongest predictors of suicide ideation, the important transition from ideation to suicide attempt is most strongly associated with disorders characterized by anxiety or agitation and problems with aggression or impulsiveness (Nock et al. 2009). These findings may be particularly relevant to the military, with up to 25% of service members reporting postdeployment psychological problems (Hoge et al. 2004, 2006). Despite the consistency of such findings, most individuals with a mental disorder will never engage in suicidal behaviors (Harris and Barraclough 1997; Nock 2009; Nock et al. 2009), making the consideration of additional risk factors critically important.

Previous Suicidal Behaviors

As is the case with many behavioral phenomena, past suicidal behavior is the strongest predictor of future suicide-related outcomes (Nock 2009), and this association remains significant even after accounting for other well-established risk factors (Joiner et al. 2005). Specifically, persons with a previous suicide attempt are around 40 times more likely to eventually die by suicide than those who have never attempted suicide (Harris and Barraclough 1997). Multiple previous suicide attempts are a particularly strong risk factor for future suicidal behavior (Oquendo et al. 2007), and subsequent attempts tend to increase in severity (Carter et al. 2005).

Psychological Factors

Researchers have also identified more specific psychological risk factors, including personality traits, temperament, and other cognitive-affective states. There is strong evidence for the role of impulsiveness (Zouk et al. 2006), aggressiveness (Nock and Marzuk 2000), hopelessness (Brezo et al. 2006), anhedonia (Nock and Kazdin 2002), and high emotional reactivity (Nock et al. 2008b). Additionally, vulnerabilities related to executive functioning, including difficulties with decision making, problem solving, cognitive flexibility, and verbal fluency (Jollant et al. 2005), appear to be particularly important.

Demographic Factors

Certain demographic factors are associated with an increased risk for suicidal behavior. Although women in the United States are more likely to attempt suicide, men are four times more likely to die by suicide (Nock et al. 2008a). The increased fatality rate among men is likely due to the use of more lethal methods, more aggressiveness, and greater intent to die (Nock and Kessler 2006). In the United States, individuals identified as non-Hispanic white are at greater risk for dying by suicide than other racial or ethnic groups. The suicide rate increases during late adolescence and early adulthood, particularly for white men, and continues at an elevated rate throughout the lifespan (Nock et al. 2008a).

Family History

A family history of mental disorders and suicidal behavior increases risk for suicidal behavior, even after controlling for presence of mental disorders in the offspring (Brent and Mann 2006; Brent et al. 2002). There appears to be a familial predisposition for high-risk traits that is not fully accounted for by psychiatric diagnosis. A parental history of panic disorder, antisocial personality disorder, and suicidal behavior, which are characterized by impulsive aggression and/or high emotional reactivity, are especially predictive of suicidal behavior in offspring (Gureje et al. 2011).

Stressful Life Experiences

Consistent with a *vulnerability-stress model*, the occurrence of suicidal behaviors often follows stressful life events, including recent conflict with a family member or romantic partner, bereavement, and legal or disciplinary problems (Brent et al. 1993; Ritchie et al. 2003; Yen et al. 2005). More chronic stressors, such as pain or illness, are also associated with increased risk (Braden and Sullivan 2008; Druss and Pincus 2000). The role of stressful experiences may be particularly salient in the military, where individuals are likely to be exposed to numerous military-specific stressors during training, deployment, and combat in addition to the life stressors and traumatic events commonly experienced in the general population (Kuehn 2009).

Situational Factors

Specific situations, such as ready access to lethal means (Lester 1998), may interact with vulnerabilities and environmental stressors to further elevate the risk of suicidal behaviors. As a consequence of their training and environment, military service members often have access to and experience with firearms, which are used in more suicides than homicides each year in the United States (Miller and Hemenway 2008) and are the most common method of suicide across all branches of the military (Department of Defense Task Force on the Prevention of Suicide by Members of the Armed Forces 2010). Acute alcohol use is another situational factor that greatly increases the risk and lethality of suicidal behavior (Sher 2006), likely because of disinhibitory effects on cognition and behavior.

Protective Factors

The identification of factors that protect against suicidal behaviors (i.e., those that decrease the probability of suicidal behaviors) has received far less empirical attention than risk factors. Nevertheless, findings from several studies suggest promising targets for intervention and future research.

Psychological Factors

There is a rapidly growing body of research on psychological factors that may protect against negative health outcomes. High emotional intelligence, or the ability to perceive, understand, and manage one's emotions, has been found to nearly eliminate the association between stressful life events and subsequent suicide attempt (Cha and Nock 2009). Among factors that may be protective are stoicism, character strength, hardiness, resilience, world-view, well-being, self-esteem, autonomy, hope, zest, gratitude, and love (i.e., the ability to form reciprocated relationships). There is evidence that such characteristics are associated with posttraumatic growth following exposure to extreme stressors (Peterson et al. 2008).

Social Support

Most research into factors that protect against suicidal behaviors has focused on aspects of the social environment. Religious affiliation (Dervic et al. 2004), responsibility to family members (Oquendo et al. 2005), and being pregnant or having children (Marzuk et al. 1997a; Qin and Mortensen 2003) are all protective against suicidal behavior. Social support within one's unit may be an especially important factor for service members. Perceived unit cohesion (e.g., supportive leadership, strong peer relations) is associated with decreased likelihood of leaving the Army and enhanced perceptions of combat readiness (Griffith 2002; Halverson 1995) and may protect against posttraumatic stress disorder (PTSD) and other psychiatric symptoms (Brailey et al. 2007; Halverson 1995).

Mental Health Treatment

Access to mental health treatment, particularly certain psychotherapies, has also been shown to protect against suicidal behaviors (Mann et al. 2005). However, the effectiveness of such services will likely depend on such factors as the type and adequacy of treatment, the probability and speed of entering treatment, and the perceived barriers to receiving or remaining in treatment (Hoge et al. 2004; Wang et al. 2005, 2007a, 2007b). Although a majority of individuals who die by suicide have contact with a primary care provider in the year before death (Luoma et al. 2002), cross-national population-based data indicate that most individuals with a history of suicide thoughts, plans, or attempts never receive any type of mental health treatment (Bruffaerts et al. 2011).

Suicide Prevention Strategies and Programs

Despite increased focus on suicide prevention within the U.S. Department of Defense (DOD) and the VA, published findings on the effectiveness of suicide prevention programs in these organizations are sparse and inconsistent (Bagley et al. 2010). Prevention programs are generally *universal* (primary), *selected* (secondary), or *indicated* (Mrazek and Haggerty 1994). Universal programs are delivered to an entire population (e.g., all sailors), selected programs are delivered to groups considered at high risk (e.g., postdeployment sailors), and indicated programs are delivered to people with detectable symptoms (e.g., postdeployment sailors with PTSD symptoms). These three categories are not mutually exclusive. For example, the

Army implemented the Applied Suicide Intervention Skills Training for chaplains, behavioral health professionals, and other gatekeepers to teach them to identify soldiers with suicidal thoughts, assess risk, create a safety plan, and follow up (Ramchand et al. 2011). Targeting those who often come in contact with these professionals is *selected prevention* (groups considered high risk), and assessment and intervention with those who report suicidal thoughts is *indicated prevention*.

Many universal programs are implemented online and can be accessed via the DOD/VA Suicide Outreach Web site (http://www.suicideoutreach.org/). On the Marine Corps' suicide prevention Web site, the National Suicide Prevention Lifeline's telephone number is given (http://www.mccsmcrd.com/BehavioralHealth/SuicidePrevention/index.html). Also, training such as the Leaders Guide for Managing Marines in Distress, information on suicide risk factors, and training videos are provided. Other universal programs are provided in person. The Marine Corps' entry-level training in suicide prevention is given to all Marines at boot camp, officer candidate school, and basic school. For enlisted Marines, training on signs, symptoms, and resources is delivered by a drill instructor via two short courses and an interactive discussion. Whether online or in person, these programs aim to teach basic information and/or skills broadly and at a low cost per participant (Ramchand et al. 2011).

Similarly, the VA has universal, selected, and indicated prevention programs. A major difference is that the VA suicide prevention programs target only health professionals, veterans, and veterans' families because the VA, unlike the military, does not have leadership or peers (e.g., fellow soldiers) who can be interventionists. Much of the information on VA programs can be found on the VA's suicide prevention Web site (http://www.mentalhealth.va.gov/suicide_prevention/). There are several practical resources on the Web site, including a suicide risk assessment guide, a veterans' crisis line, and a safety plan treatment manual. All of this information can be accessed and used by providers in the VA system and by those working with veterans in other settings.

Assessment of Suicidal Thoughts and Behaviors

Identifying past and present suicidal thoughts and behaviors has important implications for risk assessment, case conceptualization, and treatment planning. SITB should be assessed as part of a comprehensive evaluation of all patients, not just those believed to be at elevated risk (American Academy of Child and Adolescent Psychiatry 2001; American Psychiatric Association 2003; Nock et al. 2008b). It is recommended that clinicians begin by assessing less sensitive aspects of the patient's history or psychiatric presentation, then proceeding through a hierarchy of SITB severity, from suicide ideation to suicide plans to suicide attempts (Bryan and Rudd 2006; Nock et al. 2008b).

Assessment Instruments

It is recommended that, whenever possible, clinicians conduct the SITB assessment using a structured or semistructured interview with strong psychometric support. For example, the Self-Injurious Thoughts and Behaviors Interview (SITBI; Nock et al. 2007) is a comprehensive structured interview assessing presence and characteristics (e.g., frequency, age of onset) of suicide ideation, plans, gestures, and attempts, as well as nonsuicidal self-injury. The Suicide Attempt Self-Injury Interview (SASII; Linehan et al. 2006a) is a structured interview assessing past episodes of self-injurious behavior (both suicidal and nonsuicidal), including intent, outcome expectations, planning and preparations, contextual and behavioral factors, antecedent events, method, lethality, functional outcomes, and resulting injuries and medical treatment. As a final example, the Scale for Suicide Ideation (SSI; Beck et al. 1979) is a semistructured interview assessing the presence of suicide ideation, including frequency and severity, as well as suicide plans. Additionally, there are a number of self-report (patient-administered) measures that are also useful for assessing SITB, including the Beck Scale for Suicide Ideation (BSSI; Beck and Steer 1991), Adult Suicide Ideation Questionnaire (ASIQ; Reynolds 1991), and Suicidal Behaviors Questionnaire (SBQ; Linehan 1981).

Suicide Attempt Versus Nonsuicidal Self-Injury

Clinicians should attempt to determine whether a patient's self-injurious behavior was actually suicidal. Suicide attempts and nonsuicidal self-injury (NSSI) have distinct clinical features and require different approaches to management. Relative to NSSI, suicidal behaviors are more likely to result in death, and there is increased risk that patients who engage in such behaviors subsequently die by suicide (Harris and Barraclough 1997). By comparison, NSSI is typically less severe, and research suggests that it most often serves an emotion regulatory function (Nock 2009) but may also be performed as a "suicide gesture" (Nock 2008; Nock and Kessler 2006; Tucker and Gorman 1967). In either case, the key feature distinguishing NSSI from suicidal behavior is the absence of intent to die as a result of the behavior. Clinicians are encouraged to assess intent to die with all patients who have engaged in self-injurious behavior. Importantly, a patient's behavior should be considered NSSI only if there is absolutely no evidence of intent to die (Nock and Favazza 2009). Making this determination can be complex, and there is likely to be a significant degree of variability across patients.

Suicide Attempt Versus Accident

In some instances, it may be unclear whether patients' injuries resulted from a suicidal behavior or an accident. Although such uncertainty is more likely following a fatal event, where investigators must infer causality on the basis of clues from records and the report of individuals familiar with the deceased, it may also occur following nonfatal events. Because of the severity of their injuries (e.g., traumatic brain injury) or situational factors present during the event (e.g., severe alcohol intoxication), patients may be unable to communicate or remember whether the event was intentional. Alternatively, some patients may be uncooperative or evasive in discussing the event because of concerns over legal or disciplinary repercussions. In such cases, the clinician will likely have to rely on whatever historical or objective indicators of intent are available.

Assessing Future Risk

Clinicians cannot reliably predict suicidal behaviors regardless of training or clinical experience. Therefore, they must work to find a balance between overestimating risk, which is costly in terms of clinical resources, and underestimating risk, which may threaten patient safety (Bryan and Rudd 2006). These difficult decisions must be informed by thorough assessment that integrates a variety of clinical data. At a minimum, the clinician should collect the following information (American Psychiatric Association 2003; Bryan and Rudd 2006):

- History of SITB, particularly suicide attempts
- Severity of current or recent self-injurious thoughts, particularly intent to die
- Presence of a suicide plan, including articulation of a specific method, lethality of the method, availability of the means to carry it out, and any preparatory acts
- Situational stressors, such as family discord, the breakup of a romantic relationship, financial concerns, and legal or disciplinary problems
- Psychiatric symptoms, such as anxiety, depression, mania, and psychosis
- Psychological factors, with special attention to the presence of hopelessness, impulsiveness, and aggression
- Protective factors, such as the availability of social support and willingness to access it, current treatment involvement and history of treatment compliance, and patient-identified reasons for living

Management of the Suicidal Patient

Hospitalization

Patients who arrive in an emergency department following self-injurious behavior will likely not receive psychiatric aftercare unless a member of the psychiatric service is notified and conducts an adequate evaluation. Thus, it is critical for emergency department staff to have awareness of and basic training in the identification of self-injurious behavior and psychiatric status so that consultations with psychiatric services can be made whenever needed (Hawton 2000). Similarly, given evidence that most individuals who die by suicide have had contact with a primary care provider but not a mental health provider (Luoma et al. 2002), primary care presents an important opportunity to identify and intervene with patients at risk. The VA has begun moving in this direction via primary care screening procedures for depression, PTSD, and substance abuse, with all veterans who screen positive being offered a mental health referral.

Continuity of Care

Psychiatric patients are at especially high risk for suicidal thoughts and behaviors in the weeks and months immediately following discharge from the hospital (Goldacre et al. 1993; Links et al. 2012). Problems with continuity of care in the military have been highlighted in previous reports (Department of Defense Task Force on the Prevention of Suicide by Members of the Armed Forces 2010). Similar breakdowns in care have been identified as influencing civilian suicide deaths (King et al. 2001). For patients who do not follow up with treatment, outreach efforts may be particularly important. A recent study found that among veterans with serious mental illness who had dropped out of VA care, those who returned to treatment after being recontacted by the VA had a significantly lower mortality rate (Davis et al. 2012).

Pharmacotherapy

Although pharmacotherapy is effective in treating many of the psychiatric conditions associated with SITB, it does not appear to be effective at preventing suicidal behaviors (Mann et al. 2005). Clinicians prescribing psychotropic medications for a co-occurring psychiatric disorder should also be mindful of potential misuse. The risk of intentional overdose may be managed through controlling when and how medications are dispensed, including coordination with the patient's family.

Psychotherapy

Certain psychotherapies present promising approaches to preventing suicidal behaviors in persons at risk (Mann et al. 2005). There is evidence that psychological interventions aimed at improving such factors as problem-solving ability and distress tolerance can reduce the likelihood of future suicide attempts in high-risk patients (Brown et al. 2005; Linehan et al. 2006b). A randomized controlled trial found that individuals receiving cognitive-behavioral treatment following a suicide attempt were 50% less likely to reattempt suicide and reported reduced depression and hopelessness (Brown et al. 2005).

Weapons Management

Clinicians should consider ways to restrict access to lethal means for suicidal patients. Ready access to weapons, in particular, poses a threat to patient safety. This is especially challenging in the military, where possession of firearms is not only common but may be an operational requirement. In situations in which firearms restrictions may be stigmatizing, alternatives should be considered, such as removing the firing pin but allowing the service member to maintain possession of the weapon. Command leadership must be involved in such decisions because of their operational impact. In addition to the patient's personal weapons, access to others' weapons must also be considered and may require coordination with family members and unit leadership.

Safety Planning and Contracts

When hospitalization is not clinically indicated, suicidal patients presenting to emergency departments and other acute care settings will typically be referred to outpatient mental health treatment (Allen et al. 2002). Unfortunately, many patients will not follow up on these referrals after being discharged (Krulee and Hales 1988), creating a need for very brief interventions that are deliverable during acute care. One brief intervention, commonly referred to as a "no suicide" or "no harm" contract, is a written or verbal agreement between the patient and clinician whereby the patient agrees not to engage in suicidal behaviors. Despite their use in treatment settings, contracts lack empirical support in the prevention of suicidal behavior (Kelly and Knudson 2000; Reid 1998; Stanford et al. 1994). Safety plans, on the other hand, may offer a more robust option for intervention that provides patients with prioritized strategies and resources for managing suicidal thoughts. Stanley and Brown developed a 20- to 45-minute safety planning intervention and subsequently adapted it for use with veterans under the name SAFE VET. This treatment manual is available at http://www.mentalhealth.va.gov/docs/VA_Safety_planning_manual.pdf (accessed March 26, 2012). In developing a safety plan, clinicians work collaboratively with the patient to identify internal and external warning signs that may trigger suicidal thoughts and behaviors, develop a hierarchical plan for managing these warning signs and any suicidal thoughts, and develop a plan for restricting access to lethal means (Stanley and Brown 2008).

Clinical Documentation

Although mental health providers are accustomed to documenting their clinical decisions and treatment plans, thorough documentation is especially important for patients who are suicidal or believed to be at high risk for suicidal behaviors. Clinicians should clearly explain their decisions related to hospitalization, pharmacological and psychotherapeutic interventions, restriction of lethal means, consultation with other providers and/or military commanders, discharge, aftercare, and safety plans. They should also document whether and how family and friends have agreed to support the patient's care (e.g., as the custodian of the patient's firearms). Clinicians should remain mindful that such documentation must hold up under legal scrutiny.

Clinical Practice Guidelines

There are several professional resources for providers looking for further guidance in the assessment and management of suicidal thoughts and behaviors. Clinical practice guidelines have been developed by the American Psychiatric Association (2003) and the American Academy of Child and Adolescent Psychiatry (2001). The VA and DOD have collaborated on the development of clinical practice guidelines for numerous physical and mental health conditions, including suicidality (available online at www.healthquality.va.gov). Additionally, the *Air Force Guide for Managing Suicidal Behavior* offers DOD-relevant guidance as well as tools and resources for providers (available at http://www.airforcecounseling.com/downloads/misc-guides/air-force-guide-for-managing-suicidal-behavior/).

Conclusions

Suicidal behaviors are a significant concern for clinicians, military and veteran organizations, and society as a whole. These phenomena have multiple determinants, and the interactions among preexisting vulnerabilities, stressors, and protective factors appear to be complex. Thorough assessment is important for identifying the presence and future risk of self-injurious thoughts and behaviors; however, accurate prediction is and likely will remain an elusive goal. Mitigation of suicidal behaviors is possible through the continued development and dissemination of evidence-based prevention and treatment strategies. Pharmacological interventions have yet to demonstrate efficacy in preventing future suicidal behavior, but several psychotherapeutic interventions show promising results.

SUMMARY POINTS

- It is important for both clinicians and researchers to distinguish between the various types of self-injurious thoughts and behaviors, which have different base rates, risk and protective factors, courses, and treatment outcomes.

- Within a *vulnerability-stress model*, predisposing factors (*vulnerabilities*) are thought to interact with environmental events (*stressors*) to trigger suicidal behaviors.

- Vulnerability factors that contribute to suicidal behavior include mental disorders, previous suicidal behaviors, psychological factors, demographic factors, family history, stressful life experiences, and situational factors.

- The DOD and the VA have developed a variety of universal, selected, and indicated prevention programs to address higher rates of suicidal behavior in service members and veterans.

- Effective management of suicide risk requires thorough assessment of all patients, knowledgeable medical staff, continuity of care, empirically supported interventions, weapons management, accurate clinical documentation, and familiarity with clinical practice guidelines.

References

Allen MH, Forster F, Zealberg J, et al: Report and recommendations regarding psychiatric emergency and crisis services: a review and model program descriptions. Washington, DC, American Psychiatric Association Task Force on Psychiatric Emergency Services, 2002

American Academy of Child and Adolescent Psychiatry: Practice parameter for the assessment and treatment of children and adolescents with suicidal behavior. J Am Acad Child Adolesc Psychiatry 40 (suppl 7):24S–51S, 2001

American Psychiatric Association: Practice guideline for the assessment and treatment of patients with suicidal behaviors. Am J Psychiatry 160 (suppl 11):1–60, 2003 [erratum Am J Psychiatry 16(4):776, 2004]

Bagley SC, Munjas B, Shekelle P: A systematic review of suicide prevention programs for military or veterans. Suicide Life Threat Behav 40(3):257–265, 2010

Barber ME, Marzuk PM, Leon AC, et al: Aborted suicide attempts: a new classification of suicidal behavior. Am J Psychiatry 155(3):385–389, 1998

Beck AT, Steer RA: Manual for the Beck Scale for Suicide Ideation. San Antonio, TX, Psychological Corporation, 1991

Beck AT, Kovacs M, Weissman A: Assessment of suicidal intention: the Scale for Suicide Ideation. J Consult Clin Psychol 47(2):343–352, 1979

Blow FC, Bohnert ASB, Ilgen MA, et al: Suicide mortality among patients treated by the Veterans Health Administration from 2000 to 2007. Am J Public Health 102 (suppl 1):S98–S104, 2012

Boardman AP, Grimbaldeston AH, Handley C, et al: The North Staffordshire Suicide Study: a case-control study of suicide in one health district. Psychol Med 29(1):27–33, 1999

Borges G, Angst J, Nock MK, et al: Risk factors for the incidence and persistence of suicide-related outcomes: a 10-year follow-up study using the National Comorbidity Surveys. J Affect Disord 105(1–3):25–33, 2008

Braden JB, Sullivan MD: Suicidal thoughts and behavior among adults with self-reported pain conditions in the National Comorbidity Survey Replication. J Pain 9(12):1106–1115, 2008

Brailey K, Vasterling JJ, Proctor SP, et al: PTSD symptoms, life events, and unit cohesion in U.S. soldiers: baseline findings from the neurocognition deployment health study. J Trauma Stress 20(4):495–503, 2007

Brent DA, Mann JJ: Familial pathways to suicidal behavior: understanding and preventing suicide among adolescents. N Engl J Med 355(26):2719–2721, 2006

Brent DA, Perper JA, Moritz G, et al: Stressful life events, psychopathology, and adolescent suicide: a case control study. Suicide Life Threat Behav 23(3):179–187, 1993

Brent DA, Oquendo M, Birmaher B, et al: Familial pathways to early-onset suicide attempt; risk for suicidal behavior in offspring of mood-disordered suicide attempters. Arch Gen Psychiatry 59:801–807, 2002

Brezo J, Paris J, Turecki G: Personality traits as correlates of suicidal ideation, suicide attempts, and suicide completions: a systematic review. Acta Psychiatr Scand 113(3):180–206, 2006

Brown GK, Ten Have T, Henriques GR, et al: Cognitive therapy for the prevention of suicide attempts: a randomized controlled trial. JAMA 294(5):563–570, 2005

Bruffaerts R, Demyttenaere K, Hwang I, et al: Treatment of suicidal people around the world. Br J Psychiatry 199(1):64–70, 2011

Bryan CJ, Rudd MD: Advances in the assessment of suicide risk. J Clin Psychol 62(2):185–200, 2006

Carter G, Reith DM, Whyte IM: Repeated self-poisoning: increasing severity of self-harm as a predictor of subsequent suicide. Br J Psychiatry 186:253–257, 2005 doi:10.1192/bjp.186.3.253

Cha C, Nock M: Emotional intelligence is a protective factor for suicidal behavior. J Am Acad Child Adolesc Psychiatry 48(4):422–430, 2009 doi:10.1097/CHI.0b013e3181984f44

Davis CL, Kilbourne AM, Blow FC, et al: Reduced mortality among Department of Veterans Affairs patients with schizophrenia or bipolar disorder lost to follow-up and engaged in active outreach to return for care. Am J Public Health 102 (suppl 1):S74–S79, 2012

Department of Defense Task Force on the Prevention of Suicide by Members of the Armed Forces: The challenge and the promise: strengthening the force, preventing suicide and saving lives. Washington, DC, U.S. Department of Defense, 2010

Dervic K, Oquendo MA, Grunebaum MF, et al: Religious affiliation and suicide attempt. Am J Psychiatry 161(12):2303–2308, 2004 doi:10.1176/appi.ajp.161.12.2303

Druss B, Pincus H: Suicidal ideation and suicide attempts in general medical illnesses. Arch Intern Med 160(10):1522–1526, 2000

Fisch M: The suicidal gesture; a study of 114 military patients hospitalized because of abortive suicide attempts. Am J Psychiatry 111(1):33–36, 1954

Goldacre M, Seagroatt V, Hawton K: Suicide after discharge from psychiatric inpatient care. Lancet 342(8866):283–286, 1993

Griffith J: Multilevel analysis of cohesion's relation to stress, well-being, identification, disintegration, and perceived combat readiness. Mil Psychol 14(3):217–239, 2002

Gureje O, Oladeji B, Hwang I, et al: Parental psychopathology and the risk of suicidal behavior in their offspring: results from the World Mental Health surveys. Mol Psychiatry 16(12):1221–1233, 2011

Halverson RR: Psychological well-being and physical health symptoms of soldiers deployed for Operation Uphold Democracy: a summary of human dimensions research in Haiti. Fort Belvoir, VA, Defense Technical Information Center, 1995

Harris EC, Barraclough B: Suicide as an outcome for mental disorders. A meta-analysis. Br J Psychiatry 170:205–228, 1997

Hawton K: General hospital management of suicide attempters, in The International Handbook of Suicide and Attempted Suicide. Edited by Hawton K, van Heeringen, K. Chichester, UK, Wiley, 2000, pp 519–537

Hawton K, Houston K, Haw C, et al: Comorbidity of Axis I and Axis II disorders in patients who attempted suicide. Am J Psychiatry 160(8):1494–1500, 2003

Hill JV, Johnson RC, Barton RA: Suicidal and homicidal soldiers in deployment environments. Mil Med 171(3):228–232, 2006

Hoge CW, Castro CA, Messer SC, et al: Combat duty in Iraq and Afghanistan, mental health problems, and barriers to care. N Engl J Med 351(1):13–22, 2004 doi:10.1056/NEJMoa040603

Hoge CW, Auchterlonie JL, Milliken CS: Mental health problems, use of mental health services, and attrition from military service after returning from deployment to Iraq or Afghanistan. JAMA 295(9):1023–1032, 2006

Joiner TE Jr, Conwell Y, Fitzpatrick KK, et al: Four studies on how past and current suicidality relate even when "everything but the kitchen sink" is covaried. J Abnorm Psychol 114(2):291–303, 2005 doi:10.1037/0021-843X.114.2.291

Jollant F, Bellivier F, Leboyer M, et al: Impaired decision making in suicide attempters. Am J Psychiatry 162(2):304–310, 2005 doi:10.1176/appi.ajp.162.2.304

Kaplan MS, Huguet N, McFarland BH, et al: Suicide among male veterans: a prospective population-based study. J Epidemiol Community Health 61(7):619–624, 2007 doi:10.1136/jech.2006.054346

Kelly KT, Knudson MP: Are no-suicide contracts effective in preventing suicide in suicidal patients seen by primary care physicians? Arch Fam Med 9(10):1119–1121, 2000

Kessler RC, Borges G, Walters EE: Prevalence of and risk factors for lifetime suicide attempts in the National Comorbidity Survey. Arch Gen Psychiatry 56(7):617–626, 1999

Kessler RC, Berglund P, Borges G, et al: Trends in suicide ideation, plans, gestures, and attempts in the United States, 1990–1992 to 2001–2003. JAMA 293(20):2487–2495, 2005 doi:10.1001/jama.293.20.2487

King EA, Baldwin DS, Sinclair JMA, et al: The Wessex Recent In-Patient Suicide Study, 1. Case-control study of 234 recently discharged psychiatric patient suicides. Br J Psychiatry 178:531–536, 2001

Krulee DA, Hales RE: Compliance with psychiatric referrals from a general hospital psychiatry outpatient clinic. Gen Hosp Psychiatry 10(5):339–345, 1988

Kuehn BM: Soldier suicide rates continue to rise: military, scientists work to stem the tide. JAMA 301(11):1111–1113, 2009 doi:10.1001/jama.2009.342

Lande RG: Felo De Se: soldier suicides in America's Civil War. Mil Med 176(5):531–536, 2011

Lester D: Preventing suicide by restricting access to methods for suicide. Arch Suicide Res 4:7–24, 1998

Linehan MM: Suicidal behaviors questionnaire. Unpublished inventory. Seattle, University of Washington, 1981

Linehan MM, Armstrong HE, Suarez A, et al: Cognitive-behavioral treatment of chronically parasuicidal borderline patients. Arch Gen Psychiatry 48(12):1060–1064, 1991

Linehan MM, Comtois KA, Brown MZ, et al: Suicide Attempt Self-Injury Interview (SASII): development, reliability, and validity of a scale to assess suicide attempts and intentional self-injury. Psychol Assess 18(3):303–312, 2006a doi:10.1037/1040-3590.18.3.303

Linehan MM, Comtois KA, Murray AM, et al: Two-year randomized controlled trial and follow-up of dialectical behavior therapy vs therapy by experts for suicidal behaviors and borderline personality disorder. Arch Gen Psychiatry 63(7):757–766, 2006b doi:10.1001/archpsyc.63.7.757

Links P, Nisenbaum R, Ambreen M, et al: Prospective study of risk factors for increased suicide ideation and behavior following recent discharge. Gen Hosp Psychiatry 34(1):88–97, 2012

Luoma JB, Martin CE, Pearson JL: Contact with mental health and primary care providers before suicide: a review of the evidence. Am J Psychiatry 159(6):909–916, 2002

Mann JJ, Apter A, Bertolote J, et al: Suicide prevention strategies: a systematic review. JAMA 294(16):2064–2074, 2005 doi:10.1001/jama.294.16.2064

Marzuk PM, Tardiff K, Leon AC, et al: Lower risk of suicide during pregnancy. Am J Psychiatry 154(1):122–123, 1997a

Marzuk PM, Tardiff K, Leon AC, et al: The prevalence of aborted suicide attempts among psychiatric in-patients. Acta Psychiatr Scand 96(6):492–496, 1997b

Miller M, Hemenway D: Guns and suicide in the United States. N Engl J Med 359(10):989–991, 2008 doi:10.1056/NEJMp0805923

Mrazek PJ, Haggerty RJ: Reducing Risks for Mental Disorders: Frontiers for Preventive Intervention Research. Washington, DC, National Academy Press, 1994

National Center for Injury Prevention and Control: Web-based Injury Statistics Query and Reporting System (WISQARS). Centers for Disease Control and Prevention, 2005. Available at: www.cdc.gov/ncipc/wisqars. Accessed June 28, 2012

Nelson R: Suicide rates rise among soldiers in Iraq. Lancet 363(9405):300, 2004 doi:10.1016/S0140–6736(03)15428-1

Nock MK: Actions speak louder than words: an elaborated theoretical model of the social functions of self-injury and other harmful behaviors. Appl Prev Psychol 12(4):159–168, 2008 doi:10.1016/j.appsy.2008.05.002

Nock MK: Why do people hurt themselves? New insights into the nature and functions of self-injury. Curr Dir Psychol Sci 18(2):78–83, 2009 doi:10.1111/j.1467-8721.2009.01613.x

Nock MK, Favazza AR: Nonsuicidal self-injury: definition and classification, in Understanding Nonsuicidal Self-Injury: Origins, Assessment, and Treatment. Edited by Nock MK. Arlington, VA, American Psychological Association, 2009, pp 9–18

Nock MK, Kazdin AE: Examination of affective, cognitive, and behavioral factors and suicide-related outcomes in children and young adolescents. J Clin Child Adolesc Psychol 31(1):48–58, 2002

Nock MK, Kessler RC: Prevalence of and risk factors for suicide attempts versus suicide gestures: analysis of the National Comorbidity Survey. J Abnorm Psychol 115(3):616–623, 2006 doi:10.1037/0021-843X.115.3.616

Nock MK, Marzuk PM: Suicide and violence, in The International Handbook of Suicide and Attempted Suicide. Edited by Hawton K, van Heeringen K. Chichester, UK, Wiley, 2000, pp 437–456

Nock MK, Holmberg EB, Photos VI, et al: Self-injurious thoughts and behaviors interview: development, reliability, and validity in an adolescent sample. Psychol Assess 19(3):309–317, 2007 doi:10.1037/1040-3590.19.3.309

Nock MK, Borges G, Bromet EJ, et al: Suicide and suicidal behavior. Epidemiol Rev 30:133–154, 2008a doi:10.1093/epirev/mxn002

Nock MK, Wedig MM, Janis IB, et al: Self-injurious thoughts and behaviors, in A Guide to Assessments That Work. Edited by Hunsley J, Mash EJ. New York, Oxford University Press, 2008b, pp 158–177

Nock MK, Hwang I, Sampson N, et al: Cross-national analysis of the associations among mental disorders and suicidal behavior: findings from the WHO World Mental Health Surveys. PLoS Med 6(8):e1000123, 2009 doi:10.1371/journal.pmed.1000123

Oquendo MA, Dragatsi D, Harkavy-Friedman J, et al: Protective factors against suicidal behavior in Latinos. J Nerv Ment Dis 193(7):438–443, 2005

Oquendo MA, Bongiovi-Garcia ME, Galfalvy H, et al: Sex differences in clinical predictors of suicidal acts after major depression: a prospective study. Am J Psychiatry 164(1):134–141, 2007 doi:10.1176/appi.ajp.164.1.134

Peterson C, Park N, Pole N, et al: Strengths of character and posttraumatic growth. J Trauma Stress 21(2):214–217, 2008 doi:10.1002/jts.20332

Petronis KR, Samuels JF, Moscicki EK, et al: An epidemiologic investigation of potential risk factors for suicide attempts. Soc Psychiatry Psychiatr Epidemiol 25(4):193–199, 1990

Posner K, Oquendo MA, Gould M, et al: Columbia Classification Algorithm of Suicide Assessment (C-CASA): classification of suicidal events in the FDA's pediatric suicidal risk analysis of antidepressants. Am J Psychiatry 164(7):1035–1043, 2007 doi:10.1176/appi.ajp.164.7.1035

Qin P, Mortensen PB: The impact of parental status on the risk of completed suicide. Arch Gen Psychiatry 60(8):797–802, 2003 doi:10.1001/archpsyc.60.8.797

Ramchand R, Acosta J, Burns RM, et al: The War Within: Preventing Suicide in the U.S. Military. Santa Monica, CA, RAND, 2011

Reid WH: Promises, promises: don't rely on patients' no-suicide/no-violence "contracts." J Pract Psychiatry Behav Health 4:316–318, 1998

Reynolds W: ASIQ, Adult Suicidal Ideation Questionnaire: Professional Manual. Odessa, FL, Psychological Assessment Resources, 1991

Ritchie EC, Keppler WC, Rothberg JM: Suicidal admissions in the United States military. Mil Med 168(3):177–181, 2003

Sher L: Alcohol consumption and suicide. QJM 99(1):57–61, 2006 doi:10.1093/qjmed/hci146

Silverman MM, Berman AL, Sanddal ND, et al: Rebuilding the tower of Babel: a revised nomenclature for the study of suicide and suicidal behaviors, part 1: background, rationale, and methodology. Suicide Life Threat Behav 37(3):248–263, 2007 doi:10.1521/suli.2007.37.3.248

Stanford EJ, Goetz RR, Bloom JD: The No Harm Contract in the emergency assessment of suicidal risk. J Clin Psychiatry 55(8):344–348, 1994

Stanley B, Brown GK: The safety plan treatment manual to reduce suicide risk: Veteran version. Washington, DC, U.S. Department of Veterans Affairs, 2008

Tucker GJ, Gorman ER: The significance of the suicide gesture in the military. Am J Psychiatry 123(7):854–861, 1967

Wang PS, Berglund P, Olfson M, et al: Failure and delay in initial treatment contact after first onset of mental disorders in the National Comorbidity Survey Replication. Arch Gen Psychiatry 62(6)603–613, 2005

Wang PS, Aguilar-Gaxiola S, Alonso J, et al: Use of mental health services for anxiety, mood, and substance disorders in 17 countries in the WHO world mental health surveys. Lancet 370(9590):841–850, 2007a doi:10.1016/S0140-6736(07)61414-7

Wang PS, Angermeyer M, Borges G, et al: Delay and failure in treatment seeking after first onset of mental disorders in the World Health Organization's World Mental Health Survey Initiative. World Psychiatry 6(3):177–185, 2007b

Yen S, Pagano ME, Shea MT, et al: Recent life events preceding suicide attempts in a personality disorder sample: findings from the collaborative longitudinal personality disorders study. J Consult Clin Psychol 73(1):99–105, 2005 doi:10.1037/0022-006X.73.1.99

Zouk H, Tousignant M, Seguin M, et al: Characterization of impulsivity in suicide completers: clinical, behavioral and psychosocial dimensions. J Affect Disord 92(2–3):195–204, 2006 doi:10.1016/j.jad.2006.01.016

Chapter 11

Collaborative Care

Mitigating Stigma and Other Barriers to Care Through Mental Health Service Delivery in Primary Care Settings

Justin Curry, Ph.D.
Charles Engel, M.D., M.P.H.
Doug Zatzick, M.D.

MENTAL HEALTH DISORDERS and associated psychosocial problems are endemic among civilian and active duty military and veteran populations in the United States (Kessler et al. 2005a, 2005b) and worldwide (WHO International Consortium in Psychiatric Epidemiology 2000; World Health Organization 2001). There is a growing evidence base, however, suggesting that common mental health disorders respond to both pharmacological and psychotherapeutic interventions. Curiously, a large proportion of individuals with mental health disorders who would likely benefit from such interventions neither seek out nor receive treatment.

In these high-risk active duty military and veteran populations, current research indicates that between 23% and 57% of psychiatric needs go unmet (Chermack et al. 2008; Fikretoglu et al. 2008; Hankin et al. 1999; Hoge et al. 2004, 2006; Seal et al. 2010; Taniellan and Jaycox 2008). Moreover, when care is received, it is frequently suboptimal as a result of treatment dropout and/or nonadherence to medication regimens (Seal et al. 2010; Taniellan and Jaycox 2008). This is particularly concerning when one considers that active duty service members and military veterans with mental health disorders have access to some of the nation's most comprehensive health care. This striking gap between needs and services has led to calls for changes in health service delivery systems and reform of current models of health care delivery (Burman et al. 2009).

In this chapter, we draw attention to the link between barriers to care (particularly stigma associated with mental health care) and suppressed treatment seeking and service delivery rates. We discuss the emerging rubric of collaborative care health service models and argue that such models offer a promising solution to fill the gap between needs and services by directly addressing actual and perceived barriers to care. Finally, we present specific case studies of collaborative care implementation in both active duty military and U.S. Department of Veterans Affairs (VA) settings illustrating the effectiveness of health systems innovation that expands the reach of service delivery without compromising treatment efficacy.

Barriers to Care

The concept of barriers to care has been used to explain, at least in part, the striking disparity between observed psychiatric need and actual service utilization (Burman et al. 2009; Hoge et al. 2004; Seal et al. 2011). Fundamentally, *barriers to care* may be defined as any factor or collection of factors, either endogenous or exogenous, that tend to exert an inhibitory effect on treatment-seeking behavior and/or treatment adherence. Consequently, barriers to care make it less likely that persons in need of treatment will actually receive it.

Broadly speaking, barriers to care fall into two general categories: 1) those that are internal and have to do with the patients' attitudes, beliefs, or knowledge; and 2) those that are external and have more to do with access, logistics, and policy. Of course, some barriers to care do not neatly parse into such arbitrary categories and consist of an amalgamation of both internal and external factors.

Barriers to care may apply to any sort of treatment or health condition and across population groups. External barriers to care may include distance to appropriate treatment facilities, availability of child care, ability to take time off of work, access to qualified specialty health care providers, wait times at specialty care clinics, insurance and managed care policies controlling referrals to specialty care, and availability of after-hours or weekend appointment times, among others. Common general internal barriers to care include distrust of medical professionals or systems, a lack of awareness of one's illness or condition, a lack of knowledge of treatment options, inaccurate beliefs regarding the treatability of an illness, a belief that one can address the health issue without assistance, or an unwillingness to acknowledge that a health condition exists. Stigma (to be discussed in greater detail in the following section) around having a health condition is an especially common barrier to care that has both internal and external characteristics, is particularly relevant to the question of mental health issues, and may disproportionately impact military and veteran populations.

As with stigma, certain barriers to care regarding mental health issues may be particularly relevant in military and veteran populations. Burman et al. (2009, p. 775) pointed out that military culture "promotes pride in inner strength, self-reliance, toughness, and being able to 'shake off' ailments or injuries." Consequently, help-seeking behavior may be particularly difficult for military populations, and this cultural bias may extend into civilian life as active duty service members transition to veteran status. Research suggests that the single largest barrier to care among military service members is an unwillingness to acknowledge the existence of a mental health issue. In U.S. service members who screened positive for targeted mental disorders, only between 17.1% and 19.5% acknowledged having a problem (Hoge et al. 2004). Similarly, in Canadian peacekeepers, researchers found that an even smaller proportion (4.5%–16%) of those screening positive for a mental health condition actually endorsed the presence of a psychiatric concern (Fikretoglu et al. 2008).

In addition to this observed reluctance to acknowledge reported symptoms as problematic and therefore worthy of care, some of the other most common barriers to care cited by military personnel include a lack of trust in military health care, administration, or social services (Fikretoglu et al. 2008; Hoge et al. 2004; Maguen and Litz 2006); not knowing where to go for mental health treatment (Hoge et al. 2004; Maguen and Litz 2006); the cost of mental health care (Fikretoglu et al. 2008; Hoge et al. 2004; Maguen and Litz 2006); the perceived inconvenience of seeking mental health care (Fikretoglu et al. 2008; Hoge et al. 2004; Maguen and Litz 2006); a belief that mental health care is ineffective (Hoge et al. 2004; Maguen and Litz 2006); concern about what others might think or how they might act if they knew that one was in treatment for a psychiatric issue (Fikretoglu et al. 2008; Hoge et al. 2004; Maguen and Litz 2006); and concern regarding the impact that mental health care may have on one's career (Burman et al. 2009; Hoge et al. 2004). Strikingly, military service personnel with self-reported psychiatric symptoms are significantly more likely to endorse a greater number of barriers to care than are those military personnel without such symptoms (Hoge et al. 2004; Maguen and Litz 2006).

Although internal barriers to care seem to be most prevalent in active duty populations, veterans and their providers appear to recognize a greater number of external barriers to care while also endorsing several internal concerns (many of the latter related to stigma) (Table 11–1). Research suggests that important external barriers to care endorsed by veterans include lack of access to services (particularly for rural veterans), lack of time to travel to and attend health care appointments, difficulty securing child care during scheduled treatment visits, and financial constraints (Sayer et al. 2009b). Researchers have noted that younger veterans, including those who have served in Iraq or Afghanistan, frequently view the VA health system as designed for and catering to older and more visibly injured veterans (Sayer et al. 2009a; Taniellan and Jaycox 2008).

TABLE 11-1. Frequently endorsed barriers to care

General population

Internal	External
Distrust of medical professionals or systems	Travel or distance to treatment facilities
Lack of awareness of one's illness or condition	Unavailability of child care
Lack of knowledge of treatment options and inaccurate beliefs regarding the treatability of an illness	Work schedule conflicts
	Unavailability of qualified specialty health care providers
	Wait times
Belief that one can address the health issue without assistance	Insurance and managed care policies
	Unavailability of after-hours or weekend appointment times
Unwillingness to acknowledge that a health condition exists	**Stigma**
Stigma	

Military and veteran populations

Internal	External
Unwillingness to acknowledge the existence of a mental health issue	Military culture promoting self-reliance and self-sufficiency
Avoidance of trauma-related feelings and memories	Invalidating posttrauma sociocultural environment
Values and priorities that conflict with treatment seeking	Travel or distance to treatment facilities[a]
	Real career impacts
Lack of trust in military health care, administration, or social services	Work schedule conflicts[a]
Knowledge barriers	Unavailability of qualified specialty health care providers[a]
Perceived inconvenience of seeking mental health care	Access barriers[a]
	Cost of mental health care[a]
Belief that mental health care is ineffective	**Stigma**
Concern regarding the impact that mental health care may have on one's career	
Other treatment-discouraging beliefs	
Stigma	

[a]Particularly relevant to veteran populations.

Sayer et al. (2009a) described seven major categories of barriers to care endorsed by veterans with posttraumatic stress disorder (PTSD). These categories include both endogenous and exogenous factors and help illustrate the complexity of the relationship between barriers to care and treatment-seeking behavior. They include avoidance of trauma-related feelings and memories, values and priorities that conflict with treatment seeking, treatment-discouraging beliefs, health care system concerns, knowledge barriers, access barriers, and an invalidating posttrauma sociocultural environment.

Clinician Notes on Barriers to Care and Mental Health

- Barriers to care inhibit treatment-seeking behavior and include both contextual or environmental (i.e., external) factors and psychological or interpersonal (i.e., internal) factors.

- Clinicians can mitigate the impact of barriers to care through adjustments to practice structure.

- Clinicians have more ability to influence external barriers to care than they do internal barriers to care:

  - Consider adjusting clinic hours to accommodate "after-hours" appointments.

  - Consider providing on-site child care services at clinics.

- Clinicians can also influence internal barriers to care:

  - Remind patients that mental health treatments are effective and are supported by research.

  - Listen to patients' concerns about mental health treatment and discuss them.

  - Remind patients that mental illness is not a character flaw and that treatment seeking is a sign of strength and resilience.

- Consider adopting collaborative care models of practice:

  - Address external barriers to care by colocating specialty care within primary care settings or by extending service delivery through telephone case management services.

  - Address internal barriers to care by reducing reliance on specialty care referrals and allowing more issues to be addressed in the primary care setting.

  - Enhance patients' experience of care and care continuity by creating robust primary care clinic service delivery models.

Stigma

Stigma, particularly as it relates to individuals with mental illness, and its effects on access to mental health services have been the subject of frequent study. Conceptually, stigma may be described as a theoretical construct consisting of four critical elements: cues, stereotypes, prejudice, and discriminatory behavior (Corrigan 2004) (Figure 11–1). At the same time, stigma may be further categorized by the functional space in which it is operative: public stigma (the influence of stigma as it is applied by others to a stigmatized individual or group) and self-stigma (the influence of stigma as it is internalized by one with a certain condition).

Of course, stigma is more than a theoretical construct. It is a process with actual consequences for both those who are stigmatized and those who hold stigmatizing beliefs. People who are stigmatized have a lower overall quality of life (Alonso et al. 2009; Rüsch et al. 2010), lower self-esteem (Marcussen et al. 2010), and lower sense of mastery (Marcussen et al. 2010) and experience significant work and role limitations (Alonso et al. 2009) and greater social limitations (Alonso et al. 2009).

Generally, attempts at stigma reduction have fallen into three categories: 1) protest (presenting information that is discordant with or is inconsistent with stigmatizing beliefs or self-image), 2) education (providing accurate information about psychiatric conditions at a public or population level, often through public health campaigns), and 3) contact (providing direct interpersonal contact with people with mental illness (often through taped media but also through in vivo exposure) in an effort to enhance opinions and dispel stereotypes. Of these intervention categories, protest strategies appear to be ineffective, education strategies appear to have meaningful but transient impacts, and contact strategies appear to offer the greatest promise (Brown et al. 2010).

Today, there is abundant evidence that stigma remains a significant impediment to treatment-seeking behavior in U.S. and allied active and Reserve components (Hoge et al. 2004; Iversen et al. 2011; Stecker et al. 2007) and that service members with psychiatric conditions are less likely to self-report psychiatric symptoms (Warner et al. 2011) or seek assistance and are more likely to endorse other barriers to care. Furthermore, preference for and access to mental health treatment are insufficient facilitators to overcome the inhibitory effects of stigma on service utilization (Stecker et al. 2007). Finally, the negative effects of stigma appear not to decrease as service members transition to veteran status (Iversen et al. 2011).

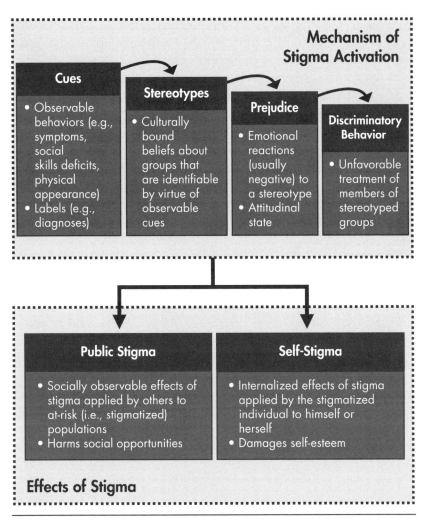

FIGURE 11–1.   Corrigan's theoretical model of stigma.

Within the military setting, stigma is reinforced by the very real potential consequences of receiving psychiatric diagnoses, including early separation, suspension of security clearances, and duty restriction prohibiting certain military job requirements (e.g., loss of flight status for aviators and aviation crew members). However, the impacts of stigma on military personnel appear to be at least partially mediated by certain military-specific variables. In particular, the perceived quality of unit leadership (Greene-Shortridge et al. 2007; Wright et al. 2009), the presence of a "family friendly" unit environment (Greene-Shortridge et al. 2007), and positive perceptions of unit support for treatment (Pietrzak et al. 2009) and unit cohesion (Wright et al. 2009) are all associated with lower levels of perceived stigma. Furthermore, if service members do engage in treatment, there is some evidence to suggest that perceived stigma is reduced (Greene-Shortridge et al. 2007).

Although interventions aimed at reducing stigma appear to have promise, they are likely to be slow to develop, and service members and veterans with problems now can ill afford to wait for treatment. Which interventions, then, can be implemented immediately that will both increase the reach of military and veteran health services to include those currently not being served and likely decrease important barriers to care that not only inhibit treatment initiation but also adversely affect treatment adherence and completion? A promising set of solutions to this question can be found in collaborative care.

Clinician Notes on Stigma and Mental Health

- The term *stigma* refers to the constellation of negative attitudes, beliefs, and behaviors that surround socially undesirable conditions.

- Stigma, or, more accurately, the fear of stigma, is an important barrier to care that assumes added significance in military and veteran populations.

- Clinically, stigma is most relevant as an impediment to identification and treatment initiation for mental health issues.

- To a lesser extent, stigma may also contribute to early discontinuation of therapeutic services.

- Because stigma is a complex and socially constructed issue, clinicians are limited in their ability to mitigate its effects.

- Clinicians can take steps, however, to limit the effects of public stigma:

  - Engage clinic staff in in-service instruction efforts providing education about mental illness and people with psychiatric diagnoses.

  - Dispel myths among clinic staff that mental illness is dangerous, unchangeable, and/or treatment resistant.

  - Provide training to staff on how to engage patients with mental health conditions in a sensitive and supportive manner.

- Clinicians can structure provider-patient interactions to reduce the impact of self-stigma:

  - Institute universal confidential screening for common mental health disorders to counteract stigma-driven underreporting of mental health symptoms.

  - Emphasize that treatments for psychiatric conditions are effective.

  - Encourage patients to discuss their experience dealing with psychiatric symptoms.

- Consider adopting collaborative care models of practice:

  - Colocating mental health services in primary care settings mitigates stigma associated with being seen in a specialty care setting.

  - Collaborative care models support negotiated diagnoses that can effectively minimize patients' perception of stigma.

  - Collaborative care models employing telephone contacts and symptom-oriented care enhance patient privacy and focus on symptoms (typically not stigmatized directly) over diagnostic labels.

Collaborative Care

Collaborative care, an important subset of integrative care initiatives, is defined as a disease management strategy that identifies optimal roles for primary care providers, practice nurses, mental health specialists, and other allied health professionals in the treatment of chronic conditions and psychiatric illness (Katon et al. 2001; Zatzick et al. 2004). Essential elements of collaborative care include shared patient-provider treatment planning; the provision of medical support services such as care management; and active, sustained follow-up that promotes continuity in care delivery. A key feature of the collaborative care approach for psychiatric conditions is the establishment of a continuous healing relationship by a mental health treatment team. The team performs an initial evaluation and then treats the patient longitudinally, facilitating care provision across service delivery sectors (e.g., primary care and mental health specialty care). Collaborative care relies on the flexible integration of patient perspectives into the delivery of care so as to facilitate shared patient-provider treatment planning and ensure active patient participation in care. Finally, collaborative care is multifaceted, combining care management and psychopharmacological and psychotherapeutic interventions. Early combined interventions are thus ideal for patients with complex comorbid presentations (Katon et al. 2010; Roy-Byrne et al. 2010; Unützer et al. 2002; Zatzick et al. 2004).

The Veterans Health Administration has taken a leading role in promoting and developing integrated models of behavioral health and primary health care. In 2007, under the framework of its Primary Care–Mental Health Integration (PC-MHI) initiative, the VA issued a call for proposals to individual medical centers and Veterans Integrated Service Networks (VISNs) to develop integrated care models addressing the most common mental health concerns that present for treatment in primary care settings (i.e., depression, substance abuse, and PTSD) (Post and Van Stone 2008; Post et al. 2010; Zeiss and Karlin 2008). By early 2010, the VA had funded 137 distinct integrated primary care mental health programs under the PC-MHI initiative. These programs fell into three broad model categories: depression care management, behavioral health laboratories, and colocated collaborative care. Recently, the VA health system has come to the conclusion that the most successful integrated programs are those that blend components of these three core models (Pomerantz and Sayers 2010).

Not only have collaborative care models shown themselves to be effective at reducing symptoms of depression, they also demonstrate superiority over usual (i.e., noncollaborative) care. In one study, researchers determined that a collaborative care model was superior to usual care in reducing depression symptoms between baseline and 3 months but showed no significant difference when compared with outcomes at the 9-month mark, suggesting that collaborative care models are associated with more rapid recovery. Subjects receiving collaborative care interventions were also more likely to receive a wider range of treatment interventions to address depression concerns, including pharmacotherapy and cognitive-behavioral therapy (Hedrick et al. 2003).

What, then, are the key elements of collaborative models that make them so effective? The first and, arguably, most important seems to be the presence of a care facilitator or case manager (Bower et al. 2006; Upshur 2005; Williams et al. 2007). Other key factors include specialist supervision of case managers (Bower et al. 2006; Williams et al. 2007), systematic identification of patients, professional background of staff (Bower et al. 2006), inclusion of patient education and self-management interventions, monitoring of symptom severity and treatment adherence, and regular decision support to primary care providers around medication management (Williams et al. 2007).

In addition to these key factors that contribute to the success of collaborative care programs, it is important to note that such programs are well received by providers, who report high levels of satisfaction with collaborative care models (Gallo et al. 2004; Reiss-Brennan et al. 2006), prefer them to usual care, perceive improved coordination of services, perceive less stigma for patients, and endorse significantly improved communication between primary care and mental health services (Gallo et al. 2004). There is also evidence to support that once established, collaborative care systems can be replicated, sustained effectively, and extended to other mental health concerns (Katon et al. 2006; Oxman et al. 2005; Rubenstein et al. 1999). These findings are of particular relevance to the current discussion because they speak directly to the ability of collaborative care models to eliminate certain barriers to care and, perhaps, to reduce the stigma associated with mental illness.

Given the potential impact on reducing barriers to care and stigma, both the VA and the military have adopted system-wide collaborative care approaches to the treatment of depression and PTSD. In part because of its organizational and administrative structure, the VA has launched a number of different collaborative care interventions operating in different geographic locations, including the Colocated Collaborative Care Model active in VISN 2 in upstate New York (Funderburk et al. 2010), the White River Model of Colocated Collaborative Care active in Vermont (Pomerantz et al. 2010), and the Translating Initiatives for Depression into Effective Solutions (TIDES) model active in over 50 VA primary practices across the United States (Luck et al. 2009; Smith et al. 2008). To date, the

Army is the only service branch to implement a system-wide collaborative care approach. The Re-Engineering Systems of Primary Care Treatment of Depression and PTSD in the Military (RESPECT-Mil; Engel et al. 2008) is currently active in more than 90 Army primary care clinics around the world and is structurally analogous to the TIDES initiative in the VA.

Clinician Notes on Collaborative Care and Mental Health

- Collaborative care models appear to be the most effective among integrative care approaches.

- Collaborative care effectively mitigates the effects of stigma and other barriers to care while offering improved or more rapid symptom resolution.

- Both patients and primary care providers prefer collaborative care approaches to treatment over usual care.

- Optimized collaborative care performance is associated with several key elements:

  - Inclusion of care facilitators or case managers in the treatment team

  - Provision of clinical supervision of care facilitators by specialty care providers

  - Systematic identification of patients with targeted health concerns

  - Incorporation of patient education materials and self-management strategies in the treatment milieu

  - Ongoing monitoring of symptom severity and treatment adherence

  - Routine decision support to primary care providers around management of psychotropic medications

- Collaborative care models are effective in stand-alone clinic settings and are scalable across large health care systems.

- Collaborative care modalities avoid structural, policy, and institutional impediments frequently observed in other approaches to integrative care.

- Up-front costs to establish collaborative care practices may be significant (depending on existing medical personnel on staff) but pay dividends in quality and continuity of care.

The RESPECT-Mil Program

Building on the work of the MacArthur Initiative on Depression and Primary Care and the civilian Re-Engineering Systems of Primary Care Treatment of Depression (RESPECT-D) program (Dietrich et al. 2004), the RESPECT-Mil program employs the three-component model (Oxman et al. 2002) to support collaborative care interventions. The three components include 1) a primary care practice that has been prepared (through education, training, and the provision of appropriate clinical tools) to recognize and provide treatment for depression and PTSD; 2) a care facilitator to enhance the quality and frequency of collaborative communication between primary care providers, mental health specialists, and patients and to monitor and support patient treatment progress; and 3) ready access to a psychiatrist who will provide informal consultative and medication management advice to primary care physicians and who will provide behavioral health clinical supervision to care facilitators in their ongoing contact with patients. In this model, service members identified as having either depression or PTSD are afforded the opportunity to receive care for these disorders within the primary care clinic and to have that care managed by their primary care physician, whose reach, scope of practice, and functional competencies have been extended by the addition of the care facilitator and the consulting psychiatrist. The RESPECT-Mil program is a two-phase systems level intervention that includes 1) an initial primary prevention element consisting of population level screening for depression and PTSD at each clinic visit and 2) the more important element of facilitated primary care treatment of identified mental illness.

Setting up a RESPECT-Mil implementation site begins with preparing the primary care clinic for collaborative care practice. This involves brief standardized Web-based training for clinic providers and staff, hiring of one or more registered nurses to serve as care facilitators, and coordinating with local behavioral health systems to identify at least one psychiatrist to provide consultation and supervision services. Other logistical concerns include the preparation of patient education materials and printing program forms and scales.

After collaborative care is established, all service members who present for routine primary care services complete a six-item screening tool consisting of a two-item depression screen and a four-item PTSD screen. Service members who screen positive for depression are asked to complete the Patient Health Questionnaire-9 (PHQ-9; Kroenke et al. 2001), a nine-item depressive disorder diagnostic aid with demonstrated validity and sensitivity. Service members screening positive for PTSD are asked to complete the PTSD Checklist (Blanchard et al. 1996), a 17-item PTSD diagnostic tool with excellent psychometric properties. Both measures include an item assessing suicidal ideation. The primary care provider reviews all screening measures with the patient. If the provider confirms a likely diagnosis of depression or PTSD, then he or she offers at-risk patients a variety of treatment options, including referral to RESPECT-Mil care facilitation, referral directly to specialty mental health care, or continued disease management within primary care but without the additional assistance of the RESPECT-Mil program.

RESPECT-Mil care facilitators are expected to make telephone contact with all new service members referred to the RESPECT-Mil program within 7–10 business days following entry into the program. Thereafter, the care facilitator contacts enrolled service members at least once per month, at which times psychoeducation services are provided and appropriate diagnostic aids are readministered to assist with outcome monitoring and psychosocial interventions such as self-management. Care facilitators review cases as needed with consulting psychiatrists and serve a critical feedback function to primary care by communicating with the primary care provider regarding recommended therapeutic changes and patient status updates.

The feasibility of implementing the RESPECT-Mil program was assessed in a 16-month trial carried out at a busy primary care clinic at Fort Bragg, North Carolina. Results of this feasibility study showed that RESPECT-Mil could be implemented with little or no disruption to clinic workflow and that added time requirements for primary care physicians and staff were, on average, minimal. Moreover, this initial trial demonstrated increased diagnostic identification, increased rates of treatment initiation for depression and PTSD, and moderate to high rates of treatment efficacy (Engel et al. 2008).

As of February 2012, the RESPECT-Mil program was operating in 93 clinics at 35 Army installations and one Marine Corps air station. More than 1.7 million primary care visits have been screened, and in nearly 13% of those visits, the patient screened positive for depression and/or PTSD, with roughly 6% of all screen positive visits resulting in a presumptive diagnosis of PTSD or depression. Just over 55% of visits associated with a presumptive diagnosis reflect the detection of previously unrecognized illness or previously unmet needs. For the remaining visits, patients were not offered a referral because they were already receiving some form of behavioral health service to address identified need. This suggests that RESPECT-Mil is an effective mechanism for both increasing the recognition of unreported depression and PTSD and facilitating enhanced service utilization for these disorders. Almost 16,500 service members have been enrolled in RESPECT-Mil care facilitation since its inception in 2007, and initial analyses of outcome metrics appear promising. However, there is some indication that more efforts are required to maintain service members in active care-facilitated treatment and to reduce the proportion of cases lost to follow-up.

Conclusions

Underreporting of common mental illnesses and resistance to utilizing proven interventions to treat these conditions remains a significant problem. This is true both in the general populace and in military service member and veteran populations, where the problem is exacerbated by an increased risk for these mental disorders and other negative sequelae of trauma exposure. The needs-service gap and the increased risk among military and veteran groups can be accounted for, in part, by general and military- or veteran-specific culturally defined and logistic barriers to care. Most notable of such barriers to treatment-seeking behavior and treatment maintenance is the stigma associated with mental illness.

Collaborative care models of integrated treatment offer a promising way forward in increasing both access to and utilization of services through providing superior treatment efficacy while concomitantly introducing structural and systemic changes that directly address barriers to care. RESPECT-Mil is a specific case example that includes several successful program elements, and studying that endeavor provides a context for understanding how such programs are implemented.

The introduction of collaborative care initiatives with the military and veteran health systems may, in some ways, be more easily accomplished than in civilian settings because of common structures, administrative policies, and information management systems throughout the organization. The megalithic nature of these systems of care, however, may also impart a certain system level momentum that must be overcome in order to effect change. Furthermore, as health care policies continue to shift in nature in both the private and public sectors, the health care environments in which collaborative care programs are implemented must remain flexible, continue to adjust to enterprise level changes, and stand ready to continue to demonstrate their relevance and effectiveness.

SUMMARY POINTS

- Current research indicates that between 23% and 57% of psychiatric needs of combat-exposed active duty service members and veterans go unmet.

- Barriers to care may be defined as any factor or collection of factors, either endogenous or exogenous, that tend to exert an inhibitory effect on treatment-seeking behavior and/or treatment adherence, ultimately limiting access to care.
- Service members and veterans with psychiatric conditions are less likely to self-report psychiatric symptoms or seek assistance and are more likely to endorse other barriers to care.
- People who are stigmatized have a lower overall quality of life, lower self-esteem, and lower sense of mastery and experience significant work and role limitations and greater social limitations.
- Collaborative care is an effective management strategy that coordinates roles for primary care providers, practice nurses, mental health specialists, and other allied health professionals in the treatment of chronic conditions and psychiatric illness.
- RESPECT-Mil is a promising collaborative care program currently employed in military health care facilities designed to identify and treat depression and PTSD in service members.

References

Alonso J, Buron A, Rojas-Farreras S, et al: Perceived stigma among individuals with common mental disorders. J Affect Disord 118(1–3):180–186, 2009

Blanchard EB, Jones-Alexander J, Buckley TC, et al: Psychometric properties of the PTSD Checklist (PCL). Behav Res Ther 34(8):669–673, 1996

Bower P, Gilbody S, Richards D, et al: Collaborative care for depression in primary care. Making sense of a complex intervention: systematic review and meta-regression. Br J Psychiatry 189:484–493, 2006

Brown SA, Evans Y, Espenschade K, et al: An examination of two brief stigma reduction strategies: filmed personal contact and hallucination simulations. Community Ment Health J 46(5):494–499, 2010

Burman MA, Meredith LS, Taniellan TL, et al: Mental health care for Iraq and Afghanistan war veterans. Health Aff 28(3):771–782, 2009

Chermack ST, Zivin K, Valenstein M, et al: The prevalence and predictors of mental health treatment services in a national sample of depressed veterans. Med Care 46(8):813–820, 2008

Corrigan P: How stigma interferes with mental health care. Am Psychol 59(7):614–625, 2004

Dietrich AJ, Oxman TE, Williams JW Jr, et al: Re-engineering systems for the treatment of depression in primary care: cluster randomised controlled trial. BMJ 2004:329, 2004 doi:10.1136/bmj.38219.481250.55

Engel CC, Oxman T, Yamamoto C, et al: RESPECT-Mil: feasibility of a systems-level collaborative care approach to depression and post-traumatic stress disorder in military primary care. Mil Med 173(10):935–940, 2008

Fikretoglu D, Guay S, Pedlar D, et al: Twelve month use of mental health services in a nationally representative, active military sample. Med Care 46(2):217–223, 2008

Funderburk JS, Sugarman DE, Maisto SA, et al: The description and evaluation of the implementation of an integrated healthcare model. Fam Syst Health 28(2):146–160, 2010

Gallo JJ, Zubritsky C, Maxwell J, et al: Primary care clinicians evaluate integrated and referral models of behavioral health care for older adults: results from a multisite effectiveness trial (PRISM-e). Ann Fam Med 2(4):305–309, 2004

Greene-Shortridge TM, Britt TW, Castro CA: The stigma of mental health problems in the military. Mil Med 172(2):157–161, 2007

Hankin CS, Spiro A III, Miller DR, et al: Mental disorders and mental health treatment among U.S. Department of Veterans Affairs outpatients: the Veterans Health Study. Am J Psychiatry 156(12):1924–1930, 1999

Hedrick SC, Chaney EF, Felker B, et al: Effectiveness of collaborative care depression treatment in Veterans' Affairs primary care. J Gen Intern Med 18(1):9–16, 2003

Hoge CW, Castro CA, Messer SC, et al: Combat duty in Iraq and Afghanistan, mental health problems, and barriers to care. N Engl J Med 351(1):13–22, 2004

Hoge CW, Auchterlonie JL, Milliken CS: Mental health problems, use of mental health services, and attrition from military service after returning from deployment to Iraq or Afghanistan. JAMA 295(9):1023–1032, 2006

Iversen AC, van Staden L, Hughes JH, et al: The stigma of mental health problems and other barriers to care in the UK Armed Forces. BMC Health Serv Res 11:31, 2011

Katon W, Von Korff M, Lin E, et al: Rethinking practitioner roles in chronic illness: the specialist, primary care physician, and the practice nurse. Gen Hosp Psychiatry 23(3):138–144, 2001

Katon WJ, Zatzick D, Bond G, et al: Dissemination of evidence-based mental health interventions: importance to the trauma field. J Trauma Stress 19(5):611–623, 2006

Katon WJ, Lin EHB, Von Korff M, et al: Collaborative care for patients with depression and chronic illnesses. N Engl J Med 363(27):2611–2620, 2010

Kessler RC, Berglund P, Demler O, et al: Lifetime prevalence and age-of-onset distributions of DSM-IV disorders in the National Comorbidity Survey Replication. Arch Gen Psychiatry 62(6):593–602, 2005a

Kessler RC, Chiu WT, Demler O, et al: Prevalence, severity, and comorbidity of 12-month DSM-IV disorders in the National Comorbidity Survey Replication. Arch Gen Psychiatry 62(6):617–627, 2005b

Kroenke K, Spitzer RL, Williams JB: The PHQ-9: validity of a brief depression severity measure. J Gen Intern Med 16(9):606–613, 2001

Luck J, Hagigi F, Parker LE, et al: A social marketing approach to implementing evidence-based practice in VHA QUERI: the TIDES depression collaborative care model. Implement Sci 4:64, 2009 doi:10.1186/1748-5908-4-64

Maguen S, Litz BT: Predictors of barriers to mental health treatment for Kosovo and Bosnia peacekeepers: a preliminary report. Mil Med 171(5):454–458, 2006

Marcussen K, Ritter C, Munetz MR: The effect of services and stigma on quality of life for persons with serious mental illnesses. Psychiatr Serv 61(5):489–494, 2010

Oxman TE, Dietrich AJ, Williams JW Jr, et al: A three-component model for re-engineering systems for the treatment of depression in primary care. Psychosomatics 43(6):441–450, 2002

Oxman TE, Dietrich AJ, Schulberg HC: Evidence-based models of integrated management of depression in primary care. Psychiatr Clin North Am 28(4):1061–1077, 2005

Pietrzak RH, Johnson DC, Goldstein MB, et al: Perceived stigma and barriers to mental health care utilization among OEF-OIF veterans. Psychiatr Serv 60(8):1118–1122, 2009

Pomerantz AS, Sayers SL: Primary Care–Mental Health Integration in healthcare in the Department of Veterans Affairs. Fam Syst Health 28(2):78–82, 2010

Pomerantz AS, Shiner B, Watts BV, et al: The White River Model of Colocated Collaborative Care: a platform for mental and behavioral health care in the medical home. Fam Syst Health 28(2):114–129, 2010

Post EP, Van Stone WW: Veterans Health Administration Primary Care–Mental Health Integration initiative. N C Med J 69(1):49–52, 2008

Post EP, Metzger M, Dumas P, et al: Integrating mental health into primary care within the Veterans Health Administration. Fam Syst Health 28(2):83–90, 2010

Reiss-Brennan B, Briot P, Cannon W, et al: Mental health integration: rethinking practitioner roles in the treatment of depression: the specialist, primary care physicians, and the practice nurse. Ethn Dis 16(suppl 3):S3/37–S3/43, 2006

Roy-Byrne P, Craske MG, Sullivan G, et al: Delivery of evidence-based treatment for multiple anxiety disorders in primary care: a randomized controlled trial. JAMA 303(19):1921–1928, 2010

Rubenstein LV, Jackson-Triche M, Unützer J, et al: Evidence-based care for depression in managed primary care practices. Health Aff (Millwood) 18(5):89–105, 1999

Rüsch N, Corrigan PW, Todd AR, et al: Implicit self-stigma in people with mental illness. J Nerv Ment Dis 198(2):150–153, 2010

Sayer NA, Friedemann-Sanchez G, Spoont M, et al: A qualitative study of determinants of PTSD treatment initiation in veterans. Psychiatry 72(3):238–255, 2009a

Sayer NA, Rettmann NA, Carlson KF, et al: Veterans with history of mild traumatic brain injury and posttraumatic stress disorder: challenges from provider perspective. J Rehabil Res Dev 46(6):703–716, 2009b

Seal KH, Maguen S, Cohen B, et al: VA mental health services utilization in Iraq and Afghanistan veterans in the first year of receiving new mental health diagnoses. J Trauma Stress 23(1):5–16, 2010

Seal KH, Cohen G, Bertenthal D, et al: Reducing barriers to mental health and social services for Iraq and Afghanistan veterans: outcomes of an integrated primary care clinic. J Gen Intern Med 26(10):1160–1167, 2011 doi:10.1007/s11606-011-1746-1

Smith JL, Williams JW Jr, Owen RR, et al: Developing a national dissemination plan for collaborative care for depression: QUERI series. Implement Sci 3:59, 2008 doi:10.1186/1748-5908-3-59

Stecker T, Fortney JC, Hamilton F, et al: An assessment of beliefs about mental health care among veterans who served in Iraq. Psychiatr Serv 58(10):1358–1361, 2007

Taniellan TL, Jaycox LH (eds): Invisible Wounds of War: Psychological and Cognitive Injuries, Their Consequences, and Services to Assist Recovery. Santa Monica, CA, RAND, 2008

Unützer J, Katon W, Callahan CM, et al: Collaborative care management of late-life depression in the primary care setting: a randomized controlled trial. JAMA 288(22):2836–2845, 2002

Upshur CC: Crossing the divide: primary care and mental health integration. Adm Policy Ment Health 32(4):341–355, 2005

Warner CH, Appenzeller GN, Grieger T, et al: Importance of anonymity to encourage honest reporting in mental health screening after combat deployment. Arch Gen Psychiatry 68(10):1065–1071, 2011

Williams JW Jr, Gerrity M, Holsinger T, et al: Systematic review of multifaceted interventions to improve depression care. Gen Hosp Psychiatry 29(2):91–116, 2007

WHO International Consortium in Psychiatric Epidemiology: Cross-national comparisons of the prevalences and correlates of mental disorders. Bull World Health Organ 78(4):413–426, 2000

World Health Organization: The World Health Report 2001: mental health: new understanding, new hope. Geneva, Switzerland, World Health Organization, 2001

Wright KM, Cabrera OA, Adler AB, et al: Stigma and barriers to care postcombat. Psychol Serv 6(2):108–116, 2009

Zatzick D, Roy-Byrne P, Russo J, et al: A randomized effectiveness trial of stepped collaborative care for acutely injured trauma survivors. Arch Gen Psychiatry 61(5):498–506, 2004

Zeiss AM, Karlin BE: Integrating mental health and primary care services in the Department of Veterans Affairs health care system. J Clin Psychol Med Settings 15(1):73–78, 2008

PART III

Meeting the Needs of Military
and Veteran Children
and Families

Chapter 12

Deployment-Related Care for Military Children and Families

Kris Peterson, M.D.
Patricia Lester, M.D.
Jesse Calohan, DNP, PMHNP-BC
Alvi Azad, D.O., M.B.A., Maj USAF MC

DURING THE PAST DECADE, active duty, Reserve, and National Guard servicemen and servicewomen of the U.S. Army, Air Force, Navy, Marines, and Coast Guard have borne the brunt of multiple wars in various combat environments. Behind all military service members are their families, which are a critical part of our nation's military; without their support, our service members could not accomplish all that they do. Much of the focus of military medicine has been on treating service members for both their psychological and their physical wounds, but military families and children have also been affected and are in need of both community and health care services.

At the beginning of the wars in Afghanistan and Iraq, there were few data outlining the effect of combat deployment on military families. Existing prewar data suggested that military families are strong and resilient. The data also suggested that compared with nonmilitary community samples, there are fewer mental health issues and better overall coping within the military community (Jensen et al. 1986). As a result, the war-related

needs of military families and individual family members were not anticipated to be overly demanding at the onset of the current war. The earlier
findings, however, are from studies of military family separations during
noncombat sea duty, the Persian Gulf War, and other contingency operations that were very different in scope and length than Operations Enduring Freedom (OEF), Iraqi Freedom (OIF), and New Dawn (OND).

Resources within the military health care system are targeted to meet
the mental health needs of service members who have been returning from
deployment with increasingly prevalent combat stress–related challenges.
Resources in the military health care system originally allocated for family
issues were largely refocused to meet the needs of the service members at
the beginning of combat operations. Families with mental health needs are
being referred to the civilian network of care, which is provided through
the military health care program TRICARE. An assessment of mental
health care in the community performed in 2006 (M. Faran et al., unpublished data, May 2006) identified a significant shortfall that left many families struggling to find adequate services to meet their needs. As
deployment-related needs of military families were more clearly identified,
additional resources, services, and programs (both community based and
clinical) were developed to effectively target those needs.

In this chapter we examine the effect of deployment on military families
and children and outline some of the ongoing efforts to further understand
and address the needs of this critical population through continued research and expanded systems of care.

Military Families and Their Impact on Military Readiness

> It struck me that the best wasn't good enough. We have not, until this
> point, treated Families as the readiness issue that they are.
>
> Gen George W. Casey Jr., Chief of Staff of the Army, quoted in
> Army.mil news October 17, 2007 article by Elizabeth M. Lorge

Both military and political leadership have come to understand that the
health of service members' families has a profound impact on military readiness. Understanding the impact of the current war on military families requires an appreciation of the shift in demographics of the military population
as well as several unique characteristics of OEF/OIF. The demographics of
the military force now include a significantly higher percentage of married
service members and service members with children than in the past. The
Department of Defense Report on Community Demographics (Deputy Un-

der Secretary of Defense 2009) reported that more than 50% of service members are married and that 40% of them have children, much higher percentages than in previous conflicts.

Not only are the demographics of the military family different but so is the nature of the current conflict, which has continued for more than a decade. As a result, deployments have been more frequent, with less at-home or "dwell" time (time between deployments). The U.S. Army's desired dwell time is roughly 2 years for active duty members and approximately 4 years for Reserve component soldiers. Although this has been the goal, the Army has been far short of reaching those targets (Schogol 2009). National Guard and Reserve forces, an all-volunteer fighting force, have been heavily engaged in the current conflicts, making up roughly half of the total combat force and about a third of all service members deployed (Deputy Under Secretary of Defense 2009). The deployment operations tempo has been similar for Marines. Although the operations tempo is less for the Air Force and Navy, all military service families have experienced increased demands, stress, and deployment challenges over the past decade. The repeated crescendo and decrescendo of operational intensity have led to unpredictable demands on service members and their families.

Service members self-report that their own readiness for combat is affected by their family's well-being. The service members interviewed throughout OIF and OND as well as in Afghanistan have consistently reported that one of their top concerns is the well-being of their families and the challenges related to deployment separations (Mental Health Advisory Team V 2008). Mental health assessment teams (MHATs) that have interviewed service members in combat settings found that family well-being is viewed as either a combat readiness enhancer or a detractor, depending on how the family is functioning. "The well-being of military families is essential to the health of soldiers deployed to OIF. Soldiers continue to express many concerns about the ability of rear detachment commanders and family readiness groups (FRG's) to adequately support families" (Mental Health Advisory Team II 2005, p. 22). When military families do poorly, service members' ability to focus and complete missions is eroded.

Surveys of spouses of deployed soldiers also identified concerns about the ability of the military to adequately care for their needs (Mental Health Advisory Team II 2005). A consistent theme in recent military suicide data suggests that relationship and family issues are often identified as precipitating stressors. Greater access to resources or supportive services for in-trouble families or relationships was deemed critical. As a result, MHAT V recommended that TRICARE rules be amended to cover marital and family counseling as a medical benefit as a strategy to reduce soldier suicide risk (Mental Health Advisory Team V 2008). In addition, Military OneSource started offering counseling services to service members and spouses in order to address these untreated family concerns.

In recognition of the important role of the military family as a critical support to service members and the military mission, the Army Family Covenant was developed and signed in 2007 by senior leaders (Lorge 2007). In the Family Covenant, Secretary of the Army Pete Geren stated,

> the health of our all-volunteer force, our Soldier-volunteers, our Family-volunteers, depends on the health of the Family. The readiness of our all-volunteer force depends on the health of the Families.... I can assure you that your Army leadership understands the important contribution each and every one of you makes. We need to make sure we step up and provide the support Families need so the Army Family stays healthy and ready (Lorge 2007).

Gen George W. Casey Jr., then Chief of Staff of the Army, similarly described the stress on families: "[they] were the most stretched, and as a result, the most stressed, part of the force, and that what we are asking those families was a quantum different than anything I expected we would ask" (Lorge 2007). The Army Family Covenant states,

> We recognize the commitment and increasing sacrifices that our families are making every day. We recognize the strength of our Soldiers comes from the strength of their Families. We are committed to providing Soldiers and Families a Quality of Life that is commensurate with their service. We are committed to providing our Families a strong, supportive environment where they can thrive. We are committed to building a partnership with Army families that enhances their strength and resilience (Lorge 2007).

The Army Family Covenant (Lorge 2007) focuses on five programmatic goals:

- Standardizing and funding existing family programs and services
- Increasing accessibility and quality of health care
- Improving soldier and family housing
- Ensuring excellence in schools, youth services, and child care
- Expanding education and employment opportunities for family members

Support of the Army Family Covenant was put at the center of the Army's strategic health care initiative map, with other military service branches also focusing on similar issues. The Air Force and the Navy and Marines have also adopted similar focuses for their services in recognition of the demands on their communities (Lorge 2007).

The Effect of War on Military Families and Children

> It would be destructive to assume either widespread pathology or uniform resilience in children, as a result of wartime experience.
>
> Stephen J. Cozza, ret COL (Cozza et al. 2005, p. 372)

At the outset of OEF/OIF/OND, studies on the impact of deployment and combat stress on military families and children were limited largely to cross-sectional or clinical samples or were based on retrospective accounts. Additionally, the research that had been completed was conducted during conflicts of much shorter duration and lesser intensity. In general, prior data suggested overall family resilience to combat deployments, with mild to moderate impact on family members, including children. The data led many people to assume that OEF/OIF/OND impact on military families would be subclinical in nature. Despite limitations, prior research on military families and children facing deployment stress provided a foundation to guide the emerging pictures of both risk and resilience in military families affected by OEF/OIF/OND wartime service.

Scientific literature has reported that military families must contend with ongoing stressors extending from repeated relocation and parental absence, as well as wartime deployments (Palmer 2008). Although some studies of the effects of wartime deployment on children and families point to apparent resilience exhibited by military children despite these demands (Cozza et al. 2005; Jensen et al. 1996), such reports are tempered by other OEF/OIF studies that indicate increased child distress during parental deployment (Chartrand et al. 2008; Flake et al. 2009), risk for child maltreatment (McCarroll et al. 2008), and increased anxiety and school problems in adolescents (Chandra et al. 2010a). In general, extant scientific studies of military children are extremely limited and challenge our ability to draw firm conclusions. Studies conducted during OEF/OIF suggest that the impact of deployment at different developmental stages is unique and significant.

Chartrand and colleagues (2008) studied the effect of wartime military deployments on the behavior of young children in military families. In this study, the authors collected data from the parents and child care providers of children ages 1½–5 years of deployed military service member parents. In the study, children were enrolled at child care centers at a large Marine base with a high deployment rate. The research reported "that children aged between 1½ and 3 years appear to react differently to parental deployments than children ages 3 to 5 years (by parental report)" (Chartrand et al. 2008, p. 1012). Children between 3 and 5 years of age with a deployed parent evidenced the highest reported behavioral symptoms, and children between 1½ and 3 years of age evidenced significantly lower externalizing symptoms scores as reported by their caregiver parents. The authors hypothesized that these younger children may have benefited from greater amounts of time with their attachment figures (mothers) during their fathers' deployments, "thereby providing a continuous secure base for them during the parental separation. This hypothetical effect may be attenuated for older children, who are more aware of the absence of their other parent and are more involved in relationships outside the family" (Chartrand et al. 2008, p. 1013).

An additional study looked at the emotional and behavioral adjustment problems in school-age children (6–12 years) whose active duty Army and Marine Corps parents were deployed (Lester et al. 2010). Findings showed that although many children did well, parental distress in both service members and at-home civilian spouses and cumulative length in months of parental combat-related deployments during the child's lifetime were independently correlated with increased child depression and externalizing symptoms. Child anxiety symptoms were elevated both during and following a parent's wartime deployment. Overall, this research suggested that parental combat deployments have an effect that lasts beyond the duration of deployment and are associated with outcomes in children predicted by both the length of deployment and the level of psychological distress in both civilian and service member parents.

Flake and colleagues (2009) reported similar findings in military children ages 5–12 years. This study surveyed military spouses of deployed service members with children in this age group and looked at psychosocial health measures. The authors found that a third of the participants showed "high risk" for psychosocial morbidity, and 42% reported "high risk" for parenting stress. The latter significantly predicted worse child psychosocial morbidity. Similar to Lester and colleagues (2011), this group also identified higher distress and poorer outcomes in the deployed group.

A larger study (Chandra et al. 2010a) reporting on the effects of deployment on adolescents looked at the effect of deployment on child social and emotional functioning in the school setting. Staff at military schools were questioned about the "academic, behavioral, and emotional issues faced by children of deployed soldiers" (Chandra et al. 2010a, p. 218). The conclusions of the study elucidated school staff perceptions of the negative social and emotional impacts on military youth. This study was followed by additional research on children of military service members who were deployed, looking at social, emotional, and academic parameters (Chandra et al. 2010a). Findings in this study similarly showed the negative effects of cumulative deployments on families as well as the positive relationship between child outcomes and nondeployed parent outcomes. The authors suggested the benefit of programs for caregivers and children, especially those experiencing poorer mental health.

In addition to the impact of separation during deployments, reunification challenges can develop as a result of service member combat-related stress disorders. Military servicemen and servicewomen who have been exposed to combat and have resultant mental health disorders have increased risk of maladaptive relationships with their family. The impact of war on combat participants is well known and potent. It varies with the intensity, duration, and frequency of combat. Service members returning from Iraq and Afghanistan who have been exposed to traumatic, life-threatening events are at increased risk for posttraumatic stress disorder (PTSD) and other mental health disorders (Hoge et al. 2004). Studies looking at the scope of mental health and cognitive issues faced by service members returning from Iraq and Afghanistan estimated that about a third have stress-related difficulties. A RAND study estimated that roughly 18% of soldiers having deployed to OEF/OIF had PTSD or major depression and that 20% "experienced probable TBI during deployment. About one-third of those previously deployed have at least one of these three conditions, and about 5% report symptoms of all three" (Adamson et al. 2008, p. xxi).

Parent and partner psychopathology strongly affect family relationships. PTSD contributes to impaired relations with service members' families and aggression toward intimate partners and children. The severity of the violence correlated with the severity of PTSD as did behavioral patterns of "aggressive responding" and socioeconomic status (Grieger et al. 2010). One study of Vietnam veterans found that negative satisfaction with parenting, as defined as a lack of "perceived efficacy, enjoyment, quality of the relationship, satisfaction, and problems presented by the children," was associated with the severity of their PTSD symptoms (Samper et al. 2004, p. 312). "A study by Ruscio and colleagues (2002) found that of the PTSD symptom clusters, emotional numbing was most positively associated with child misbehavior and disagreement with children and most negatively associated with sharing experiences, contact, and overall quality of the parent-child relationship" (Benedek and Wynn 2001, p. 210). These studies and findings illustrate that the mental health and well-being of service members returning from combat and their spouses will have a direct effect on their children.

Distinct from the effects of PTSD, three studies have identified increased rates of child maltreatment associated with combat deployment. Rentz and colleagues (2008) examined rates of child maltreatment in military and nonmilitary families in Texas from 2000 to 2003, finding doubled rates of child maltreatment in military families, with no change in child maltreatment in nonmilitary families during the same period. Gibbs et al. (2007) examined the association of child maltreatment and deployment timing in a large sample of substantiated Army enlisted family maltreatment cases and found that rates of maltreatment were greater during combat deployment than nondeployment periods. In an examination of Army child maltreatment rates from 1991 to 2004, McCarroll et al. (2008) found the highest child neglect rates during two large-scale deployments to the Middle East in1991 and in 2002–2004, with the greatest neglect rates being reported in the youngest children.

Clinical Support for Military Families During Deployment

> We need to make sure that we give our Soldiers and families all the support they need to make them successful.
>
> Delores Johnson, director of Family Programs,
> U.S. Army Community and Family Support Center

At the beginning of OEF and OIF there were a limited number of psychiatrists and other mental health providers available to meet the mental health needs of dependent spouses and children. Even though trained to treat families and children, many providers serve in assignments that are dedicated to the care of active duty military service members. All military service branches saw an increased need for mental health support for military servicemen and servicewomen at the start of the war, resulting in shortages in available behavioral health providers. As a result, dependent spouses, children, and adolescents were referred out to the civilian network through TRICARE. In a survey done in 2009, 21% of the Army's child and adolescent psychiatrists identified the lack of meaningful clinical support of children and adolescents on their military installations as impeding access to care (K. Peterson, unpublished survey, March 2009).

The military is still struggling to increase its child and adolescent behavioral health expertise. Despite tremendous efforts to address shortfalls, the problem reflects a national shortage. The American Academy of Child and Adolescent Psychiatry (AACAP) reported that there is a significant shortage of child and adolescent psychiatrists in the United States, stating

> there is a dearth of child psychiatrists.... Furthermore, many barriers remain that prevent children, teenagers, and their parents from seeking help from the small number of specially trained professionals.... This places a

burden on pediatricians, family physicians, and other gatekeepers to identify children for referral and treatment decisions (U.S. Department of
Health and Human Services 1999, p. 138).

The AACAP reported that in 2009 there were roughly 7,400 child psychiatrists in the nation treating clients part time (20 hours per week) (American Academy of Child and Adolescent Psychiatry 2013). Exacerbating the
situation further, military installations are often located in rural areas
where there is a severe shortage of child psychiatric services, adding to the
challenge of hiring child psychiatrists or finding those in the civilian community who can provide the required care.

Innovative Programs to Meet Needs of Military Children and Families

With the needs of military children being recognized, innovative programs
have been developed, ranging in scope from community support programs to
access to clinical services. Military OneSource (www.militaryonesource.mil),
a military-contracted community support program, offers a broad range of
online services, providing resources to families, telephone support, and access
to nonmedical counseling services for short-term problems. Military communities also make available military family life consultants, who provide on-site
support services and counseling to military families in the worldwide communities in which they live. Other nongovernmental programs, such as Give an
Hour (www.giveanhour.org), have effectively developed a cadre of national
volunteers who donate their time to provide support and clinical services to
military members and their families. A comprehensive discussion of all programs is beyond the scope of this chapter. Several programs are included in
this section to describe some of the efforts within the U.S. Department of Defense to support military children and families using innovative prevention
and treatment strategies.

Child, Adolescent and Family Behavioral Health Office (CAF-BHO)

The Child, Adolescent and Family Behavioral Health Office (CAF-BHO) was
initially designed as a pilot program to further assess the impact of deployment
on families and to build subject matter expertise to identify best practices and
export them across the U.S. Army Medical Command (MEDCOM). CAF-
BHO was designed to train primary health care managers in mental health
evaluations and treatment of common psychiatric disorders. It sought to estab-

lish centers at each installation designed to strengthen, coordinate, and integrate delivery of care and to introduce methods and techniques based on the best practices of military and civilian clinicians, researchers, and academicians.

Since its inception, CAF-BHO has implemented school-based behavioral health programs as best practice on installations and in local communities to expand access to evaluation services and provide earlier detection of mental disorders. The CAF-BHO has promoted evidence-based treatments and built an assessment system that allows installations to measure the effectiveness of their methods and programs against standards drawn from analyses of an Army-wide database. The CAF-BHO has implemented programs at a number of sites, including Fort Lewis in Washington, Schofield Barracks in Hawaii, Fort Campbell in Kentucky, Fort Meade in Maryland, and multiple installations in Germany, with full implementation at all Army installations scheduled by FY2016.

CAF-BHO focuses on six key tasks:

- Act as the lead office for MEDCOM for child, adolescent, and family behavioral health matters and for developing a behavioral health system of care for Army children and families using the public health model
- Promote the coordination and integration of child and family behavioral health programs in the Army through the implementation of child and family assistance centers and school behavioral health programs at installation level
- Provide training and coaching to behavioral health providers in evidence-based, modularized cognitive-behavioral therapy, use of standardized clinical instruments, and other clinically relevant measures
- Provide evidence-informed training programs for primary care clinicians in the evaluation and management of common behavioral health disorders, as well as resiliency and other intervention and prevention training for nonprofessionals
- Serve as a repository of knowledge and a clearinghouse for state-of-the-art and evidence-based behavioral health care for Army children and families
- Centralize and standardize data collection for needs identification, outcome measurement, and performance improvement

School Behavioral Health

In 2010 the National Defense Authorization Act (H.R. 2647, sec. 722) provided funding to expand services for military children and adolescents out of the traditional treatment settings. Over the past couple of years, school-based behavioral health programs have been taking shape and providing support to military children, teachers, and counselors within the school setting.

The School Behavioral Health Program uses a public health model, providing a continuum of care from prevention through early intervention to behavioral health treatment. The overarching goal is to facilitate access to care by embedding behavioral health within the school setting and to provide state-of-the-art prevention, intervention, evaluation, and treatment through standardization of school behavioral health services and programs. Services are directed at improving academic achievement, maximizing wellness and resilience of children and families, and ultimately promoting optimal military readiness.

The program provides direct and nondirect clinical services in the schools. A full array of behavioral health care services are provided with behavioral health staff fully integrated within the school and community. Nondirect care services emphasize prevention and resiliency building through educational programs available to students, families, and the community, promoting "help-seeking behavior," reducing stigma, optimizing resiliency and well-being, and providing support and coping strategies for dealing with deployment and other military stressors.

Child and Family Assistance Centers

Child and Family Assistance Centers (CAFACs) were originally implemented at Schofield Barracks in Hawaii as a model for caring for military families. The design was identified as a best practice by the CAF-BHO, which sought to export it to targeted medical centers in the MEDCOM. CAFACs provide a cost-effective, comprehensive, integrated behavioral health system of care to support military children, military families, and the Army community throughout the Army Force Generation (ARFORGEN) and Family Life Cycle models at large-deployment platforms. CAFACs are aligned with the Army's Services and Infrastructure Core Enterprise (SICE) initiative. CAFACs, like SICE, focus on coordinating, integrating, and synchronizing resources to eliminate duplication of effort and to maximize care delivery.

The overarching goals of CAFACs are to facilitate access to care by having one point of entry for behavioral health concerns and to provide state-of-the-art prevention, evaluation, and treatment through standardization of behavioral health services and programs. The programs use a public health model of continuum of care, focusing on prevention and early intervention to promote wellness and resilience and providing a higher level of behavioral health care when needed. Programs that are preventive and seek to decrease stigma, providing support and coping strategies for dealing with such military stressors as deployment, are available to children, families, and the community. Direct care programs include screening, early intervention, evaluation, and treatment.

The outpatient interventions are coordinated throughout the disciplines; social work, family and marital therapists, psychologists, and psychiatrists work together in a multidisciplinary format that facilitates optimal care.

Families Overcoming Under Stress (Project FOCUS)

Project FOCUS (Families Overcoming Under Stress) is one of the first trauma-informed, skill-based preventive interventions designed to address families dealing with traumatic stress and other adversities (Lester et al. 2010; Saltzman et al. 2011). The conceptual model for the intervention drew on prior family-based programs that had been evaluated through randomized controlled trials to improve child and family level psychological health and coping outcomes over time. Core elements from three previously developed intervention models (Beardslee et al. 2011; Layne et al. 2008; Lester et al. 2008) were incorporated into a standardized preventive intervention that could be applied to a range of challenging child and family stressors. This program was recognized for its potential to support the military family through deployment stress and was implemented in the Navy, Army, and Air Force over the course of OEF/OIF/OND.

FOCUS teaches practical skills to meet the challenges of deployment and reintegration, to communicate and solve problems effectively, and to successfully set goals and create a shared family narrative. It does this by bringing the family together to create a family deployment narrative. This is often the first time parents hear their child's version of what the deployment meant to them. FOCUS integrates research on traumatic stress and prevention programs that have been proven effective and combines these elements to specifically meet the needs of military families. FOCUS addresses a family's wartime deployment stress and helps the family better understand and deal with combat stress–related reactions, when present. The FOCUS program targets parent and child distress and supports effective coparenting through individual and family level training in such skills as emotion regulation, managing trauma and loss reminders, problem solving, narrative sharing, and empathy building. FOCUS is designed to build on existing family strengths; to increase family cohesion, communication, and support; and to support the maintenance of consistent care routines in the home: all core characteristics of resilient families.

Implementation and process outcomes have shown that the program is well received, and FOCUS recipients believe the program addresses relevant issues (Lester et al. 2012, 2013). Both parents and children in FOCUS demonstrate significant improvement in emotional and behavioral adjustment. Further, children's prosocial behaviors and positive coping skills increase from the time they begin the program to when they end their participation. Reductions in anxiety, depression, and global distress for both service members and civilian parents are noteworthy given the brevity of the intervention and the importance of parental psychological health and effective parenting.

Conclusions

During the past 10 years the impact of war on service members and their families has become better understood. Resources initially focused on the individual needs of the service member, but communities and professionals quickly learned that providing resources for military families is just as critical. Military family health and well-being are essential to the deployment readiness of service members. As the understanding of military family risk and resilience has grown, programs have been developed to assist these families. Although many resources are found to be helpful to military families, the greatest challenge continues to be synchronizing, synergizing, and integrating these resources in a fashion that allows for accessibility and ease of use. In addition, future research must identify best practices and programs in order to promote the best outcomes. Essential to this process is the continued education of practitioners who work with military families on a daily basis, in schools, in medical offices, or in community settings.

When working to support today's fighting force, clinicians should no longer focus only on the service member as an individual; they must identify and engage the military family as similarly affected and critical to maintaining military readiness. As has been highlighted throughout this chapter, a service member's overall health and duty performance is directly correlated to the health of his or her family. It is clear that although many military families have struggled, and continue to do so, our nation is committed to supporting and providing the necessary resources to assist them in their wellness and resilience.

SUMMARY POINTS

- Studies of military children prior to the Iraq and Afghanistan wars have largely documented their health and high functioning.
- Both military and political leadership have come to understand that the health of service members' families has a profound impact on military readiness.
- Recent scientific literature has reported that military children and families must contend with ongoing stressors ex-

tending from repeated relocation and parental absence, as well as wartime deployments.

- In addition to the effects of PTSD, several studies have identified increased rates of child maltreatment associated with combat deployment.

- With the increasing needs of military children being recognized, innovative programs have been developed, ranging in scope from community support programs to greater access to clinical services.

References

Adamson D, Burnam A, Burns L, et al: Invisible Wounds of War: Psychological and Cognitive Injuries, Their Consequences, and Services to Assist Recovery. Santa Monica, CA, RAND, 2008

American Academy of Child and Adolescent Psychiatry: Child and adolescent psychiatry workforce crisis: solutions to improve early intervention and access to care. Washington, DC, American Academy of Child and Adolescent Psychiatry, 2013. Available at: http://www.aacap.org/App_Themes/AACAP/docs/resources_for_primary_care/workforce_issues/workforce_brochure_2013.pdf.

Beardslee W, Lester P, Klosinski L, et al: Family-centered preventive intervention for military families: implications for implementation science. Prev Sci 12(4):339–348, 2011

Benedek D, Wynn G (eds): Clinical Manual for Management of PTSD. Washington, DC, American Psychiatric Publishing, 2011

Chandra A, Martin LT, Hawkins SA, et al: The impact of parental deployment on child social and emotional functioning: perspectives of school staff. J Adolesc Health 46(3):218–223, 2010a

Chandra A, Lara-Cinisomo S, Jaycox LH, et al: Children on the homefront: the experience of children from military families. Pediatrics 125(1):16–25, 2010b

Chartrand MM, Frank DA, White LF, et al: Effect of parents' wartime deployment on the behavior of young children in military families. Arch Pediatr Adolesc Med 162(11):1009–1014, 2008

Cozza SJ, Chun RS, Polo JA: Military families and children during Operation Iraqi Freedom. Psychiatr Q 76(4):371–378, 2005

Deputy Under Secretary of Defense: Demographics 2009: profile of the military community. U.S. Department of Defense, 2009. Available at: http://www.militaryonesource.com/MOS/ServiceProviders/2007DemographicsProfileofthe MilitaryCommuni.aspxd. Accessed May 27, 2011.

Flake EM, Davis BE, Johnson PL, et al: The psychosocial effects of deployment on military children. J Dev Behav Pediatr 30(4):271–278, 2009

Gibbs DA, Martin SL, Kupper LL, et al: Child maltreatment in enlisted soldiers' families during combat-related deployments. JAMA 298(5):528–535, 2007

Grieger T, Benedek D, Ursano R: Violence and aggression, in Clinical Manual for Management of PTSD. Edited by Benedek D, Wynn G. Washington, DC, American Psychiatric Publishing, 2010, pp 205–225

Hoge CW, Castro CA, Messer SC, et al: Combat duty in Iraq and Afghanistan, mental health problems, and barriers to care. N Engl J Med 351(1):13–22, 2004

H.R. 2647, 111th Cong., 1st Sess. sec. 722 (2010)

Jensen PS, Lewis RL, Xenakis SN: The military family in review: context, risk, and prevention. J Am Acad Child Psychiatry 25(2):225–234, 1986

Jensen PS, Martin D, Watanabe H: Children's response to parental separation during Operation Desert Storm. J Am Acad Child Adolesc Psychiatry 35(4):433–441, 1996

Layne CM, Saltzman WR, Poppleton L, et al: Effectiveness of a school-based group psychotherapy program for war-exposed adolescents: a randomized controlled trial. J Am Acad Child Adolesc Psychiatry 47:1048–1062, 2008

Lester P, Rotheram-Borus MJ, Elia C, et al: TALK: teens and adults learning to communicate, in Evidence-Based Treatment Manuals for Children and Adolescents. Edited by LeCroy CW. New York, Oxford University Press, 2008, pp 170–285

Lester P, Peterson K, Reeves J, et al: The long war and parental combat deployment: effects on military children and at-home spouses. J Am Acad Child Adolesc Psychiatry 49(4):310–320, 2010

Lester P, Mogil C, Saltzman W, et al: Families overcoming under stress: implementing family-centered prevention for military families facing wartime deployments and combat operational stress. Mil Med 176(1):19–25, 2011

Lester P, Saltzman WR, Woodward K, et al: Evaluation of a family-centered prevention intervention for military children and families facing wartime deployments. Am J Public Health 102(suppl 1):S48–S54, 2012

Lester P, Stein JA, Saltzman W, et al: Psychological health of military children: longitudinal evaluation of a family-centered prevention program to enhance family resilience. Mil Med, 178(8):838–845, 2013

Lorge E: Army leaders sign covenant with families. U.S. Army, 2007. Available at: http://www.army.mil/article/5641/army-leaders-sign-covenant-with-families. Accessed October 2, 2013.

McCarroll JE, Fan Z, Newby JH, et al: Trends in US Army child maltreatment reports 1990–2004. Child Abuse Review 17:108–118, 2008

Mental Health Advisory Team II: Operation Iraqi Freedom (OIF-II) Mental Health Advisory Team (MHAT-II) report. Rockville, MD, Office of the U.S. Surgeon General, 2005

Mental Health Advisory Team V: Operation Iraqi Freedom 06-08: Iraq Operation Enduring Freedom 8: Afghanistan. Rockville, MD, Office of the U.S. Surgeon General, 2008

Palmer C: A theory of risk and resilience factors in military families. Mil Psychol 20:205–217, 2008

Rentz ED, Marshall SW, Martin SL, et al: Occurrence of maltreatment in active duty military and nonmilitary families in the State of Texas. Mil Med 173(6):515–522, 2008

Ruscio AM, Weathers FW, King LA, et al: Male war-zone veterans' perceived relationships with their children: the importance of emotional numbing. J Trauma Stress 15(5):351–357, 2002

Samper RE, Taft CT, King DW, et al: Posttraumatic stress disorder symptoms and parenting satisfaction among a national sample of male Vietnam veterans. J Trauma Stress 17(4):311–315, 2004

Saltzman WR, Lester P, Beardslee WR, et al: Mechanisms of risk and resilience in military families: theoretical and empirical basis of a family-focused resilience enhancement program. Clin Child Fam Psychol Rev 14(3):213–230, 2011

Schogol J: Deployments will delay Army's dwell time goal. Stars and Stripes, December 5, 2009

U.S. Department of Health and Human Services: Mental health: A report of the Surgeon General. Rockville, MD, U.S. Department of Health and Human Services, 1999. Available at: http://profiles.nlm.nih.gov/ps/access/NN-BBHS.pdf. Accessed June 2, 2011.

Chapter 13

Children and Families of Ill and Injured Service Members and Veterans

Susan L. Van Ost, Ph.D.
Gregory A. Leskin, Ph.D.
Tricia D. Doud, Psy.D.
Stephen J. Cozza, M.D.

U.S. MILITARY children and families serve their country together with their military service members. As part of military life, these families endure multiple transitions between residences, communities, and schools as well as separation from their service member parent during repeated deployment. When service members are physically injured as a result of military service, long-term care is often provided by their families, who must then deal with the challenges resulting from these health conditions. In addition to obvious bodily injury, many service members exhibit psychological injuries, including posttraumatic stress disorder (PTSD), adjustment problems, and the detrimental cognitive effects of traumatic brain injury (TBI). These conditions can profoundly disrupt family relationships over subsequent months and years.

In this chapter we examine how military-related injuries and combat stress disorders can negatively influence a service member or veteran's relationships with spouse, children, and family of origin. Professional guidance is provided on how best to support these families through the acute and longer-term rehabilitation phases of the recovery period. Families must be prepared for more obvious or "visible" injury as well as for "invisible" psychological injuries that may not become apparent until the later course of reintegration into the family and community. With proper care, even powerfully impacted families can integrate new knowledge and skills to better address the injury, support one another, and learn new roles and routines to function more successfully.

Background: Characteristics of the Wars

In response to the terrorist attacks of September 11, 2001, the U.S. military engaged in conflicts in the Middle East, with combat operations beginning in Afghanistan in October 2001 and in Iraq in March 2003. Since then, more than 47,000 men and women have sustained varying levels of injury severity in theater (iCasualties.org 2009), and approximately 19,000 have incurred an injury severe enough to require medical evacuation. Because of improved in-theater medical treatment and immediate transportation to tertiary care facilities (Gawande 2004), service members now survive with more extensive and serious physical injuries than was true in prior wars.

The most common cause of physical injury is blasts, often caused by improvised explosive devices (Owens et al. 2008). Musculoskeletal injuries, spinal cord injuries, amputations, burns, other disfiguring injuries, and ocular injuries are commonly reported (Spelman et al. 2012). Given its variable severity and the potential for delayed diagnosis, the incidence of TBI is inconsistently reported in the literature, with estimates ranging from 250,000 (Defense and Veterans Brain Injury Center, http://www.health.mil/Research/TBI_Numbers.aspx) to as high as 19% of all Operation Enduring Freedom and Operation Iraqi Freedom combat veterans.

Twenty percent of returning combat veterans endorse symptoms consistent with a combat-related stress disorder, such as PTSD, depression, or substance use disorder (Hoge et al. 2004). In addition, high rates of comorbid physical and mental disorders can significantly complicate individual functioning as well as clinical diagnosis and treatment. Because 43% of active U.S. military service members have children, the numbers of children and families affected by these conditions are compelling.

Course of Injury Recovery

Recovery from injury can be conceptualized as a trajectory organized into four phases (Cozza and Guimond 2011): 1) acute care, when life-saving, life-sustaining medical interventions are provided in or near the combat theater and the family is initially notified; 2) medical stabilization, when specialized medical and surgical care occurs and the service member is prepared for function outside the hospital; 3) transition to outpatient care, which begins prior to discharge and includes the planning of follow-up care and ongoing rehabilitation; and 4) long-term rehabilitation and recovery, in which physical recovery continues to progress and service members learn to adapt to their injury. Each phase presents a different set of family challenges and corresponding need for professional intervention and support. Family members experience considerable distress and turmoil during the initial days and weeks after notification of their service member's injury. Because most spouses visit the hospitalized service member, decisions must be made about how best to inform the children, whether children should be included in the visit, and how to arrange for child care and maintenance of the family household. For more serious injuries, hospitalizations can frequently extend over many months. Because these injuries require intensive and long-term medical and rehabilitative care, visiting spouses and children must travel far from home to one of the Level 1 military treatment facilities where comprehensive medical and rehabilitative care is available. Some families (parents and spouses) eventually decide to move their households to the vicinity of the facility, which disrupts their connections to supportive jobs, schools, friends, and communities.

Acute Care

Family disruption and distress are experienced equally by the parents and siblings of single service members. These family members will have their lives disrupted by travel to the hospital and subsequent participation in longer-term care. Although a young service member may have successfully emancipated from the family of origin, both the service member and relatives must now adjust to an extended period of unexpected dependent care. When the service member is married with children, distraught spouses and other adult relatives must describe the injury in a way that is appropriate to the developmental level of each child.

Table 13–1 references key aspects of injury communication during the acute care phase of recovery. Ideally, notification should first occur with adults alone so that children can be protected from unnecessarily traumatic information and from the distressed adult emotional response to news of injury. The most important communication to children of any age is that despite news of the injury, their service member parent will be cared for and important adults will remain available to provide care and comfort (Cozza et al. 2011). All children require calm adult assistance to better integrate their understanding of serious injuries. This support should include age-appropriate explanation of the injury so that children can better understand the emotions and behavior of adults around them. The amount and type of information that adults share should be based on their children's developmental, emotional, and cognitive capacities.

TABLE 13-1. Professional interventions to guide injury communication

Notify adults when they are alone so that children are protected from the adult emotional response and adults can later communicate with greater calm.

Educate parents on the expected reactions from children at different ages.

Help parents gauge what to tell their children on the basis of their ages and cognitive and emotional capacities.

Ensure that all children know that important adults will remain available to them.

Ensure that all children know that the injured parent is receiving care.

If children visit in the hospital, carefully prepare them for the altered appearance and behavior of the injured parent.

Encourage family members to conduct an ongoing dialogue about the injury.

Encourage a shared understanding among family members about the impact of the injury on them and the service member.

Alter and revise communication about the injury as children mature.

Teach the family to discuss the injury with people outside the family (service providers, teachers, coaches, community professionals, extended family members).

Infants and toddlers (0–2 years), although not cognitively capable of understanding the injury of a service member parent, will quickly respond to perceived changes in the availability of adult caretakers, differences in the emotional climate of the household, and shifts in daily routine. Their distress may manifest in disturbances of sleep, eating, self-regulation, and attachment. The primary source of protection for young children is in the comfort, consistency, and routine that is provided by their caregivers.

Preschoolers (3–6 years) may have a greater awareness of the injury but are normally prone to egocentric and "magical" thinking. For example, they might worry that the injury could happen to them or that it is punishment for misdeeds committed by themselves or the parents. It is essential to explain, using developmentally appropriate language, that the injury is not their fault and to reassure them that they are still safe and protected and are free to share any feelings that may arise.

School-age children (7–12 years) demonstrate less egocentric thinking but may harbor feelings of guilt and anxiety. Although often eager to contribute, they can be confused about how to act and what to do. They may feel uneasy about bringing up questions. It may be necessary to check in with them on a regular basis about how they are feeling regarding the changes that have occurred in the home.

Older children and teens (13+ years) are generally capable of understanding and accepting more detail, including the cause of the injury, the nature and severity of physical wounds, the plan for treatment, and likely adjustments to be made by the family (e.g., expected separations for hospital visits, changes in child care arrangements). However, teenagers who are becoming more independent from their families may be confused or frustrated by the sudden need to once again be intensely involved. They can be ambivalent or resentful about increased chores and child care responsibilities.

Medical Stabilization

During the indeterminate period of hospitalization, children may be left under the supervision of other adults either at home or at the homes of family members and friends in local or distant communities. Siblings may be split up to live at different locations. Sometimes children are uprooted to join their parents at the hospital. All of these options, with their attendant disruption of schedules, caretakers, and relationships, are unsettling for children and may add to the existing stress of the noninjured spouse.

For some families, the occurrence of a combat injury can compound whatever conflicts (separation, divorce, infidelity, or disputes between spouses and in-laws) may have preceded it. Behavioral health providers must therefore negotiate with concerned parties to ensure that their communication and visitation with the service member are calming and supportive. In addition, the behavioral health providers may choose to implement educational, psychological, and practice supports designed to stabilize the family's adjustment and reduce interpersonal conflict.

During the hospital-based phase of recovery, the levels of necessary intervention include the following:

1. *Hospital-based accommodations* to develop child- and family-friendly environments for visiting and living. Facilities should establish policies that will limit younger children's unnecessary exposures to upsetting images and experiences. Parents should be informed about the expected reactions by children of different ages (see the section "Course of Injury Recovery") and guided on how to prepare children for visiting the hospital and their injured military parent.

2. *Provision of practical resources* to help stabilize the family through extended combat injury treatment. Services should include assistance with financial support, housing, travel, child care, and educational needs. Medical staff must be familiar with military regulations and able to refer families to both military and civilian resources.

3. *Family education, monitoring, and counseling* to support family members through recovery. A major goal is to support appropriate coping skills and monitor and prevent development of individual and family dysfunction. Multifamily or spouse groups are useful for education and supportive sharing. Families should be informed about likely changes in the service member's behavior due to PTSD or TBI and alerted to the effect of these injuries on parenting and marital relationships (Grieger et al. 2006). Table 13–2 describes risk factors for which children and families should be monitored.

Transition to Outpatient Care

Even when families are resilient, combat injury is likely to complicate family members' daily routine, increase stress, and diminish hopes for the future. Although most family members would prefer to have their former lives back and therefore aspire to a complete recovery, many will have to adjust to a long-term and possibly permanent change in their loved one. Professionals must therefore help family members acknowledge their sense of loss while at the same time developing optimism about the possibility of a different but satisfactory future.

As hospitalization comes to an end, families become more vulnerable as they move home or to less structured facilities. The transition to at-home and outpatient care can mean loss of connections made with other combat-injured families while at the hospital, loss of supportive hospital services, and renegotiation of family relationships around the changed physical and psychological status of the injured service member. Daily responsibilities and routines must be resumed while managing an injured service member whose function in previous roles of spouse and parent are restricted by physical pain, sleeplessness, and emotionally distant or irritable behavior. Additionally, the service member and family may be stressed by the possible end of a cherished military career and the associated loss of military housing, friends, schools, and community connections.

Long-Term Rehabilitation and Recovery

Previous research has demonstrated the long-term challenges associated with recovery from combat injury. For example, focus groups were conducted with combat-injured families who were 1–5 years postinjury (Cozza and Guimond 2011). The majority of families reported that 1) their service members continued to experience physical and posttraumatic stress symptoms related to their injuries; 2) all family members experienced universally high distress with ongoing anxiety, shame, and sadness; 3) transitions from military to Department of Veterans Affairs or civilian treatment were accom-

TABLE 13-2. Risk factors for child and family postinjury adjustment problems

At-home (nondeployed) parent is functioning poorly (isolated, angry, depressed, or anxious).

Nondeployed parent and/or children have limited or absent social network.

Family has no contact or limited contact with military families undergoing similar transitions.

Children have a history of learning, behavioral, or "difficult temperament" symptoms.

There is a history of neglect, abuse, or other trauma.

Injured service member exhibits irritability, hypersensitivity, emotional numbing, substance abuse, or violence.

The family has limited access to instrumental supports such as financial resources, child care, and coordination with schools.

There is a history of marital or family tension prior to the injury.

---

panied by frequent disappointment with service delivery and care; 4) family roles were disrupted as some service members (particularly those with PTSD or TBI) often remained unable to resume full parental and household responsibilities; and 5) they needed help in communicating with children about the injury and its consequences.

Service members diagnosed with PTSD or TBI often exhibit a broad range of behavioral changes, resulting in significant impact on family relationships. Because families are usually responsible for the bulk of long-term care and caregiver distress is strongly predictive of poor patient outcome, the service member's recovery can be heavily influenced by the degree of family support received (Perlesz et al. 2000). Certain key features of both PTSD and TBI can significantly disrupt a service member's family and interpersonal relationships. These symptoms include impaired self-awareness, behavioral rigidity, reduced self-control, apathy, withdrawal, emotional lability, irritability, impulsivity, concentration problems, and sleep dysregulation (Kennedy et al. 2007). Family members, both adults and children, can feel criticized, trapped, isolated, and confused by the interactions that may result from these symptoms.

Assessing the Family

When first conducting a family assessment, it is necessary to obtain the patient's permission to invite other family members to discuss their experiences through the injury recovery and resultant changes in family relationships.

Most service members and veterans are likely to be resistant if they believe that they or their injuries will be "blamed" for problems in their family. Efforts should be made to help them minimize such perceptions by emphasizing that all injured families are faced with challenges and that the goal of family assessment and intervention is to develop a shared understanding of the injury and recovery experience and to use effective strategies to maintain health and strength within their families.

A family assessment may be conducted through more informal discussion and consultation by the treatment team or include use of clinical measures when deemed appropriate. An assessment of the combat-injured family includes an inventory of 1) their active concerns about family members' physical health and emotional status; 2) the family's ability to access required resources and services (including health care, child care, and education); and 3) assessment of family structure, discipline, emotional support, communication, problem solving, and capacity to manage distress and interpersonal conflict.

Interventions With Combat-Injured Families

The principles that guide appropriate intervention have developed from an integration of literature on resilience, trauma, and prior work with families coping with combat and TBI. The following is a brief review of these key investigations into strategies for coping with postinjury stress. The ultimate goal of intervention is to sustain and improve resilience in the face of trauma and stress. In this regard, Saltzman et al. (2011) emphasized that resilient adaptation requires maintenance of nurturing interactions between family members, which, in turn, requires support from a larger, extrafamilial social network.

The Workgroup on Intervention with Combat Injured Families (Cozza 2009) made recommendations regarding key elements of intervention with the children and families of the combat injured. Emphasis was placed on 1) developmentally sensitive and age-appropriate injury communication; 2) delivery of care that is longitudinal in scope, culturally sensitive, and specific to the needs of individual families; and 3) promotion of an interconnected community of care requiring coordination between the family, health care providers, and military and civilian community resources.

The Families Overcoming Under Stress (FOCUS) program developed at the University of California, Los Angeles is a family-centered resiliency training founded on interventions previously shown to improve the psychological health of traumatized children and families (Lester et al. 2011). Begun in 2008 and currently serving military installations worldwide, this program provides evidence-informed preventive intervention to military families with emphasis on development of goal setting, emotional regulation, communication skills, and family-based narrative. Recent evaluative data (Lester et al. 2012) have indicated the effectiveness of this approach in preventing the development of psychological problems in at-risk military and injured families. FOCUS-CI, a refinement of FOCUS, is currently being studied in a randomized controlled intervention trial with families of combat-injured service members.

Psychological First Aid (PFA) is an evidence-informed intervention for early level to midlevel mass trauma recovery (Hobfoll et al. 2007). The National Child Traumatic Stress Network and the National Center for PTSD (2006) have developed a PFA Field Operations Guide that includes recommendations for dealing with traumatized individuals of all ages. Key elements include promotion of safety, calm, connectedness, self-efficacy, and hope, all of which apply to the needs of combat-injured families as well. In addition, there is growing literature on the impact of TBI on nonmilitary family members (Kreutzer et al. 2010) as well as description and evaluation of model programs. The Brain Injury Family Intervention (BIFI; Kreutzer et al. 2009) is one example and highlights several key areas for family intervention: recognition of the patient's changed behavior, instruction about the typical course of recovery, development of stress management techniques, and emphasis on self-care and planning for the future.

Critical Strategies

Table 13–3 summarizes intervention goals for the children and families of injured service members and veterans. As suggested by the literature and established programs cited in the previous section, behavior health providers must employ the following strategies in order to work toward these goals: 1) reduce individual and family distress, 2) expand strategies for effective emotion regulation, 3) provide information about the impact of combat injury using child guidance approaches, 4) instill principles of helpful injury communication, 5) create a sense of shared understanding, and (6) problem solve and set goals that support a sense of hopefulness. In the following sections we describe the application of these principles to the treatment of families of combat-injured service members.

Reducing Individual and Family Distress

By collaborating with the family to obtain necessary support and services, clinical providers can gain the family's trust and promote a sense of safety. The initial stages of intervention must therefore include an assessment of basic needs in the areas of work and finance, medical care, military status,

TABLE 13-3. Critical strategies and interventions for the children and families of injured service members

Critical Strategy	Interventions
Reduce individual and family distress	Facilitate the physical and emotional stability of caregivers and children Develop consistent child discipline and predictable routines for household maintenance
Promote emotion regulation	Encourage individual, couple, and family identification of feelings and development of calming strategies Encourage mutually enjoyable couple and family activity
Provide practical information	Link the service member's changed behavior to the injury Educate regarding the expected course of recovery Recognize family strengths
Child guidance	Promote an age-appropriate understanding of the injury and course of recovery Teach that the child did not create the problems seen in the family and that the injured parent may be different but is still the child's parent; promote hopefulness about the future Teach the child to acknowledge and cope with sadness, grief, and anxiety related to the injury
Injury communication	Train parents to use age-appropriate language to discuss the injury and its implications Develop strategies for communication with extrafamilial support systems
Shared understanding	Develop a shared family narrative about the impact of the injury on the service member's behavior and the expected course of recovery Correct misunderstandings Develop coparenting by facilitating mutual understanding and emotional regulation
Problem solving and goal setting	Encourage the family to identify current challenges, break them into components, and formulate steps leading to attainment

housing, education, and child care. After the family's needs are identified, the provider's role is to give simple, accurate information about how to obtain needed services and then develop a shared action plan by which both the provider and the family will take steps toward accessing resources. The family is empowered to reach out and self-advocate while the provider remains present to support and supplement the family's efforts. Because guilt and frustration are natural reactions when feeling helpless to relieve the suffering of an injured family member (Kreutzer et al. 2010), caretakers are at risk for exhaustion and self-neglect. Clinical providers must therefore make strenuous efforts to ensure that the emotional and physical needs of those who care for the injured service member are being met. To ensure the stability of the household and safety of the children, providers must be ready to intervene at the earliest signs of depression, excessive worry, or suicidal ideation in any family member. Counseling caretakers about the importance of respite and self-care is an essential element of intervention.

Because children feel safer and calmer when their daily routines are predictable and consistent, families dealing with multiple transitions (residence, schools, and community) will need help achieving a more organized lifestyle. Through discussion and introduction of supportive services, the clinical provider's role is to develop systems for household maintenance, regular meals, money management, medical care, and child management.

Effective Emotion Regulation

Overwhelmed family members, especially caretakers, may not realize the degree to which chronic daily stress is disrupting their interactions with the children and injured service member. An important step toward improvement of family function is to ensure that members have identified and can practice personally effective stress-reduction strategies. As family members achieve greater calm, they will be able to communicate more clearly and effectively.

A first step toward effective emotion regulation is to recognize stress reactions and the situations that provoke them. Children and adults can be taught to monitor changes or extremes in their emotional states by first learning to label and express their feelings, then to identify when and how positive or negative responses are triggered. One example is the FOCUS program's association of colors with different intensities of feeling (Lester et al. 2011). By pooling information about feelings, preferred forms of relaxation, and situations that provoke discomfort, families can identify mutually acceptable activities and times when they are most likely to be enjoyed. Individuals can be taught to reduce worry and tension by engaging in positive self-talk, allowing themselves breaks as needed, developing more realistic expectations, and setting priorities. Couples and parent-child dyads can be encouraged to jointly engage in activities that are calming for both participants.

Practical Information and Child Guidance

Adult distress is observed by the children. Table 13–3, adapted from Cozza et al. (2011), lists intervention goals for the distressed children of families of combat-injured service members. In general, these interventions emphasize appropriate injury communication, acceptance of changed family circumstances, and hopeful development of goals for the future. When the clinical practitioner is able to reassure and realistically orient adults in the family, the children are able to achieve greater calm and stability. Specifically, the practitioner must work toward the following:

1. All family members should be taught to link the service member's changed behavior to the injury rather than to some action of their own. Encourage recognition that everyone, parents and children alike, are affected by the injury. This might include description of expected reactions from children at different developmental levels (see the section "Course of Injury Recovery"). For example, school-age children must be reminded that the tensions they see at home are not their fault and that it is not their responsibility to "fix" them. Adolescents should be relieved of excessive adult responsibilities and deterred from impulsive risk-taking behavior.
2. To further normalize the family's sense of confusion and distress, provide information about the typical course of family recovery from combat injury (see the section "Course of Injury Recovery"). Propose realistic expectations about the length of the recovery process, suggesting that recovery might require months or years, with the ultimate goal of achieving a "new normal" in which the family's adjustment will be different from before the injury although still satisfactory.
3. With genuine regard, the provider must describe, summarize, and compliment the family's efforts up to this point in the recovery process, expressing confidence in their fundamental ability to maintain strength and cohesion in the face of adversity. For example, the practitioner might express admiration for a family member's courage in making significant adjustments to be with her husband, her ongoing efforts to address the needs of both her husband and her children, and her courage in making the difficult move to a new city. The practitioner should be alert to the family's willingness to attempt challenging tasks in order to cope more effectively with the injury.

Injury Communication

Injury communication is an essential component of injured family care. In its broadest sense, "injury communication" refers both to the *exchange of information*—provision and delivery of information related to the injury—and to the *impact of information*—the family's capacity to process information and its behavioral impact on individual members. Effective injury communication involves the timely, appropriate, and accurate sharing of information from the moment of injury notification and continuing throughout treatment and rehabilitation (see Table 13–1).

A primary goal of injury communication, to be achieved over time, is to help family members integrate the injury experience through a process of *shared understanding.* To this end, ongoing dialogue about the injury and its implications is extremely important. Clinicians must demonstrate, and encourage parents to use, developmentally appropriate language when speaking with children about the injury.

Effective injury communication (Cozza and Guimond 2011) also requires communication with parties outside of the home. The family should be encouraged to reach out to family, friends, the community, and professional providers by describing their unique struggle with the service member's injury and related behavioral issues. For example, parents can teach and encourage their children to speak with teachers, coaches, and counselors. Developing relationships with health care providers, counselors, ministers, and community organizers makes it more likely that adults and children in the family will seek and receive help when needed.

Shared Understanding

An important goal during the later phases of injury recovery is to promote the family's shared understanding of the injury and its effect on relationships. This normalizes and contextualizes the service member's behavior and helps children understand what to expect in the current circumstances and over time. Development of shared understanding requires an *ongoing* dialogue about the injury, what aspects of the service member's behavior can be attributed to the injury, and how the service member's recovery and behavior are likely to fluctuate and change over time. Because children are able to process more information about the injury as they get older, the ongoing and continual nature of this dialogue becomes important.

The family narrative (Lester et al. 2011; Saltzman et al. 2011) and Family Talk (Beardslee et al. 2003) interventions are procedures designed to facilitate an exchange of views between parents and children about their individual reactions to the service member's injury. In a chronological format, each family member is encouraged to describe his or her individual emotional reactions before, during, and after the injury. Engaging in this structured exchange has several benefits: 1) Misinterpretations and misunderstandings about why people behave as they do can be identified and corrected. 2) After they are freed from misconceptions about each other, family members are able to communicate with greater empathy and work as a team toward common goals. 3) The service member's recovery is facilitated as information about the condition and his or her own efforts to cope are revealed and family members are drawn closer to him or her in mutual support.

Problem Solving and Goal Setting

After a foundation of mutual understanding and ongoing dialogue about the injury are established, the family is ready to engage in a process of identifying and addressing current challenges. This process provides a sense of priority, prevents working on too many things at once, and provides a framework from which to recognize and evaluate progress. For example, the FOCUS program helps families analyze broader goals and break them down into manageable components, think through alternative ways of addressing these goals, select the best option, and then formulate a step-by-step action plan for accomplishment (Lester et al. 2011). Issues that were formerly overwhelming can be broken down into smaller and more manageable parts, which leads to a sense of self-efficacy and hope. Couples and families learn to break larger problems into smaller and more immediately achieved components. As steps leading to partial achievement are realized, the family becomes more optimistic about moving forward in a hopeful fashion.

Conclusions

Combat injury can profoundly affect the lives of service members and veterans, their families, and their children. Although any injury will require substantial adjustment and accommodation, the signature injures of the current wars—PTSD and TBI—can profoundly alter service members' behavior and are particularly disruptive of family and interpersonal relationships. Clinical providers must be prepared to help families with differing challenges at each phase of the recovery process. Critical intervention strategies include reduction of distress, development of emotional regulation, facilitated injury communication and shared communication, and promotion of strategies for problem solving and goal setting. The ultimate goal of these interventions is to assist the family in gaining acceptance of a "new normal" that includes both acceptance of their changed service member and hopefulness about the future.

SUMMARY POINTS

- Many physically injured service members exhibit symptoms of PTSD, adjustment problems, and the detrimental cognitive effects of TBI that can profoundly disrupt family relationships and function.
- The injury recovery trajectory can be organized into four phases: acute care, medical stabilization, transition to outpatient care, and long-term rehabilitation and recovery.
- Children in combat-injured families are particularly vulnerable, and clinicians must be aware of and attentive to their unique developmental needs.

- Family disruption and distress are likely consequences of combat injuries and require family-centered intervention strategies.

- Family-centered care should incorporate the following strategies: 1) reduce individual and family distress, 2) expand strategies for effective emotion regulation, 3) provide information about the impact of combat injury using child guidance approaches, 4) instill principles of helpful injury communication, 5) create a sense of shared understanding, and 6) problem solve and set goals that support a sense of hopefulness.

References

Beardslee WR, Gladstone TRG, Wright EJ, et al: A family-based approach to the prevention of depressive symptoms in children at risk: evidence of parental and child change. Pediatrics 112(2):e119–e131, 2003

Cozza SJ (ed): Proceedings: Workgroup on Intervention with Combat Injured Families. Bethesda, MD, Center for the Study of Traumatic Stress, Uniformed Services University of the Health Sciences, 2009

Cozza SJ, Guimond JM: Working with combat-injured families through the recovery trajectory, in Risk and Resilience in U.S. Military Families. Edited by MacDermin-Wadsworth S, Riggs D. New York, Springer, 2011, pp 259–277

Cozza SJ, Chun RS, Miller C: The children and families of combat-injured service members, in War Psychiatry. Edited by Richie EC. Washington, DC, Borden Institute, 2011, pp 503–533

Gawande A: Casualties of war: military care for the wounded from Iraq and Afghanistan. N Engl J Med 351(23)2471–2475, 2004

Grieger TA, Cozza SJ, Ursano RJ, et al: Posttraumatic stress disorder and depression in battle-injured soldiers. Am J Psychiatry 163(10):1777–1783, quiz 1860, 2006

Hobfoll SE, Watson P, Bell CC, et al: Five essential elements of immediate and mid-term mass trauma intervention: empirical evidence. Psychiatry 70(4):283–315, 2007

Hoge CW, Castro CA, Messer SC, et al: Combat duty in Iraq and Afghanistan, mental health problems, and barriers to care. N Engl J Med 351(1):13–22, 2004

iCasualties.org: Iraq coalition casualty count, 2009. Available at: http://www.icasualties.org. Accessed October 1, 2012.

Kennedy JE, Jaffee MS, Leskin GA, et al: Posttraumatic stress disorder and posttraumatic stress disorder-like symptoms and mild traumatic brain injury. J Rehabil Res Dev 44(7):895–920, 2007

Kreutzer JS, Stejskal TM, Ketchum JM, et al: A preliminary investigation of the brain injury family intervention: impact on family members. Brain Inj 23(6)535–547, 2009

Kreutzer JS, Marwitz JH, Godwin EE, et al: Practical approaches to effective family intervention after brain injury. J Head Trauma Rehabil 25(2):113–120, 2010

Lester P, Mogil C, Saltzman W, et al: Families overcoming under stress: implementing family-centered prevention for military families facing wartime deployments and combat operational stress. Mil Med 176(1):19–25, 2011

Lester P, Mogil C, Saltzman W, et al: Evaluation of a family-centered prevention intervention for military children and families facing wartime deployments. Am J Public Health 102(suppl 1):S48–S54, 2012

Owens BD, Kragh JF Jr, Wenke JC, et al: Combat wounds in Operation Iraqi Freedom and Operation Enduring Freedom. J Trauma 64(2):295–299, 2008

Perlesz A, Kinsella G, Crowe S: Psychological distress and family satisfaction following traumatic brain injury: injured individuals and their primary, secondary, and tertiary carers. J Head Trauma Rehabil 15(3):909–929, 2000

National Child Traumatic Stress Network and National Center for PTSD: Psychological First Aid: Field Operations Guide, 2nd Edition. Washington, DC, U.S. Department of Veterans Affairs, 2006

Saltzman WR, Lester P, Beardslee WR, et al: Mechanisms of risk and resilience in military families: theoretical and empirical basis of a family-focused resilience enhancement program. Clin Child Fam Psychol Rev 14(3):213–230, 2011

Spelman JF, Hunt SC, Seal KH, et al: Post deployment care for returning combat veterans. J Gen Intern Med 27(9):1200–1209, 2012

Chapter 14

Caring for Bereaved Military Family Members

Jill Harrington-LaMorie, D.S.W., LCSW
Judith Cohen, M.D.
Stephen J. Cozza, M.D.

UNIQUE FEATURES of military death may pose distinctive risks or serve as protective factors to family survivors. Surprisingly, there is little empirical evidence on the impact of a service member's death on the family and how best to understand and support survivors (Harrington-LaMorie and McDevitt-Murphy 2011). Despite the paucity of scientific study, clinicians can benefit from a review of what is known about military deaths, the communities in which they occur, and information about death and loss in the civilian community that is pertinent to grief in military families and the interventions that will support their health.

Demographics of the Deceased and Their Survivors

U.S. Service Member Death in the Past Decade

Since September 11, 2001, nearly 16,000 military service members have died on active duty status, with more than one-third of these deaths attributed to the wars in Iraq and Afghanistan (S. Cozza, J. Fisher, C. Ortiz, J. LaMorie, C. Fullerton, and R.J. Ursano, "Military Service Member Death in a Decade of War," manuscript in preparation, 2014). The U.S. Department of Defense (DOD) classifies military deaths into eight broad categories: accident, hostile action, homicide, illness, self-inflicted, terrorist attack, pending, and undetermined. The overwhelming majority of active duty military deaths are sudden and violent in nature and include homicide, friendly fire, suicide, accidental overdose, suffocation or asphyxiation, vehicular accidents, training accidents, aviation accidents, sniper fire, drowning, engine fires, death by improvised explosive devices, impalement, mutilation by rocket-propelled grenades, torture, and falling as well as sudden or unexpected natural deaths, including myocardial infarction, aneurysm, stroke, and cancer (Cozza et al., "Military Service Member Death" 2014).

Suicide rates have increased across all service branches, especially in the Army and Marine Corps, where the greatest increase in suicide rates has occurred in the past decade. One-third of military suicides have been inflicted by service members who have never been deployed to a war zone (Department of Defense Task Force on the Prevention of Suicide by Members of the Armed Forces 2010). Firearms are the most commonly used method of self-inflicted death, with 41% of military suicides using a non-military-issued firearm (Department of Defense Task Force on the Prevention of Suicide by Members of the Armed Forces 2010). Equally distressing is the number of veterans (service members no longer on active duty) who die by suicide each year. Twenty percent of the 36,000 U.S. suicide deaths each year are of veterans (Congressional Quarterly 2010).

More than 95% of all service members who died while on active duty in the past decade were male. The largest proportion of deaths was of enlisted men under the age of 30. Similarly, officers who died on active duty were primarily male but represent a smaller percentage of the total deceased (Cozza et al., "Military Service Member Death" 2014). Just over half of all service members who have died were married with at least one child, often of young age. All branches of the military (Army, Navy, Air Force, and Marines) have incurred casualties in combat theater, with the greatest number occurring in the Army (55%), followed by the Marine Corps (17%), the Navy (15%), and the Air Force (12%) (Cozza et al., "Military Service Member Death" 2014). Because of the size of the Army and current U.S. ground operations in theater, the Army and Marine Corps have suffered the highest percentages of overall deaths. All three components (active duty, Reserve, and National Guard) have been affected. Eighty percent of active duty status deaths are service members who serve on regular active duty; 20% are of service members who serve in the Reserves and National Guard (Cozza et al., "Military Service Member Death" 2014).

Profile of Surviving Military Families

Given the age (18–40 years) of most military casualties, the typical profile of a service member's surviving family may include young parents (who may be early middle age themselves), siblings (sometimes teens or younger), a young spouse or adult partner, children from newborn (some unborn) to young adult, and a group of extended family members and friends who vary in age from very young to elderly. Very little information is known about survivor demographics except for data kept by the DOD and U.S. Department of Veterans Affairs on surviving spouses and dependent children for the purpose of managing military and survivor benefits. Military family survivors reside in all 50 states and outside the United States. Surviving spouses and children may choose to live closer to military installations after the death in order to utilize military benefits, move to locations where they find higher social support from extended family and long-term friends, or relocate because of new employment.

Wartime Death and Bereavement in Families

Most of what we know about the impact of active duty military death and wartime bereavement on surviving families comes from studies conducted in Israel (Rubin et al. 1999). Israel's 62 years of independence in the aftermath of the Holocaust have been marked by conflict with neighboring Arab and Palestinian-Arab states. The impact of military loss has been a principal area of bereavement research in Israel, particularly since the 1973 Yom Kippur War, which lasted 20 days and resulted in the deaths of approximately 2,600 young adult Israeli military servicemen and the wounding of just over 7,200.

In a pioneering anthropological work, Palgi (1973) observed the grief and bereavement reactions of parents whose sons died in military service during the Yom Kippur War and noticed discernible responses of bereaved fathers, who seemed to be experiencing a deep sense of loss, accompanied by intense feelings of deprivation. These fathers seemed to age prematurely. Subsequent research on parents bereaved by military loss suggested that social withdrawal and isolation were a common consequence. Purisman and Maoz (1977) studied parents who had an adult son killed during the War of Attrition (1969–1970). Their study showed higher levels of depression and somatic complaints and poor self-concept among bereaved Israeli parents. Gay (1982) measured the self-concept of parents who lost their adult sons in the 1973 Yom Kippur War. She compared grief and adjustment scores of bereaved Israeli parents with the scores of nonbereaved

Israeli adults in general society. Her findings suggested that bereaved parents ranked poorly in measures of self-concept and had higher incidences of somatic complaints and depression.

Rubin (1990) investigated Israeli parents who had lost an adult son in a war, with time since loss at an average of 9 years, compared with parents who had lost a 1-year-old child to illness around the same time. He discovered that parents who had adult sons die in war demonstrated higher levels of current grief as well as higher levels of recalled grief than parents who had suffered the death of an infant child to illness. His research brought to light how the circumstances of death, age of the deceased, and age of the bereaved parent may predispose parents to potentially more intense grief reactions as well as complicated and enduring bereavement. As a follow-up to his findings, Rubin studied 102 Israeli parents who had suffered the death of their sons to war in the preceding 4–13 years. In this second study, Rubin (1992) found that bereaved parents of fallen wartime sons showed higher levels of grief and anxiety than did the control group of 73 nonbereaved Israeli adults. This study proposed that despite the length of time since the death loss, there may be a more long lasting impact of wartime death on these parents, whose grief is less inclined to subside over time.

Each war or conflict is a unique historical event, influenced by such factors as time, era, economics, technology, and culture. Anecdotal reports are available in the popular press, but surprisingly little research has explored the bereavement experiences among surviving families of service members who die in the U.S. active duty military. In spite of the paucity of research on U.S. military families, the United States can draw associations from the findings of the Israeli research to begin to conduct vitally needed studies on a population at risk for exposure to trauma and grief about which we know very little.

Military Death and the Family System

Just as the definition of survivor is broad, so too is the definition of what constitutes a surviving military family. In this section, we describe some considerations for working with bereaved military families of procreation (spouses and children) and families of origin (parents and siblings).

As stated in the section "Profile of Surviving Military Families," the majority of military deaths are of adolescents to young adults, ages 18–40 years. Distinctive problems plague families who experience the loss of a young adult. For surviving families some of these difficulties include future losses, changed roles, challenges with identity, financial issues, and changed family order.

When a young adult dies, family roles change, identity within the family may change, and familial developmental tasks are challenged as family members grieve the death of this person throughout their life span (Walter and McCoyd 2009). Grieving someone who dies an untimely death has an inherent challenge by placing the survivor in the position of a prolonged journey of grieving multiple secondary losses across the lifespan. The long-term impact of a young, untimely death is family members being confronted with grieving in their future, especially during developmental milestones.

Spouses

The death of an active duty U.S. military service member confronts the surviving spouse with a series of compounding, multiple losses associated with the death. If the couple has children, the surviving spouse is confronted with what to tell the children and how much to tell them. After the death, spouses suffer many secondary losses. They must often make immediate decisions during periods of extreme duress regarding housing or moving (where to live or relocate), benefits, schooling for children, insurance, and future employment. The military system is not always easy to navigate or compassionate to the survivor in assisting with the transition of care. Widows and widowers experience the loss of an identity as a "military spouse," a way of life as part of the "military family," loss of housing (if on base or post), loss of friends in the unit or command, and a loss of feeling connected to the greater military community. Military families live and function in the culture of the military, which has its own customs, laws, hierarchal structure, bureaucratic systems, health system, educational systems, codes of conduct, rituals, and housing. Many spouses are afforded little opportunity to develop their own careers, hobbies, and support networks outside of the military because of frequent moves and the demands of the military career on the family. This adds to the often intense feelings of having to create a new identity after the service member's death. For many surviving spouses of regular, active duty personnel, the death of their spouse is an involuntary, immediate, abrupt transition from the identity of a "military" to a "civilian" family and way of life. However, tied by benefits, many surviving spouses often feel torn between the two worlds, creating feelings of confused identity.

New dating relationships are a challenge for a vast majority of surviving spouses. One noted reason is the potential loss of benefits. War widows often relate that dating relationships can become difficult if the new person in the relationship feels threatened by "living in the shadow" or "filling the shoes" of a war hero—a larger-than-life individual. Surviving spouses with overall supportive and positive marital relationships at the time of their spouse's death often report having feelings of betrayal when they begin dating again. They may feel as though they are cheating on their spouses. Even as they recognize the reality of the death, they may still feel that they are betraying their feelings of love and marital commitment.

Children

Bereaved military children face unique challenges related to the parent's military status in addition to universal grief and traumatic grief issues addressed elsewhere (e.g., Cohen and Mannarino 2008). Confusion can arise from the nature of the deployment cycle (if the child's parent was killed in combat), military rites and rituals associated with the death, and (similar to the surviving parent) transitions from military to civilian family life.

The military honors its fallen service members through military bereavement rites and rituals. Although these rituals provide needed comfort to many military families and may be helpful to grieving adults and children, they may not perfectly meet the needs of all children. Military rituals that may affect military children include the following:

- *Death notification:* Even young military children are familiar with the ritual of death notification and are often frightened when uniformed service members come to their door, knowing they are bringing dreaded news. If there has been a divorce or marital separation, the child may find out about the parent's death from the media or a phone call, possibly without the other parent's presence to provide support.
- *Return of remains:* When service members die in combat, their remains are returned to families. However, remains may not all be recovered simultaneously or may not be recovered at all. Repeated recovery of newly identified remains may lead to resurgence of grief symptoms, distress, worsening of nightmares, or intrusive thoughts about the death.
- *Military funerals:* If the family requests a military funeral, rituals include the presence of an honor guard, draping the American flag over the casket, firing three rifle volleys, a bugler playing "Taps," folding the flag after the service, and giving the flag to the fallen service member's widow, widower, mother, or designated next of kin. Although these rituals may be comforting, some children may find these military images upsetting.
- *Political protests:* Because the media often cover funerals of Operation Enduring Freedom/Operation Iraqi Freedom combat-killed service members, these funerals sometimes attract political protesters, for example, carrying signs saying "Thank God for dead soldiers," causing confusion, anger, and sadness in children.

- *Change in status:* After a service member death, family members obtain a new service identification card that changes all of their designated military statuses to "deceased." If the family lives on a military installation, they must move off base within 12 months after the death. Like their surviving parent, children may be saddened and challenged by these losses and transitions away from military schools, activities, and friends.

Parents

The death of a child, at any age, is considered to be one of life's most devastating losses, the impact of which can be pervasive over time (Worden 2009). Because the expected natural order for parents is to precede their children in death, parents must adapt to a new and seemingly illogical reality. Strong feelings of guilt coupled with remorse over their inability to protect their child can be particularly challenging for parents whose children die young and unexpectedly. These feelings make accepting the reality of the loss most difficult and prolonged for parents. Although considerable attention has been paid to the impact of the death of a pediatric-adolescent child on parents, very little attention has been paid to the impact of the death of a young adult child.

If there were real or perceived shame or stigma associated with the death, which is often the case with suicide and homicide-suicide, parents may not receive public, community, or family support. This is especially true in cases in which a service member committed homicide-suicide. Parents may be inappropriately held accountable or may feel responsible for their service member's actions, which also can be highly stigmatizing. Grief for the death of their child is often not afforded or considered.

Reaching out to other bereaved parents who understand their loss can be a helpful and nurturing process for bereaved parents. Peer support and self-help groups have been found to be effective in aiding parents in maintaining more positive memories of their deceased child (Klass 1988).

Siblings

Bereaved siblings are often an unrecognized and disenfranchised group of survivors, who cope to survive in the shadow of their service member sibling's death. Even though bereaved siblings experience profound loss, they are often overlooked in their grief (Godfrey 2006). Society may not recognize siblings as primary grievers or acknowledge the death of an adult sibling as a significant loss (Godfrey 2006), and this can be true after military deaths, as well. Social and emotional supports for siblings who have lost a young adult brother or sister are limited.

Grief Reactions

Although the experience of grief is universal, each death is experienced individually, in its own unique way and its own unique time. This is part of what makes each person fully human and identifies individual human relationships and attachments as distinctive. There are a wide range of reactions exhibited by those who grieve. Although some people may experience many of the normal grief reactions, there may be significant individual differences. Table 14–1 presents a list of common grief reactions.

Normative Grief

Normative grief reactions include a broad range of behaviors and feelings such as sadness, crying, anger, guilt and self-reproach, anxiety, loneliness, fatigue, problems with decision making, helplessness, shock, yearning, relief, numbness, physical reactions (stomachache, shortness of breath, lack of energy), disbelief, confusion, preoccupation, sleep disturbances, appetite disturbances, social withdrawal, hyperactivity, and visiting places that remind the mourners of the deceased. Bereavement experts in the field report that approximately 80% of bereaved persons experience normative or "uncomplicated grief" with an adaptive course of adjustment (Bonanno and Lilienfeld 2008). Although there is no timeline for grief, most individuals begin to assimilate their loss and experience decreased grief reactions from 6 to 13 months after the death. The majority of survivors are able to integrate the loss into their lives with resilience (Bonanno 2004; Neimeyer et al. 2010). Unfortunately, 10%–20% of bereaved persons suffer from complications that can prolong grief reactions, impair mental and physical health, and prohibit an adaptive course of healing (Shear et al. 2005).

The literature suggests that bereaved persons affected by sudden, violent deaths caused by accident, suicide, homicide, terrorism, and war are highly vulnerable to psychological trauma (Doka 1996; Green 2003) and incur the potential of developing complicated grief (Prigerson and Jacobs 2001; Rando 1993). The impact of bereavement with trauma can be long lasting. Research finds that violent death loss predicts symptoms of posttraumatic stress disorder (PTSD), anxiety, depression, and health impairments that can further expose the survivor to a more enduring, distressing, and complicated bereavement (Rynearson 2006). Most military survivors expect to encounter grief, but they do not understand that they may suffer from symptoms of trauma, which can complicate bereavement.

TABLE 14–1. Commonly experienced grief reactions

Physical reactions	Behavioral reactions	Emotional reactions	Cognitive reactions	Spiritual reactions
Headaches	Wearing clothing of the deceased	Sorrow or overwhelming sadness	Memory problems	Emptiness
Nausea	Searching for what was lost	Fear	Inability to concentrate	Challenge of beliefs or values
Increased activity	Crying	Anxiety	Problems with decision making	Search for meaning or purpose
Decreased activity	Keeping room of deceased intact	Guilt	Confusion	Pessimism or idealism
Muscular tension	Carrying picture or object of deceased	Anger	Auditory or visual hallucinations	Acceptance
Shortness of breath	Absentmindedness	Yearning	Impaired self-esteem	Forgiveness
Heart palpitations	Distancing from people	Despair	Denial of reality of loss	Experiences of spiritual connectedness
Chest pain	Sensing the deceased	Relief	Repeated review of loss event	Compassion
Loss of motor skills	Disbelief	Numbness	Increase or decrease of dreams	Peacefulness
Dizziness	Distraction or preoccupation	Confusion	Suicidal thoughts or death wish; desire to "rejoin" the dead	Spiritual or religious affirmation
Insomnia	Seeking solitude	Release	Creativity	
Fatigue or sleep disturbances	Seeking forgiveness	Helplessness	Wisdom	
Weakness	Providing forgiveness	Hopelessness		
Choking sensation	Avoiding painful reminders	Listlessness		
Muscle weakness	Inability to sit still	Feeling lost		
Dry mouth	Intrusive thoughts	Bitterness or vengefulness		
Empty sensation in stomach	Loss of interest in regular events	Loneliness		
Weight and appetite change	Dreams	Longing		
		Lack of control		

Complicated Grief

The death of an attachment figure triggers a natural prolonged process of protest, despair, and reorganization as the survivor attempts to adapt to the loss (Bowlby 1980). It is estimated that between 10% and 20% of bereaved people experience complicated grief. Previously referred to as *traumatic grief* and renamed to avoid confusion with PTSD, the term *complicated grief* (CG) has been used to refer to a pattern of adaptation to bereavement that involves the presentation of certain grief-related symptoms at a time well beyond that which is considered adaptive. Also described as prolonged grief disorder (PGD), CG can often leave survivors feeling "stuck" or "frozen in time." CG symptoms have been shown to be distinctive from depression and anxiety clusters (Bonanno et al. 2007; Lichtenthal et al. 2004; Prigerson et al. 1996). These symptoms include marked and chronic separation distress (such as longing and searching for the deceased) and symptoms of traumatic distress (such as feelings of disbelief, mistrust, anger, shock, or detachment from others and experiencing somatic symptoms of the deceased). Individuals who suffer from CG experience a sense of unrelenting and disturbing disbelief about the death and oppose accepting the painful reality to the point of functional impairment.

Persons who suffer from CG may experience an inability to enjoy life, emotional numbness, lack of trust, intrusive thoughts about the deceased, persistent inability to perform acts of daily functioning for months or years after the death, and abuse of drugs and alcohol and may engage in high-risk behaviors. Individuals suffering from CG are also at higher risk for the development of health and mental health impairments, such as heart attack, stroke, medical neglect, depression, PTSD, and anxiety. They are also more likely to engage in self-destructive behaviors and are at a higher risk for suicide.

Warning signs and symptoms should be taken seriously and should not be dismissed by the caregiver or clinician as "just part of the grieving process" because they can be potentially life-threatening. Given the young age of the affected population, negative coping strategies, such as the abuse of alcohol, drugs, and prescription medication, may be prevalent (Tables 14–2 and 14–3).

DSM-5 Diagnostic Classification

DSM-5 contains reviewed and revised diagnoses related to bereavement (American Psychiatric Association 2013, pp. 5–25). Persistent complex bereavement disorder (PCBD) is a newly defined diagnosis included in Section III of DSM-5 that incorporates previously proposed diagnostic systems of CG

TABLE 14–2. Assessing for complicated grief

These intensive reactions, years later, may include

Constant longing, yearning, or pining for the lost person; preoccupation with sorrow

Intrusive thoughts about the deceased

Intense feelings of emotional pain and sorrow related to separation distress

Avoidance of reminders of the loss

Extreme focus on the loss and reminders of the loved one

Feeling stunned, shocked, or dazed by the loss

Confusion about role in life or a diminished sense of self

Problems accepting the death

Numbness or detachment

Difficulty trusting others since the loss

Feelings of bitterness and anger over the loss and others

Difficulty moving forward (e.g., making new friends, pursuing new interests)

Feeling emotionally numb since the loss

Feeling that life is unfulfilling, empty, or meaningless without the deceased

Inability to enjoy life since the death

and PGD. PCBD will serve as a working model for continued research and further clarification of appropriate diagnostic criteria. DSM-5 criteria that are required are the death of someone with whom the individual had a close relationship and symptoms of persistent longing, intense sorrow, preoccupation with the deceased, or preoccupation with the circumstances of death extending at least 12 months (6 months for children) beyond the death. In addition, the individual must have at least six symptoms extending beyond 12 months in the areas of reactive distress or social or identity disruption that lead to significant symptomatology or dysfunction (American Psychiatric Association 2013).

Traumatic Grief in Surviving Military Children

Military children whose parents die suddenly or violently may develop a traumatic grief reaction (Cohen et al. 2006). The shocking nature of a military death is exemplified by the image of a chaplain and notifying officer arriving at a family's front door. A traumatic reaction may follow a characteristically sudden and horrific death such as from an improvised explosive

TABLE 14–3. Complicated grief: risk and protective factors

Risk factors	Protective factors
Proximity to the death: Did the death occur at a distance or up close? Did the person witness the death? Did he or she narrowly escape death as well?	Advance preparation for the loss
	Long-standing positive social support network
Cause of death: Was the death sudden, accidental, unexpected, brutal, homicide, suicide, or from chronic illness?	Personality
	Secure attachment style
	Previous ability to cope with life stressors and adapt (positive coping skills)
Relationship to the deceased: Was the deceased a parent, a friend, a child, the spouse, a sibling, or a fellow service member?	Sociodemographic variables
	Absence of prebereavement depression
Past history of losses: Is this death one in a string of deaths? Is this the first experience of death? How were prior deaths handled?	Positive spiritual or religious beliefs
	Economic resources
	Professional intervention
Current mental health status or life stressors at the time of the death: Childhood abuse and serious neglect Childhood separation anxiety Close kinship relationship to the deceased Insecure attachment style Inadequate support Dependency Ambiguous relationship with deceased	

device, accident, or suicide. A child may also have a traumatic reaction from other types of death such as an acute injury with a prolonged hospitalization even without exposure to gruesome aspects of the course of treatment and death. Research is still determining the length of time since death and severity, duration, and interference of symptoms to distinguish the condition, but the current literature focuses on children with childhood traumatic grief (CTG) having symptoms characteristic of PTSD. When this occurs, the child is stunned and overwhelmed by emotions and reactions that interfere with normative, healthy grief reactions. Characteristic PTSD symptoms include (National Child Traumatic Stress Network 2007)

- *Intrusive memories about the death:* Intrusive memories can occur in thoughts and images, a common example of which is reliving the memories through nightmares. For military children, it may be from imagining the parent's death or suffering (e.g., from news reports, movies, or stories from others) or from reliving the notification.

- *Avoidance and numbing:* Reminders of the person who died and the death itself trigger painful and overwhelming emotions. Hence, the child may cope by becoming numb to all emotions or avoiding people, places, and events that may provoke reminders. For example, military children may withdraw from military peers or resist military ceremonies.
- *Increased arousal:* Physical and emotional reactivity can be recognized by such symptoms as difficulty sleeping, poor concentration, irritability, anger, always being on alert, being easily startled, and having new fears.

Military Community Support

Active duty military communities have the ability to lend support and services to family members, particularly spouses and dependent children, after the death of a service member. After the death, and dependent on the command structure, many members of the community are mobilized to assist the bereaved family with instrumental support by providing meals, respite child care, and assistance with other responsibilities. In addition, the military organization provides benefits to surviving dependents and/or designated beneficiaries. Survivor benefits include continued military housing (for 1 year), death benefit payment, military life insurance benefits, casualty assistance, and funerary support, as well as ongoing military family dependent benefits that provide access to health care, commissary (less expensive grocery) services, and a multitude of military and veteran support services.

Meaning Making and Commitment to Service

Interest in meaning and meaning making in the context of stressful life events continues to grow, especially in the field of bereavement. Research suggests that the greater the bereaved individual's ability to find meaning (i.e., make sense of the loss), the less intense is his or her experience of grief (Neimeyer et al. 2006). The military survivor's viewpoint of the service member's military career and the circumstance of the death may be an essential determining factor. Some family members may be angry at their loved one's choice to enlist. Those who encouraged the service member to join the military may be left with a sense of responsibility or guilt for the death. Pride in military service can be a healing factor but may be confusing when experienced alongside the devastating negative emotions of grief. For some people, there is additional anger directed at the military that sent their family member to war or the enemy who killed them.

Clinical Considerations

Within weeks of the death, clinicians should focus on providing and promoting supportive assistance, encouraging adaptive functioning, and monitoring for risk or maladaptive responses. Early after the death of a loved one, survivors benefit from empathic listening and supportive reflection that acknowledges the reality of the loss and the emotional impact on the survivor. In addition, clinicians can help survivors identify sources of support, whether the interpersonal support of caring friends and family members or the instrumental support that may be available from organizations within the military and civilian communities. Clinicians can help the bereaved prioritize the many expectations placed on them (e.g., caring for themselves and their children, completing death benefit paperwork, making funeral or memorial arrangements) and with setting limits when faced with unnecessary tasks or expectations. Clinicians should ask about health-promoting or risk behaviors, including sleeping, eating, exercise, and alcohol consumption or other substance use that may support or hinder healthy adaptation. The use of psychopharmacology (anxiolytics or sleeping aids) may be helpful in the early period after the death.

In some circumstances added risk may be present, for example, with preexisting psychiatric illness or poor function or when circumstances of death (e.g., suicide or homicide) contribute to elevated distress. In such cases clinicians should assess risk and address any problems that may arise (worsening of psychiatric conditions, suicidal thinking) through immediate intervention. Over time, or when consulted later (months or years) after the death of a loved one, clinicians should assess the longer-term course of grief and associated levels of distress and sadness and the survivor's overall function and adaptation to the grief and determine whether any clinical conditions such as complicated grief, depression, or other disorders are present that require more definitive treatment (see the next section).

Clinicians who have no experience with survivors of sudden and/or violent death would benefit from additional training before engaging in such work. Survivor cases can be complex and graphic in nature and involve an intense amount of distress and, potentially, trauma. As a reminder, if the survivor presents problems beyond one's skill set, refer the individual to a more practiced clinician. Referrals to grief therapists or practitioners competent in the treatment of grief-related disorders can be found through the Association for Death Education and Counseling (www.adec.org) and the Tragedy Assistance Program for Survivors (TAPS; www.taps.org).

Interventional Strategies and Suggested Resources

If a survivor is a parent, spouse, sibling, or child of a U.S. Armed Services member, Reservist, or National Guardsman or Guardswoman who died in active duty, he or she is eligible for bereavement counseling through the Department of Veterans Affairs Vet Centers (www.vetcenter.va.gov). Long-term support for surviving Army families can be obtained through Army Survivor Outreach Services (http://www.myarmyonesource.com/FamilyProgramsandServices/SurvivingFamilies/SurvivorOutreachServices.aspx).

Grief Counseling

The overall goal of grief counseling is to assist the survivor with normative levels of grief in adapting to the death of a loved one and adjusting to a new reality without him or her. There are three basic types of grief counseling:

1. Professional mental health counseling is provided by trained nurses, doctors, psychologists, social workers, or licensed therapists. This can be done as either individual or group counseling. Trained grief counseling professionals in the field of thanatology can be found through the Association for Death Education and Counseling at www.adec.org.
2. Trained peer or professionally facilitated counseling can take the form of one-to-one mentor programs or support groups in which volunteer peers are selected, trained, and supported under the supervision of mental health professionals. One example of this type of counseling is widow-to-widow programs.
3. Self-help or peer support consists of support programs (both individual and group) in which bereaved people offer support to other bereaved people, with or without the support of professionals. The power of peer support is an underutilized but highly recognized area of healing and support for surviving military families. TAPS, which was founded in 1994 by a military widow, provides peer-based programs for adults and children and is a considerable source of care for bereaved military-connected families, regardless of the circumstance of the death and relationship to the deceased. Congressionally chartered advocacy groups, such as American Gold Star Mothers, Inc. and Gold Star Wives of America, Inc., along with the post-9/11 American Widow Project, all provide a peer network for surviving families.

Grief Therapy

Worden (2009) stated that grief therapy is most appropriate in clinical situations that fall into one or more of four categories: grief reaction that 1) is prolonged or complicated, 2) manifests as delayed grief, 3) manifests as an exaggerated grief response, or 4) manifests through some masked somatic or behavioral symptoms. Grief therapy is typically an individual modality of treatment.

Complicated grief therapy (CGT) is a relatively new psychotherapy model designed to address symptoms of complicated grief. Drawn from attachment theory and with roots in both interpersonal therapy (IPT) and cognitive-behavioral therapy (CBT), CGT includes techniques similar to prolonged exposure (repeatedly telling the story of the death and in vivo exposure activities). The treatment also involves focusing on personal goals and relationships. CGT has been demonstrated to be effective in a trial in which participants with complicated grief were randomly assigned to CGT or IPT; individuals receiving CGT responded more quickly and were more likely to respond overall (51% versus 28%). Visit www.complicatedgrief.org for more information about complicated grief and CGT.

Children: Trauma-Focused Cognitive-Behavioral Therapy for Traumatic Grief

Although it is unclear what percentage of military children may be traumatically bereaved, effective treatment for this more symptomatic and distressed group of youngsters must be utilized when CTG is identified. Trauma-focused CBT (TF-CBT) is an evidence-based treatment for traumatized children and teens and their parents or caregivers. TF-CBT has been used successfully with children who have experienced diverse traumas, including sexual abuse, domestic violence, disaster, multiple traumas, and traumatic grief. As a family- and resilience-focused model, TF-CBT may be especially well suited for bereaved military families. TF-CBT is a components-based treatment, which implies a balance of fidelity and flexibility. Gradual exposure is a core feature of the TF-CBT model and is included in each component (Cohen et al. 2010). These components are described in more detail in the free Web-based course TF-CBTWeb, available at www.musc.edu/tfcbt, a program that clinicians are encouraged to investigate.

Conclusions and Future Directions

Similar to their civilian counterparts, bereaved military family members are a diverse group of adults and children who have suffered the death of a loved one in the military service. Multiple factors, including the age, prior function, and experience of the individual and the circumstances of death are all likely to impact the family members' emotional reactions and clinical course. In order to effectively engage this population, practitioners benefit from a clear understanding of the challenges that the family face, distinctive military cultural considerations, and important principles of care that guide grief-related treatments.

Helpful Organizations

American Gold Star Mothers, Inc., www.goldstarmoms.com
Gold Star Wives of America, Inc., www.goldstarwives.org
Got Your Back Network, www.gotyourbacknetwork.org
Hope for the Warriors, www.hopeforthewarriors.org
Military Child Education Coalition, www.militarychild.org
Military Families United, www.militaryfamiliesunited.org
National Child Traumatic Stress Network, www.nctsn.org
National Military Family Association, www.nmfa.org
Snowball Express, www.snowballexpress.org
Society of Military Widows, www.militarywidows.org
Tragedy Assistance Program for Survivors, www.taps.org
Travis Manion Foundation, www.travismanion.com
USO, www.uso.org

Bereavement Support: Children and Adolescents

National Alliance for Grieving Children, www.childrengrieve.org
The Dougy Center, www.dougy.org

Bereavement Support: Parents, Siblings, and Grandparents

The Compassionate Friends, www.compassionatefriends.org
Bereaved Parents of the USA, www.bereavedparentsusa.org

Bereavement Support: Widows, Widowers, and Partners

American Widow Project, www.americanwidowproject.org
National Widowers' Organization, www.nationalwidowers.org
Young Widow, www.youngwidow.org

Grief Counseling and Grief Therapy

Association for Death Education and Counseling, www.adec.org

Behavioral and Mental Health Care

American Academy of Child and Adolescent Psychiatry, www.aacap.org
Give-an-Hour, www.giveanhour.org
Military OneSource, www.militaryonesource.com
TRICARE, www.tricare.mil

SUMMARY POINTS

- Unique features of military death may pose distinctive risks or serve as protective factors to family survivors.
- The overwhelming majority of active duty military deaths are sudden and violent in nature.
- There is little empirical evidence on the impact of a military service member's death on families.
- There is a wide range of reactions, both normative and clinically significant, exhibited by people who grieve.
- Military communities can lend tremendous support and services to family members after the death of a service member.
- Military survivors can benefit from grief support services, grief counseling, and grief therapies that address clinically significant grief (e.g., persistent complex bereavement disorder).

References

American Psychiatric Association: Diagnostic and Statistical Manual of Mental Disorders, 5th Edition. Washington, DC, American Psychiatric Association, 2013

Bonanno GA: Loss, trauma, and human resilience: have we underestimated the human capacity to thrive after extremely aversive events? Am Psychol 59(1):20–28, 2004

Bonanno GA, Lilienfeld SO: When grief counseling is effective and when it's not. Prof Psychol Res Pr 39(3):377–378, 2008

Bonanno GA, Galea S, Bucciarelli A, et al: What predicts psychological resilience after disaster? The role of demographics, resources, and life stress. J Consult Clin Psychol 75(5):671–682, 2007

Bowlby J: Attachment and Loss, Vol 3: Loss, Sadness, and Depression. New York, Basic Books, 1980

Cohen J, Mannarino AP: Disseminating and implementing trauma-focused CBT in community settings. Trauma Violence Abuse 9(4):214–226, 2008

Cohen JA, Mannarino AP, Deblinger E: Treating Trauma and Traumatic Grief in Children and Adolescents. New York, Guilford, 2006

Cohen JA, Berliner L, Mannarino A: Trauma focused CBT for children with co-occurring trauma and behavior problems. Child Abuse Negl 34(4):215–224, 2010

Complicated Grief Program: The Complicated Grief Program. Columbia University School of Social Work, 2010. Available at: www.complicatedgrief.org. Accessed January 9, 2012.

Congressional Quarterly: Rising military suicides: The pace is faster than combat deaths in Iraq or Afghanistan. Congress.org, 2010. Available at: http://www.congress.org/news/2009/11/25/rising_military_suicides. Accessed January 9, 2012.

Department of Defense Task Force on the Prevention of Suicide by Members of the Armed Forces: The challenge and the promise: strengthening the force, preventing suicide and saving lives. U.S. Department of Defense, 2010. Available at: http://www.health.mil/dhb/downloads/Suicide%20Prevention%20Task%20Force%20report%2008-21-10_V4_RLN.pdf. Accessed January 9, 2012.

Doka K (ed): Living With Grief After Sudden Loss: Suicide, Homicide, Accident, Heart Attack, Stroke. New York, Routledge, 1996

Gay M: The adjustment of parents of wartime bereavement, in Stress and Anxiety, Vol 8. Edited by Milgram NA. New York, Hemisphere, 1982, pp 47–50

Godfrey R: Losing a sibling in adulthood. The Forum: Association of Death Education and Counseling 32(1):6–7, 2006

Green BL: Trauma Interventions in War and Peace: Prevention, Practice and Policy. New York, Kluwer Academic, 2003

Harrington-LaMorie J, McDevitt-Murphy M: Traumatic death in the United States military: initiating the dialogue on war-related loss, in Grief and Bereavement in Contemporary Society: Bridging Research and Practice. Edited by Neimeyer RA, Winokuer H, Harris D, et al. New York, Routledge, 2011, pp 261–272

Klass D: Parental Grief: Solace and Resolution. New York, Springer, 1988

Lichtenthal WG, Cruess DG, Prigerson HG: A case for establishing complicated grief as a distinct mental disorder in DSM-V. Clin Psychol Rev 24(6):637–662, 2004

National Child Traumatic Stress Network: Traumatic grief. National Child Traumatic Stress Network, 2007. Available at: http://nctsn.org/nccts/nav.do?pid=typ_tg. Accessed December 30, 2007.

Neimeyer RA, Baldwin SA, Gillies J: Continuing bonds and reconstructing meaning: mitigating complications in bereavement. Death Stud 30(8):715–738, 2006

Neimeyer RA, Burke LA, Mackay MM, et al: Grief therapy and the reconstruction of meaning: from principles to practice. J Contemp Psychother 40(2):73–83, 2010

Palgi P: The socio-cultural expressions and implications of death, mourning and bereavement arising out of the war situation in Israel. Isr Ann Psychiatr Relat Discip 11(4):301–329, 1973

Prigerson HG, Jacobs S: Traumatic grief as a distinct disorder, in Handbook of Bereavement Research: Consequences, Coping and Care. Edited by Stroebe MS, Hansson RO, Stroebe W, et al. Washington, DC, American Psychological Association, 2001, pp 613–645

Prigerson HG, Bierhals AJ, Kasl SV, et al: Complicated grief as a disorder distinct from bereavement-related depression and anxiety: a replication study. Am J Psychiatry 153(11):1484–1486, 1996

Purisman R, Maoz B: Adjustment and war bereavement: some considerations. Br J Med Psychol 50(1):1–9, 1977

Rando TA: Treatment of Complicated Mourning. Champaign, IL, Research Press, 1993

Rubin S: Death of a future: an outcome study of bereaved parents in Israel. Omega 20(4):323–339, 1990

Rubin S: Adult child loss and the two-track model of bereavement. Omega 24(3):183–202, 1992

Rubin S, Malkinson R, Witztum E: The pervasive impact of war-related loss and bereavement in Israel. International Journal of Group Tensions 28(1/2):137–154, 1999

Rynearson EK (ed): Violent Death: Resilience and Intervention Beyond Crisis. New York, Routledge, 2006

Shear K, Frank E, Houck PR, et al: Treatment of complicated grief: a randomized controlled trial. JAMA 293(21):2601–2608, 2005

Walter CA, McCoyd JLM: Grief and Loss Across the Lifespan: A Biopsychosocial Perspective. New York, Springer, 2009

Worden JW: Grief Counseling and Grief Therapy: A Handbook for the Mental Health Practitioner, 4th Edition. New York, Springer, 2009

Chapter 15

Building Resilience in Military Families

William R. Saltzman, Ph.D.
Mia Bartoletti, Ph.D.
Patricia Lester, M.D.
William R. Beardslee, M.D.

RESILIENCE is a concept that is as old as war itself. This is because it describes one of the military's fundamental tasks: to maintain or restore individual functional capacity and well-being in the face of extreme adversity. In recent years, *resilience* has become an organizing principle for program and service development across the U.S. Department of Defense and the various service branches. All of these efforts are focused on promoting individual resilience. Although these are essential military goals and are central to force readiness and force preservation, the primary focus on the individual often overlooks a growing body of research that suggests that one of the best ways to improve the resilience and well-being of all military family members, including the service member, is to enhance the health and functionality of the family as a whole (Luthar 2006; Saltzman et al. 2011; Walsh 2003). This expanding research has led to the coining of the term *family resilience* and the development of theoretical models that identify specific family level characteristics and processes that either support or undermine the protective, supportive, and healing capacities of the family (Saltzman et al. 2011; Walsh 2003).

In order to provide clinicians with theory and practical guidance on how to conduct resilience enhancement with service members and their

277

families, we first provide a description of specific family characteristics or processes that undercut family resilience. These *mechanisms of risk* are then differentiated from *mechanisms of resilience*, which include characteristics or processes associated with resilient family functioning.

Mechanisms of Risk for Military Families

Clinical and epidemiological research has identified five interrelated sets of family processes theorized to serve as risk mechanisms for families exposed to stressful circumstances. These are specific characteristics or habitual types of interaction that undercut the family's ability to function as a cohesive and supportive unit (Lester et al. 2011a; Luthar 2006; Walsh 2006). Table 15–1 presents the risk mechanisms and their theorized proximal outcomes.

Incomplete Understanding and Inaccurate Developmental Expectations

A significant portion of returning Operation Enduring Freedom/Operation Iraqi Freedom (OEF/OIF) service members and their spouses experience distress and clinically significant levels of depression and anxiety (Eaton et al. 2008; Lester et al. 2010). Accumulating research has described specific ways in which parental psychological disturbance impairs marital, parental, and, ultimately, family functioning (Galovski and Lyons 2004; Palmer 2008). For example, parents with depressive symptoms may be excessively tired, disengaged, and irritable and may be perceived by their children as distant and uncaring or by spouses as "lazy and unmotivated" (Beardslee 2002; Cummings et al. 2001). Further, parents with even subclinical levels of posttraumatic stress may have difficulty tolerating normal household stressors, reacting with anger or aggression or by psychologically or physically distancing themselves from family activities (Galovski and Lyons 2004; Sherman et al. 2005). On the positive side, research has shown that providing a family member with information on the nature, cause, and specific manifestations of deployment-related problems can enable a spouse to be more flexible and understanding (Renshaw et al. 2008) and help children to recognize that neither their parent's condition nor related family problems are their fault (Beardslee 2002; Wyman et al. 2000).

Impaired Family Communication

A second mechanism through which wartime deployment and combat operational stress can adversely affect family functioning is disruptions in family communication. Repeated prolonged separations with one parent in

TABLE 15–1. Risks and likely outcomes in families affected by wartime deployment or parental combat operational stress that are addressed by a family resilience program

Mechanisms of risk	Proximal outcomes	Program components	Expected outcomes
Incomplete understanding • Incomplete understanding of impact of deployment and combat operational stress on parent and child • Inaccurate developmental expectations	• Misinterpretation of behaviors and reactions • Anger, confusion, and frustration • Inappropriate parent reactions and support • Guilt and blame • Excessive worry about children	• Psychoeducation • Developmental guidance • Proactive family planning for deployment • Positive reframing of problem and goal statements • Training on managing trauma and loss reminders • Highlighting of family strengths	• Increased understanding, flexibility, and support • Forgiveness of self and others • Accurate expectations and parental support • Increased family confidence and optimism
Impaired family communication • Prolonged parent absence, disparate experiences, and inability to share or appreciate these differences • Lack of open emotional expression	• Isolation and estrangement • Reduced family cohesion, warmth, and timely and appropriate support • Unclear, inconsistent, or distorted information • Lack of collaborative processes (planning, problem solving, decision making) • Increased irritability and conflict	• Sharing of individual narratives and cocreation of shared family narrative • Perspective taking • Processing distortions and misattributions • Communication skills training • Family meetings	• Decreased isolation and estrangement • Clear and emotionally open communication • Increased family cohesion, warmth, and timely and appropriate support • Increased sense of coherence and meaning

TABLE 15–1. Risks and likely outcomes in families affected by wartime deployment or parental combat operational stress that are addressed by a family resilience program *(continued)*

Mechanisms of risk	Proximal outcomes	Program components	Expected outcomes
Impaired parenting • Problematic parent leadership and reactivity related to parent distress, PTSD, depression, or anxiety disorders • Reduced parental availability, engagement, and monitoring	• Inconsistent care routines • Inconsistent discipline and parenting styles • Lack of coordinated coparenting • Family or marital stress and conflict • Disruptive child behavior	• Parent narrative sharing and processing of differences and misunderstandings • Parent leadership training • Development of shared goals and support of coparenting • Skill training in collaborative decision making, problem solving, goal setting, reminder management, and emotional regulation	• Effective and coordinated parenting • Increased parental availability and monitoring • Improved care routines • Increased parental perceived competence

TABLE 15–1. Risks and likely outcomes in families affected by wartime deployment or parental combat operational stress that are addressed by a family resilience program (*continued*)

Mechanisms of risk	Proximal outcomes	Program components	Expected outcomes
Impaired family organization • Overly rigid or chaotic structure that is easily disrupted under stress	• Rigid or chaotic parenting styles • Poorly defined boundaries, roles, and responsibilities • Erratic care routines • Disengagement of family members • Decreased cohesion, confidence, and optimism	• Shared parent narratives to support effective coparenting • Activities and assignments to enhance family structure and closeness • Training on collaborative family skills and maintaining care routines • Crisis contingency planning	• Flexible family structure able to adjust to stress and change • Well-defined family boundaries, roles, responsibilities, and care routines • Effective coparenting
Lack of guiding belief systems • Lack of framework to provide coherence and make meaning out of adversity • Lack of shared beliefs to support family identity and optimism and to mobilize coping efforts • Lack of access to supportive community, rituals, and transcendent values	• Feelings of isolation, hopelessness, and pessimism • Loss of sense of coherence (life as being comprehensible, manageable, and meaningful) • Lack of common family mission and "esprit de corps"	• Family narrative creation to increase coherence and make sense of experiences • Normalizing and contextualizing adverse experiences • Highlighting strengths and past successes to support optimism • Reframing negative interpretations • Supporting family's religious or spiritual inclinations	• Development of family mission and goals and support for shared beliefs • Increased sense of coherence and meaning related to current adversities • Increased access to family, military, community, and spiritual resources and services

a war zone and the rest of the family dealing with very different stressors at home create significant discrepancies in experience and missed opportunities for parent-child bonding (Lester et al. 2011b; MacDonald et al. 1999). Bridging these gaps requires specific communication skills and attitudes that may be undercut by emotional numbing or avoidance in the service member secondary to posttraumatic stress or depression and an unwillingness to talk about wartime experiences (Lincoln et al. 2008; Riggs et al. 1998). Withholding strong emotions, pain, fear, and worry may also stem from a military family culture that enjoins members to "suck it up" and not burden others with expressions of need or hurt (Hall 2008). On the basis of our experience working with military families, we find that children of all ages understand this ethic and frequently keep their worries and fears secret from parents. The breakdown of open and emotionally responsive communication across the family frequently impairs essential sharing and parental monitoring of children's daily experiences and activities, accomplishments, and concerns and undercuts the family's ability to provide timely and appropriate support (Cozza et al. 2005; Sherman et al. 2005).

Impaired Parenting Practices

Impaired parenting practices represent a primary risk factor for military children, one that can often be addressed via short-term interventions (Gewirtz et al. 2008). A common pattern among traumatically stressed military parents often starts with disrupted sleep patterns and heightened arousal and irritability, leads to increases in spousal and family conflict, and results in parental disengagement and breakdowns in care routines and child discipline (Galovski and Lyons 2004; Lester et al. 2010). Families contending with the care and rehabilitation of an injured parent frequently experience *resource depletion* in terms of parental time, patience, and ability to maintain consistent care routines (Cozza et al. 2005). Risk may also be exacerbated by shifts toward more rigid, coercive, or authoritarian styles of parenting that may result from a parent's wartime exposure to trauma or loss (Saltzman et al. 2003).

Impaired Family Organization

Resilient families tend to develop a flexible structure that balances strong leadership and the ability to maintain consistent care routines with the adaptive capacity to accommodate to change even during stressful or disruptive family experiences (Kelley et al. 1994). In contrast, families that are overly rigid or chaotic, that provide either too much or too little structure, may slip even further toward those extremes during periods of family stress (Walsh 2006).

Lack of Guiding Belief Systems

Studies of families with one or more parents involved in OEF/OIF have found that family belief in the mission was a strong predictor of better coping and adaptation among the children (Palmer 2008). These findings are consistent with the theoretical literature that posits that resilience derives substantially from the family's ability to make sense of an experience and endow it with meaning (Antonovsky 1998), a capacity that is aided by adherence to a common set of beliefs or transcendent values (Patterson and Garwick 1994; Walsh 2006). Often, without a viable belief system to help him or her make sense of current adversities and confer meaning to daily struggles and sacrifices, the individual may become lost to bitter internal ramblings that lead to cynicism and doubt—conditions that are corrosive to individual and family resilience (McNulty 2010; Walsh 2006).

Mechanisms of Resilience in Military Families

Just as stress and adversity can initiate negative chain reactions within families that undermine resilient adjustment, positive chain reactions can be strategically set in motion to enhance individual and family resilience (Rutter 1999). In this section, we describe intervention components designed to enhance familial resilience by catalyzing adaptive family processes. These components have been described in detail elsewhere (Lester et al. 2011b; Saltzman et al. 2011) and comprise the central features of the Families Overcoming Under Stress (FOCUS) program. They are outlined in the "Program components" column of Table 15–1, accompanied by a description of targeted outcomes.

Providing Psychoeducation and Developmental Guidance

By providing a family with pragmatically detailed information about the impact of deployment, parental distress, and injury on individual family members and family functioning, clinicians can help the family avoid a number of pitfalls. Among these are excessively blaming the service member for symptoms and reactions directly related to posttraumatic stress or traumatic brain injury or the emotional sequelae of any identifiable physical or psychological injury. Providers can also help the service member desist from excessive self-blame and, most importantly, help the children to better understand a parent's symptom-driven reactions and sometimes confusing or inappropriate behavior as manifestations of the injury and not due to anything they have done. Freed from cycles of guilt and blame, family members may then be more able to engage in productive forms of self-care and problem solving with other family members (Beardslee and Knitzer 2003). After they are provided with appropriate developmental guidance, family members may also be in a better position to discriminate between benign and problematic reactions to stress and change (Mogil et al. 2010).

Developing Shared Family Narratives

After one or more wartime deployments, a gulf of time, disparate experiences, and problematic interpretations often spans between a service member and his or her family. Bridging this gulf and reestablishing familiarity and closeness is a central challenge during the extended reintegration period (Palmer 2008; Sherman et al. 2005). Unfortunately, there are numerous factors, including parent distress, psychopathology, lack of communication skills, and constraining family or cultural strictures, that may interfere with this process. By providing a family with a structured and safe forum for individual family members to share their experiences, reactions, fears, and ongoing concerns and then to collectively craft a family narrative, a number of critical family processes and capabilities can be brought online in service of improved adaptation and resilience.

Supporting Open and Effective Communication

Key hallmarks of a healthy family are direct, clear, consistent, and honest communication and the capacity to tolerate open expression of emotion (Walsh 2003, 2006). These characteristics are especially important for families experiencing stress and change, given that unclear, distorted, or vague communication can rob family members of the essential tools for successfully adapting to these challenges. Moreover, when parents withhold or "put a happy face on" communications about serious or difficult issues, they leave blanks that children fill in, often with their worst imaginings (Greene et al. 2003). As such, it is important to work within the personal and cultural framework of each family and help them to find appropriate ways to invite sharing of a wide range of feelings and extend a tolerance for differences and the expression of strong emotions (Bowen 1978; Walsh 2006).

Enhancing Selected Family Resiliency Skills

Specific parent skill sets and family level coping strategies can help families anticipate, plan for, and mitigate the impact of stressful events and improve child adjustment (Saltzman et al. 2009a; Spoth et al. 2002). Randomized controlled trials of resilience-enhancing child and family interventions have identified specific skills as being effective in improving individual and family level outcomes over time (Beardslee et al. 2007; Layne et al. 2008; Rotheram-Borus et al. 2006). These core skills include stress management and emotion regulation, collaborative goal setting and problem solving, and managing trauma and loss reminders. For optimal utility, it is important that these skills be trained at the individual and family level. For example, family members can be trained to collectively manage stress by identifying and anticipating stressful situations, monitoring idiosyncratic expressions of distress among different family members, and providing appropriate support in a timely and developmentally appropriate manner; they can be given structured opportunities to practice collaborative goal setting and problem solving; and they can be taught to work as a team to identify combat and deployment reminders and develop strategies to minimize disruptive reactions.

Supporting Effective and Coordinated Parent Leadership

Building on the military model designed to maximize "unit cohesion" and support, parents should be supported in providing clear and consistent leadership for their family unit. As noted in the section "Incomplete Understanding and Inaccurate Developmental Expectations," parental distress and psychopathology may result in impaired forms of parenting that lead to reduced parental availability, limited engagement and monitoring, inconsistent care routines and discipline, and, in many cases, disruptive or problematic child behavior. Various tools may promote consistent and coordinated parental leadership in accordance with a coparenting model. *Coparenting* refers to a set of values and practices that leads to a coequal and mutually supportive approach to parenting. In order to effectively coparent, parents must learn to communicate clearly with each other, support each other, and collaboratively negotiate childrearing decisions and disagreements along with family roles and duties (Feinberg 2002). Movement toward effective coparenting can be facilitated through the parents' sharing of their personal narratives and guided exercises to align parenting efforts (Lester et al. 2010; Saltzman et al. 2009b).

Theorized Model of Family Resilience Training

The foregoing set of intervention components designed to enhance family resilience has been operationalized within the Families Overcoming Under

Stress (FOCUS) family resiliency training program as training activities conducted with family members across a brief intervention. FOCUS is based on decades of family-centered intervention development, research, and evaluation conducted by a team from the University of California, Los Angeles and Harvard Schools of Medicine. It utilizes a theorized model of family resiliency training (see Figure 15–1) in which these training activities effect specific changes in family functioning, which, in turn, impact child and adult family member outcomes. Moreover, it is proposed that levels of distress and adaptive functioning of family members are linked both between the military and civilian caretaker parents and among parents and children. Finally, it is noted that there is a reciprocal relationship between adult and child distress and adaptive functioning and overall family functioning.

Intervention strategies guided by this model target both individual and family level change and address both the direct impact of improved resilience skills and the indirect impact of enhancing family level skills and processes. And although this model focuses on families with children, similar principles and intervention strategies have been adapted specifically for couples without children as well (Shields et al. 2010).

This model has been evaluated in primary and secondary analyses of preproject, postproject, and follow-up data collected during the first 20 months of the FOCUS large-scale demonstration project at 11 military installations in the United States and Japan. Detailed outcome data are presented elsewhere (Lester et al. 2012, 2013).

The intervention taxonomy recommended by the Institute of Medicine distinguishes prevention from treatment and divides preventive interventions into three categories on the basis of whom they target: *universal* prevention targets whole populations; *selective* prevention targets groups at increased risk relative to the rest of the population, although without identified symptoms; and *indicated* prevention targets individuals with identified but preclinical symptoms (O'Connell et al. 2009). The FOCUS program has been designed to provide *selective* and *indicated* preventive services, though it can be used to identify family members who may benefit from mental health *treatment* and can be offered concurrently to families in which a member is receiving intensive therapeutic care. A common example of selective prevention provided through the FOCUS model is proactively preparing a couple or family for an upcoming deployment. Indicated prevention is most commonly provided to couples or families in which a parent is experiencing posttraumatic stress, depression, anxiety, or difficulties secondary to traumatic brain injury or other physical injuries.

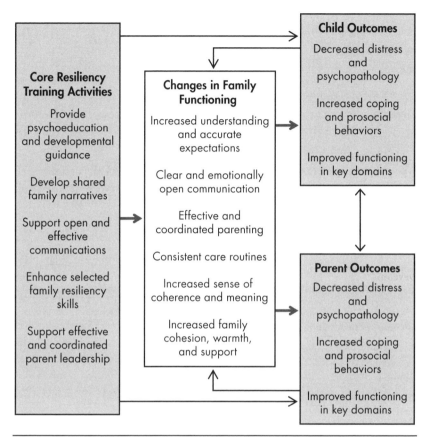

FIGURE 15–1. Theoretical model of family resiliency training.

Sequence of Core Activities for Family Resilience Training

The FOCUS intervention model has been manualized and described in detail previously (Lester et al. 2011a; Saltzman et al. 2009b). For convenience, a detailed list of core activities for each session is shown in Table 15–2 and a brief overview follows.

The program begins with two meetings with the parent(s) or couple to engage with them, translate their concerns and wishes into pragmatic goals, begin weaving in appropriate psychoeducation, and elicit and pro-

TABLE 15-2. Core activities for military family–focused intervention

Parent sessions

Session 1

Engage and elicit concerns and wishes for program participation.

Contextualize problems, highlight strengths, and praise current efforts to seek help.

Develop and prioritize family goals.

Explore gaps in relevant knowledge (impact of deployment, PTSD, or TBI; inaccurate developmental expectations; injury communication).

Begin psychoeducation in needed areas.

Develop and assign customized home activity in service of selected goal.

Session 2

Elicit individual parental narrative timelines.

Process divergences in timelines and misunderstandings or misattributions.

Summarize themes, new information, and understandings revealed in narratives and refine family goals.

Use calibrated goal sheets to identify current status and track changes on selected goals.

Continue to weave in psychoeducation and skill training (communication and support) in needed areas.

Assign customized home activity in service of selected goal.

Child sessions

Session 3

Engage and orient to program in developmentally appropriate manner.

Elicit concerns and wishes for program participation.

Develop and prioritize goals.

Explore gaps in relevant knowledge and begin psychoeducation.

Begin emotional regulation skill training as indicated (feeling identification and intensity rating, anxiety management, accessing support, etc.)

Develop and assign customized home activity.

TABLE 15–2. Core activities for military family–focused intervention *(continued)*

Session 4

Elicit narrative timeline or time map (depending on age).

Discuss themes and possible misunderstandings or misattributions.

Refine goals in light of narrative review.

Prepare child for family sessions (explain format and identify concerns and questions child would like to discuss).

Continue psychoeducation and emotional regulation training as needed.

Assign customized home activity in service of selected goal.

Parent preparation session

Session 5

Explain format and expectations for family sessions.

Review child narratives, themes, questions, and concerns.

Coach parent(s) on how best to participate in family sessions (how to supportively respond to child experiences.

Continue psychoeducation and relevant skill training (e.g., supportive listening, anger management).

Assign customized home activity in service of selected goal.

Family sessions

Session 6

Review the rationale and goals for the family meetings.

Support child in sharing narrative, questions, and concerns.

Facilitate parent-child discussion of differences in experiences, reactions, and interpretations. Support appropriate parent sharing of information and response to queries.

Address misunderstanding and misattributions, especially those regarding blame, guilt, and shame.

Help the family develop a shared understanding of the deployment experience and subsequent adversities and a shared appreciation of family strengths and past successes.

Develop and assign a home activity in service of a selected goal.

TABLE 15-2. Core activities for military family-focused intervention *(continued)*

Sessions 7 and 8

Continue to process divergent experiences and family misunderstandings and misattributions revealed in narratives.

Model and practice collaborative family discussion around identifying and prioritizing family challenges and goals.

Refine family goals and use calibrated goal sheets to identify current status and track progress.

Model and practice selected family level skills (emotional regulation, problem solving, identifying and coping with trauma or loss reminders, providing effective support, etc.).

Develop a family plan set of coping strategies to be used for anticipated stressors over the next year.

Terminate sessions and review progress and work left undone. Review goal sheets.

Explain relapse prevention skills (accurate expectations and tolerance of setbacks).

cess individual narrative timelines of their salient experiences before, during, and after deployments.

A unique aspect of this process pioneered in the FOCUS program is the use of a timeline to graphically render family members' narratives in a way that makes it easy to note differences in individual experiences and attributions. An example is provided in which the narrative timelines for both parents are superimposed (see Figure 15–2). Prior to constructing their narratives, the parents or couple are trained to use the "feeling thermometer" (shown on the left side of the timeline) as a means to describe levels of distress: higher levels on the thermometer denote higher levels of distress. The thermometer on the vertical axis of the timeline then provides a means to calibrate elevations on the personal timeline so that more stressful experiences are shown as elevations and less stressful experiences are shown as points lower down.

Following a summary of the spikes and valleys indicated in the timelines, the provider focuses the discussion on points of divergence between the two narrative lines. These discrepancies in experience and interpretation are often at the heart of ongoing misunderstandings between a husband and wife and may be clarified via discussion. In processing past and current areas of stress and conflict, the parents or couple may then revise goals for the program, and training in selected relational skills may be initiated.

In sessions with the provider and the child(ren), concerns and wishes are elicited in a developmentally appropriate and playful manner and are

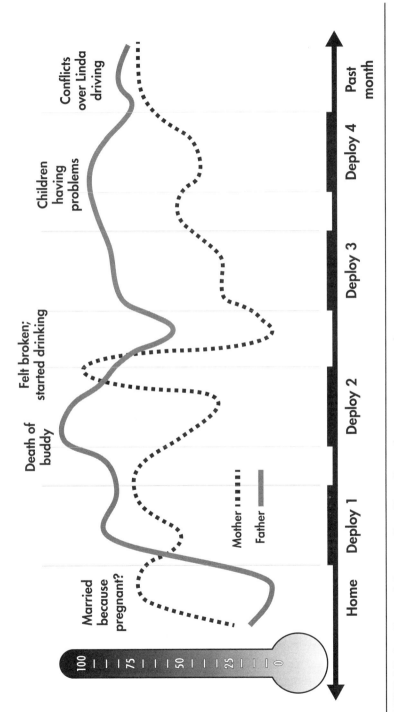

FIGURE 15–2. Parents' narrative timelines for case example.

translated into program goals. Narrative timelines are constructed, with art and play techniques employed for the younger children. Training in selected skills such as relaxation, emotion regulation, or accessing support are initiated, and discussions are held regarding which contents and materials should be shared in the family sessions.

The provider then meets with the parent(s) to prepare for the family sessions and to ensure that the adults can participate in a supportive and productive fashion. The child(ren)'s materials are reviewed, and responses to the child(ren)'s questions and concerns are reviewed.

The first of the family sessions involves the child(ren) sharing their narrative timeline and materials. The parents are then given an opportunity to comment to fill in gaps in knowledge and clarify distortions. In subsequent sessions, the family practices collaborative skills that involve problem solving, goal setting, and communicating effectively.

Application of Family Resilience Training If Working Only With Parents, Couples, or Special Populations

Parents Only

In many instances, clinicians will have the opportunity to work only with one or both parents, perhaps for a limited number of sessions, and will not have access to the children at all. In this case, family resilience enhancement may still be served by engaging the available parents in the initial parent sessions described in Table 15–2 and then using whatever additional time is available to frame current problems in family systemic terms. That is, the clinician can help parents move from a position of individual blame to a focus on reciprocal family relationships that require collaborative change. A family-centered and empathic perspective may be furthered by going through the parent narratives and repeatedly inquiring what was going on with other family members at key junctures. Sessions with the parents should also involve continued refinement and tracking of goals; family-customized psychoeducation and developmental guidance; and modeling, training, and practice of collaborative family level skills such as how to conduct a family meeting, how to engage in family problem solving, or how to collectively develop coping strategies. Many of the activities listed under the parent preparation and family sessions may also be enlisted in work with the parents alone.

Couples

Through the FOCUS demonstration project initiative through the Navy Bureau of Medicine and Surgery, demand for couples' resilience enhancement training spurred the adaptation of the program for military couples. This manualized program (Shields et al. 2010) utilizes the same theoretical model and similar core activities as the family intervention, with the addition of evidence-based couples' skill sets, and is now being adapted for veteran community-based populations as well.

Special Populations

The FOCUS family resilience training program has also been adapted for families with very young children (Mogil et al. 2010) and for families with a wounded, ill, or injured parent (Cozza et al. 2013). This latter program forms the basis of FOCUS services currently being provided at multiple installations for the U.S. Marine Wounded Warrior Regiment and is being evaluated in a multisite randomized controlled study by the Uniformed Services University of the Health Sciences (Cozza et al. 2010).

Conclusions

Converging research indicates that the family system and the primary supportive relationships within it provide a foundation for the resilience and recovery of all family members. Increasing acknowledgment of the importance of building family resilience has propelled the development of family-centered programs whose aim is to enhance specific processes and interactions within the family that support this protective and restorative capacity. The model and clinical methodology reviewed in this chapter are meant to provide scaffolding and a guide to clinicians who work with military families, couples, or individual service members. The thesis put forward here is that all levels of preventive interventions and clinical care may be guided by a family resilience–enhancing perspective, with benefit for both the individual service member and his or her family members. Even individual consultation with a service member or veteran may serve to increase knowledge and awareness of the impact of deployment and reintegration stress on family members, increase an appreciation of the distinct experiences and needs of all family members, provide developmentally appropriate communication skills to support family relationships, and develop specific coping skills that may reduce stress reactions and promote psychological health across the family system. Research and service delivery experience indicate that these core skills help the family become more cohesive and supportive and more resilient in the face of adversity. To help a family move even incrementally in this direction is a very gratifying undertaking that directly supports the nation's military men, women, and children.

SUMMARY POINTS

- One of the best ways to improve the well-being of all military family members is to enhance the health and functionality of the family as a whole.
- Research has identified five interrelated sets of family processes that serve as risk mechanisms for families exposed to stressful circumstances.
- Effective family resilience building targets these areas: inadequate knowledge, impaired communication, impaired parenting, impaired organization, and lack of guiding principles.
- These principles have been operationalized and evaluated within the Families Overcoming Under Stress (FOCUS) family resiliency training program.
- These core skills can help families become more cohesive and supportive and more resilient in the face of adversity.

References

Antonovsky A: The sense of coherence: an historical and future perspective, in Stress, Coping, and Health in Families: Sense of Coherence and Resiliency. Edited by McCubbin H, Thompson E, Thompson A, et al. Thousand Oaks, CA, Sage, 1998, pp 3–20

Beardslee WR: Out of the Darkened Room: Protecting the Children and Strengthening the Family When a Parent is Depressed, 1st Edition. Boston, MA, Little, Brown, 2002

Beardslee WR, Knitzer J: Strengths-based family mental health services: a family systems approach, in Investing in Children, Youth, Families, and Communities: Strengths-Based Research and Policy. Edited by Maton K, Schellenbach C, Leadbeater B, et al. Washington, DC, American Psychological Association, 2003, pp 157–171

Beardslee WR, Wright EJ, Gladstone TRG, et al: Long-term effects from a randomized trial of two public health preventive interventions for parental depression. J Fam Psychol 21(4):703–713, 2007

Bowen M: Family Therapy in Clinical Practice. New York, Jason Aronson, 1978

Cozza SJ, Chun RS, Polo JA: Military families and children during Operation Iraqi Freedom. Psychiatr Q 76(4):371–378, 2005

Cozza SJ, Guimond JM, McKibben JBA, et al: Combat-injured service members and their families: the relationship of child distress and spouse-perceived family distress and disruption. J Trauma Stress 23(1):112–115, 2010

Cozza SJ, Holmes AK, Van Ost SL: Family-centered care for military and veteran families affected by combat injury. Clin Child Fam Psychol Rev 16(3)311–321, 2013

Cummings EM, DeArth-Pendley G, DuRocher-Schudlich T, et al: Parental depression and family functioning: towards a process-oriented model of children's adjustment, in Marital and Family Processes in Depression: A Scientific Foundation for Clinical Practice. Edited by Beach SR. Washington, DC, American Psychological Association, 2001, pp 89–110

Eaton KM, Hoge CW, Messer SC, et al: Prevalence of mental health problems, treatment need, and barriers to care among primary care-seeking spouses of military service members involved in Iraq and Afghanistan deployments. Mil Med 173(11):1051–1056, 2008

Feinberg ME: Coparenting and the transition to parenthood: a framework for prevention. Clin Child Fam Psychol Rev 5(3):173–195, 2002

Galovski TE, Lyons J: The psychological sequelae of exposure to combat violence: a review of the impact on the veteran's family. Aggress Violent Behav 9:477–501, 2004

Gewirtz A, Forgatch M, Wieling E: Parenting practices as potential mechanisms for child adjustment following mass trauma. J Marital Fam Ther 34(2):177–192, 2008

Greene SM, Anderson E, Hetherington EM, et al: Risk and resilience after divorce, in Normal Family Processes. Edited by Walsh F. New York, Guilford, 2003, pp 96–120

Hall LK: Counseling Military Families: What Mental Health Professionals Need to Know. New York, Routledge, 2008

Kelley M, Herzog-Simmer P, Harris M: Effects of military-induced separation on the parenting stress and family functioning of deploying mothers. Women in the Navy 6:125–138, 1994

Layne CM, Saltzman WR, Poppleton L, et al: Effectiveness of a school-based group psychotherapy program for war-exposed adolescents: a randomized controlled trial. J Am Acad Child Adolesc Psychiatry 47(9):1048–1062, 2008

Lester P, Peterson K, Reeves J, et al: The long war and parental combat deployment: effects on military children and at-home spouses. J Am Acad Child Adolesc Psychiatry 49(4):310–320, 2010

Lester P, Leskin G, Woodward K, et al: Wartime deployment and military children: applying prevention science to enhance family resilience, in U.S. Military Families Under Stress. Edited by MacDermid Wadsworth S, Riggs D. New York, Springer, 2011a, pp 212–239

Lester P, Mogil C, Saltzman W, et al: FOCUS (Families Overcoming Under Stress): implementing family-centered prevention for military families facing wartime deployments and combat operational stress. Mil Med 176(1):19–25, 2011b

Lester P, Saltzman WR, Woodward K, et al: Evaluation of a family-centered prevention intervention for military children and families facing wartime deployments. Am J Public Health 102(suppl 1):S48–S54, 2012

Lester P, Stein JA, Saltzman W, et al: Psychological health of military children: longitudinal evaluation of a family-centered prevention program to enhance family resilience. Mil Med 178(8):838–845, 2013

Lincoln A, Swift E, Shorteno-Fraser M: Psychological adjustment and treatment of children and families with parents deployed in military combat. J Clin Psychol 64(8):984–992, 2008

Luthar SS: Resilience in development: a synthesis of research across five decades, in Developmental Psychopathology: Risk, Disorder, and Adaptation. Edited by Cicchetti D, Cohen DJ. New York, Wiley, 2006, pp 740–795

MacDonald C, Chamberlain K, Long N, et al: Posttraumatic stress disorder and interpersonal functioning in Vietnam War veterans: a mediational model. J Trauma Stress 12(4):701–707, 1999

McNulty PAF: Adaptability and resiliency of military families during reunification: initial results of a longitudinal study. Fed Pract March:18–27, 2010

Mogil C, Paley B, Doud T, et al: Families OverComing Under Stress (FOCUS) for early childhood: building resilience for young children in high stress families. Zero to Three 31:10–16, 2010

O'Connell M, Boat T, Warner KE: Preventing Mental, Emotional, and Behavioral Disorders Among Young People: Progress and Possibilities, 3rd Edition. Washington, DC, National Academies Press, 2009

Palmer C: A theory of risk and resilience factors in military families. Mil Psychol 20:205–217, 2008

Patterson JM, Garwick AW: Levels of meaning in family stress theory. Fam Process 33(3):287–304, 1994

Renshaw KD, Rodrigues CS, Jones DH: Psychological symptoms and marital satisfaction in spouses of Operation Iraqi Freedom veterans: relationships with spouses' perceptions of veterans' experiences and symptoms. J Fam Psychol 22(4):586–594, 2008

Riggs DS, Byrne CA, Weathers FW, et al: The quality of the intimate relationships of male Vietnam veterans: problems associated with posttraumatic stress disorder. J Trauma Stress 11(1):87–101, 1998

Rotheram-Borus MJ, Stein JA, Lester P: Adolescent adjustment over six years in HIV-affected families. J Adolesc Health 39(2):174–182, 2006

Rutter M: Resilience concepts and findings: implications for family therapy. J Fam Ther 21:119–144, 1999

Saltzman WR, Layne CM, Steinberg AM, et al: Developing a culturally and ecologically sound intervention program for youth exposed to war and terrorism. Child Adolesc Psychiatr Clin N Am 12(2):319–342, 2003

Saltzman WR, Lester P, Pynoos R, et al: FOCUS for military families: individual family resiliency training manual, 2nd Edition. Unpublished manual. Los Angeles, University of California, 2009a

Saltzman WR, Babayan T, Lester P, et al: Family-based treatment for child traumatic stress: a review and report on current innovations, in Treating Traumatized Children: Risk, Resilience and Recovery. Edited by Brom D, Pat-Horenczyk R, Ford JD. New York, Routledge, 2009b, pp 240–254

Saltzman WR, Lester P, Beardslee WR, et al: Mechanisms of risk and resilience in military families: theoretical and empirical basis of a family-focused resilience enhancement program. Clin Child Fam Psychol Rev 14(3):213–230, 2011

Sherman MD, Zanotti DK, Jones DE: Key elements in couples therapy with veterans with combat-related posttraumatic stress disorder. Prof Psychol Res Pr 36:626–633, 2005

Shields C, Saltzman W, Leskin G, et al: FOCUS for couples. Unpublished manual. Los Angeles, University of California, Los Angeles, 2010

Spoth RL, Kavanagh KA, Dishion TJ: Family-centered preventive intervention science: toward benefits to larger populations of children, youth, and families. Prev Sci 3(3):145–152, 2002

Walsh F: Family resilience: a framework for clinical practice. Fam Process 42(1):1–18, 2003

Walsh F: Strengthening Family Resilience, 2nd Edition. New York, Guilford, 2006

Wyman PA, Sandler IN, Wolchik SA, et al: Resilience as cumulative competence promotion and stress protection: theory and intervention, in The Promotion of Wellness in Children and Adolescents. Edited by Cicchetti D, Rappaport J, Sandler I, et al. Washington, DC, CWLA Press, 2000, pp 133–184

Index

Page numbers printed in **boldface** type refer to tables or figures.